Skin
Care
A *to* Z

Dear Alyshia,
Best Wishes for
Healthy Skin!
Be Well,

ALSO BY CAROLYN ASH

Timeless Skin

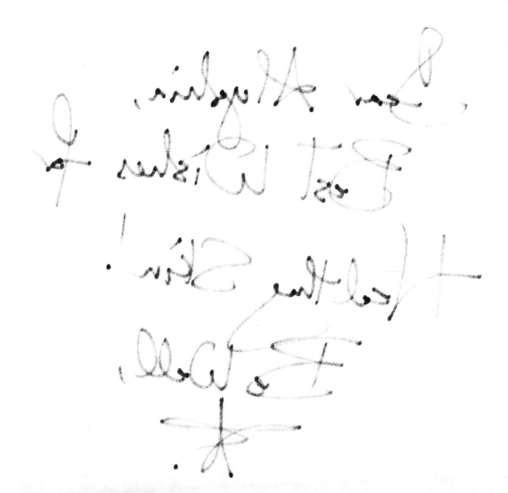

Skin Care

A *to* Z

YOUR PRACTICAL GUIDE

from America's Leading Skin Expert

Carolyn Ash

Splash
PUBLISHING

SKIN CARE A TO Z
Your Practical Guide from America's Leading Skin Expert

Splash Publishing books may be purchased for educational, business, or sales promotional use. For information please email: Special Markets Department, Splashpublishing@aol.com

Library of Congress Cataloging-in-Publication Data
Ash, Carolyn, 1961—
Skin care a to z: your practical guide from america's
leading skin expert/Carolyn Ash.—1st ed.
p. cm.
Includes index & bibliographical references
ISBN 0-9670240-1-3
1. Skin care 2. Beauty 3. Health I. Title
Library of Congress Catalog Number: 2005904682

Cover design by George Foster
Back cover photography by Larry Meiners

Printed in the United States of America

Additional permissions granted for material used in the Alcohol in Products section:

Adapted from *A Consumer's Dictionary of Cosmetic Ingredients*, 6th Edition by Ruth Winter, M.S., copyright © 2005 by Ruth Winter, M.S. Used by permission of Three Rivers Press, a division of Random House, Inc.

Adapted from *Milady's Skin Care and Cosmetic Ingredients Dictionary* 1st edition by Natalia Michalun © 2000. Reprinted with permission of Delmar Learning, a division of Thomson Learning.

Adapted and used by permission from *What's In Your Cosmetics?* by Aubrey Hampton © 2003, Organica Press. Mr. Hampton's opinion is that while naturally derived ethanol can be drying to the skin in high concentrations, it is a useful and safe ingredient in many products when used in small concentrations, especially when combined with herbal oils and vegetable glycerin to balance its drying effect. Natural ethanol is produced through the fermentation of sugar or starch; synthetic ethanol comes from the hydration of ethylene, an acrylate copolymer, and should be avoided.

Disclaimer: The author of this book is not a physician, and the ideas, procedures, and suggestions in this book are not intended as a substitute for the medical advice of a trained health professional. Neither Splash Publishing nor the author is responsible for any damages, losses, or injuries incurred as a result of any of the material contained in this book and disclaim any liability arising directly or indirectly from the use of this book. Consult your physician before adopting the suggestions in this book, as well as asking about any condition that may require diagnosis or medical attention. By following the instructions contained herein, the reader willingly assumes all risks in connection with such instructions.

C O N T E N T S

IN MEMORY OF

Gladys Brinker Ash
and
Gordon T. Lepley

Many thanks to all my clients, readers, and friends who allowed me to use your names and stories and emails in this book. Thank you to Suzanne, Walter & Fern, Allison & Marc, and Paul & Carol, for all your love and support. LAM: Thank you for all of your help, and for the lessons. Thank you Julie Flandorfer and Svetlana Potrue for taking care to make sure all the pages of this book came out looking good. Special thanks to Mel Ann Coley (please see p. 454). Thank you Bill Robinson for catching the oops (!). Additional thanks to Katie Tobias; George Foster; Ivy Charmatz; Maria Burden; Hank Schwager; Jim Flowers; Debbie Barnes; Lisa Loeb (Hello Kitty!); Lane Cawthon; Sheryl Walser; Elizabeth & Greg Wells; Blaine Fairchild; Sharolina; Archer, Grace, & Frances (my adoptees); all the authors and publishers who allowed me to use your works in this book; Sharon Kraus, Sharon Bayles, and David Sunshine for writing about your respective vocations and how they relate to healthy skin; and to all my clients and readers who have continued to support my salons and philosophies for all of these many years. **THANK YOU ALL!**

*H*appiness is nothing more than good health
and a bad memory.

– Albert Schweitzer

When I told my family and friends I was writing another book, the almost unanimous response was, "What is this one about?" It's as though writing one book about skin care was enough! Each time I heard that question, I chuckled and answered, "It's a skin care book." Then, the inevitable question that followed was, "Is there really that much more information to write about skin care?" Another chuckle emanated from deep down in my belly.

Yes, believe it or not, there is still more information to write about in regard to skin care! Halfway through writing my first book, *Timeless Skin*, I realized that I was either going to write a gargantuan book, or I was going to contain it and keep it to a certain size. I just had to stop somewhere, knowing I could always write another book some day.

Well, that day has come, and you are now holding in your hands what I consider to be a follow-up to my first effort. More than a follow-up, *Skin Care A to Z* is a continuation of *Timeless Skin*. The two books truly are siblings.

This book doesn't spend much time on trends and fads in the skin care world. I don't believe that the latest and greatest anti-aging product or procedure is really going to get you where you want to be in terms of healthy, clear skin. What I am providing in this book is the kind of interactive conversations I have with my clients. You will find many emails from readers and clients along with my responses and recommendations. You will also find several case studies from clients who were gracious enough to allow me to use their stories to illustrate different points about skin care. All of the stories and emails are used with written permission from each subject. In a few cases where I couldn't locate a client or for whatever reason could not get permission, I may have blended stories, questions, and situations together in order to make a point about a specific problem or concern.

Some of you may recognize a few things in *Skin Care A to Z* that are reminiscent of information found in *Timeless Skin*. I tried very hard to not duplicate any parts of these two books, but there were a few instances where it was necessary for clarity and because not everyone reading this book will be familiar with my first work.

The most notable instances where I have taken information directly from *Timeless Skin* are **The Basics 1-2-3** and **The Extras**. Without going into a brief description of what these programs are, new readers would be at a loss. And although I did not completely repeat myself, I did go into a description in these sections, which is similar to information found in the first book.

In *Skin Care A to Z* I refer to aestheticians (people who give facials) in the feminine. This is not to exclude the men who are in this industry, but percentage-wise there is a predominance of women compared to men who are licensed aestheticians.

Next, I want to clarify something. In my writing and in my salon practice, I am not advocating eliminating makeup altogether. I am talking about curtailing the use of foundation since it is not the best thing for your skin. Eye makeup, lips, lashes—go for it! But if your skin is clear and reflecting health (inside and out), then why cover it up? Wear as much makeup as you want to, but try not to cover up your skin with foundation.

Last but not least is the issue of product recommendations. I can almost guarantee many of you will turn to that section first to see what brand name skin care products I think you should buy. I explain the following at the beginning of that section, but it is so important I will repeat it here: I do not recommend specific product brand names in this book. In my writing I am trying to give you information about how to care for your skin and what to do and what not to do—regardless of what you are using—as well as giving you guidelines on what to look for in products.

There is no one product that is going to be right for every single person. I want to arm you with useful knowledge so you can go out into the market and select products that will work for your skin. This is very important to me, and it is the whole point of my writing. I am trying to decipher the often times confusing information that is so pervasive in the skin care world. If you can discern right from wrong, truth from hype, I believe you can use many different products with success.

I wish you well in your search for healthy, clear, and perhaps younger-looking skin. And I certainly hope that the information in this book helps you get there. I write about what I see and experience as the truth—according to me. I hope that these truths and the conversations about skin care issues contained in this book help lead you down (or up) a path to health, happiness, and freedom from worrying about your skin.

All of my best wishes to you all,

Carolyn Ash

Chicago

Waiting in line at the ticket counter at O'Hare airport, I struck up a conversation with a young man behind me. He was commenting on how unnecessary it was to still designate seat assignments on airplanes as "non-smoking." I agreed and added that I remembered when you *could* smoke on an airplane. He said he did not remember "those days;" alas, he was too young! I went one step further to say that I even remembered when you could smoke a cigarette in a movie theater! After I said that, I tried not to chuckle out loud due to the surprised look on this young man's face. I know I don't look my age, but the movie theater comment probably put me in his parent's age group. He tried not to show his shock and disbelief, but his expression, as subtle as he tried to make it, was priceless.

Since joining "The Club" (the 40-year-old club), I have had a new found sense of joy about my age. I am definitely not the person who feels a sense of loss at 40; I actually feel a sense of excitement about being older. I refuse *(refuse)* to bow to what society says about aging. There is too much that is good about getting older. These things are not physical (no kidding!), but they are profound—and real. I feel better mentally; I have a much deeper spiritual connection than I did in my 20s; I can handle complex situations with a maturity I am just now developing. Psychologically I understand myself and the world around me much better and more realistically, and I have a much deeper sense of appreciation and love for life and for the people in my life than I did even five or 10 years ago.

I want to share something with you that is an integral part of this message. The way I feel about myself, my life, and about aging *is a choice.* These positive feelings don't just happen (believe me!); I have carefully and constantly *crafted* and cultivated these feelings in order to survive in this world—this youth-driven, anti-aging world. No one is going to tell me how to feel about myself, and I am certainly not going to form my opinion about aging from magazines or commercials on TV. I choose on a daily basis to think, feel, speak, and act in ways that support myself—even as I head down the road of aging.

Over the last 10 years I have consciously and purposefully created a thought process for myself that *supports* the coming of age. It was, in a sense, a practical matter. I knew I would age (there was no stopping that train), and I knew there would be brighter, more beautiful, and *younger* people born onto the planet every day. So my choice was: will I let reality drag me down to my knees begging for mercy and perhaps less cellulite and less droopy eyelids, or will I choose to allow the inevitable and find beauty within that choice? Anyone who knows me, be it a client, friend, or family member, knows which path I have chosen to take.

Part of why I started writing in the first place was to give a voice to that choice. I wanted to add volume to my *anti*-anti-aging paradigm, knowing I couldn't possibly compete with the anti-aging world around me. But because I felt strong in my convictions about accepting aging, I also wanted to help any of you who *wanted* to feel the same way and yet might have felt like you're losing the battle. Today I am here to say *stand up strong* and don't succumb to all the hype, media attention to youth, advertising, and (even though it is my chosen industry) the skin care world.

I definitely advocate doing all the right things to keep your skin looking healthy at any age. But then, after getting enough sleep, eating right, drinking enough water, avoiding sugar, exfoliating, and applying your sunscreen, go out and face the day! Do something wonderful (or mundane). Enjoy your breath, the ability to move, and stop focusing so much time and attention on your looks. Be wise and don't belabor the task of looking good. Your looks can be taken away in an instant, or a lifetime; memories of adventures and life experiences last forever.

Taking joy in life is a woman's best cosmetic.

– Rosalind Russell

Youth is the gift of nature, but age is a work of art.

– Stanislaw J. Lee

Accutane®

Since this section is about a prescription drug, I want to reiterate that **I am not a doctor**. If you have a medical condition that requires a doctor's attention, seek his or her professional advice! I am not licensed to prescribe medications nor am I recommending bypassing getting a dermatologist's opinion for your acne problems or any other medical condition you may have. What I *do* recommend without exception is that you fully arm yourself with knowledge on the pros and cons of your particular problem areas and their solutions. I prefer taking a more wholistic approach to treating skin problems, but whether you do or not is fully your decision and responsibility. All views in this entire book are mine alone. It is up to you to decide the course of action to take in any given situation.

Throughout my career, numerous people have asked me about Accutane. It is a somewhat mysterious medication with a reputation for "curing" cystic acne. But is this true? I encourage you to read through other sections in this book to get a broader view on how you can treat and possibly stop problem skin from happening. The more you understand, the better equipped you will be to fight the good fight.

My goal is to give you some background about Accutane, a few of my clients' personal experiences, and my own thoughts concerning the use and misuse of this potentially harmful drug. I know Accutane has helped many people rid themselves of stubborn cases of acne, but I also feel too many people too much of the time reach for the quick-fix solution and neglect going deeper to the root of the problem. Like any medication, Accutane has its place in the world. I just want you to fully understand the ramifications of taking a drug to "cure" your acne problems.

What is Accutane? Accutane, or *isotretinoin*, is a derivative of vitamin A and is used for the most stubborn cases of acne. It is made and registered trademarked by Roche Laboratories. Unlike Retin-A® (retinoic acid), which is a topical product you apply to the skin, Accutane is taken internally (orally) in pill form. It comes in 10mg, 20mg, and 40mg capsules.

What are the internal and external side effects? The following information is used with permission and comes from two different sources in an attempt to give you a well-rounded view of the effects Accutane may have on your body. Although some of the information will repeat, I think this is a good thing because the more you understand about the potential risks and side effects, the more informed your decision will be.

All of the side effects listed indicate the seriousness that must be taken when considering Accutane. Remember, a quick-fix mentality focuses on now rather than looking ahead to potential consequences. Later in this section I will go over ways you can help ease the pain and annoyance of some of these effects. Know that you will experience some and maybe all of the side effects in varying degrees depending on your body's constitution, so be prepared and hope for the best.

The following is taken from *Physiology of the Skin II* by Peter T. Pugliese, M.D. If you are interested in a more technical explanation about skin and its function, you may want to read this book. It is for "professionals," but I know many of you who aren't in this profession like to read as much as possible about skin care. (See **Resources**.)

Side effects of isotretinoin may be mild or severe. Everyone on this drug will expect to have some side effects. Major side effects are:

1. *Cheilitis*, 90% of patients*
2. *Chapped, flaky skin, 90% of patients*
3. *Dry nose and eyes, 80% of patients*
4. *Loss of hair, 10% of patients*
5. *Painful joints and painful muscles, 15% of patients*
6. *Excessive peeling of the palms and soles, 10% of patients*
7. *Elevation of triglycerides in the blood, 25% of patients*
8. *Abnormal liver function tests, especially the transaminase enzymes, 15% of patients*

*Cheilitis is inflammation of the lips, usually concentrating around the corners of the mouth. This can produce anything from redness and irritation to severe cracking and scaliness.

Taken from *The Pill Book* published by Bantam Books:

Side effects [with Accutane use] increase with dosage.

Most common: Dry, chapped, or inflamed lips; dry mouth; dry nose; nosebleeds; eye irritation; conjunctivitis (pinkeye); dry or flaky skin; rash; itching; peeling skin on the face, palms, or soles; unusual sensitivity to the sun; temporary skin discoloration; brittle nails; inflammation of the nailbed or bone under toes or fingernails; temporary hair thinning; nausea; vomiting; abdominal pain; tiredness; lethargy; sleeplessness; headache; tingling in the hands or feet; dizziness; protein, blood, or white blood cells in the urine; urinary difficulties; blurred vision; bone and joint aches or pains; and muscle pain or stiffness. Isotretinoin causes extreme elevations of blood-triglyceride levels and milder elevations of other blood-fat levels including cholesterol. It also can raise blood-sugar or uric acid levels and can increase liver-function-test values.

Less common: Wound crusting caused by an exaggerated healing response stimulated by the drug, hair problems other than thinning, appetite loss, upset stomach or intestinal discomfort, severe bowel inflammation, stomach or intestinal bleeding, weight loss, visual disturbances, contact lens intolerance, pseudotumor cerebri*, mild bleeding or easy bruising, fluid retention, and lung or respiratory system infection. Several people taking isotretinoin have developed widespread herpes simplex infections.

**Pseudotumor cerebri* is one of the more dangerous (and fairly uncommon) side effects of taking Accutane. The symptoms are severe headaches followed by nausea and vomiting along with visual disturbances, which indicates an increased and intense pressure on the brain.

Easing the side effects of Accutane. If you think you have **cheilitis** or another severe lip condition, I recommend calling your dermatologist and informing him or her of this occurrence. Your doctor can prescribe a potent medication to help get rid of this uncomfortable skin problem. Keeping a non-petroleum lip balm constantly on the area will help to ease the dryness. Try not to lick your lips as this will just further the problem. For women, not wearing lipstick would help keep the lips from drying out as well.

Chapped, flaky skin is something you will probably have to contend with while on Accutane. It is the most common side effect from taking this drug. Using gentle exfoliators will help to keep the dead skin from getting out of hand. I highly recommend using body oils (vs. lotions) to keep the skin on your body from getting too flaky and dry. Generally, you want to keep your skin well lubricated to keep the dryness down to a minimum.

Dry eyes can be soothed by using eye drops. **Dry skin inside your nose** can be helped by either putting some cream there or better yet an oil or balm. Balms are thicker than oils or creams and have better sticking power.

If you are experiencing excessive **peeling of the palms and soles, brittle nails**, or **inflammation of the nailbeds**, I would recommend getting a manicure and/or pedicure. This might seem like an extravagance, but these services can really help relieve the symptoms you may be experiencing on your hands and feet. If you can't afford one of these nail services, at least get a pumice stone (very inexpensive) and get rid of the dead skin that way. Using the stone on dry skin works best, although it can be used in the tub or shower as well. Just massage the area with the stone (only on palms and soles!) and enjoy smoother skin afterwards. You could put some body oil or even oil from your kitchen on your cuticles if they are dried out.

Because being on any medication can make your skin more **photosensitive** (unusually sensitive to the sun), you must wear sunscreen on a daily basis. This is true whether you are on Accutane or not, but be especially diligent while on this medication.

What you may not know. You cannot get waxed anywhere on your body if you are currently on Accutane or even recently have been. The reason is your skin is so incredibly dried out and fragile that the wax will (or can) actually pick up several of the deeper layers of skin when it is pulled off. I have heard of people going in for facial waxing, neglecting to tell the aesthetician about the fact they are using Accutane. When the wax strip was ripped off, a good deal of skin came off with it!

Don't forget, no breast feeding your child while taking Accutane. And you also cannot give blood for at least one month after ending your treatment. This is a small fact, but an important one you may not think about. If you give blood and still have Accutane in your system, guess what? You can potentially pass this medication along to another person who might be pregnant or is about to get pregnant. I recommend waiting longer than a month to allow this powerful drug to be totally eliminated from your system. Taking supplements like chlorophyll might help to clear it from your body faster than just leaving it up to nature.

Requirements for taking Accutane. Unlike many drugs, before getting a prescription for Accutane, several requirements must be met. Why? Because Accutane carries with it significant risks. For male patients, the concerns are fewer. But for females, the potential for severe birth defects is probably the number one concern while on this medication. Because of this, no female patient is allowed to begin Accutane therapy if she is currently pregnant (no matter how far along) and definitely no pregnancies should occur while a woman is taking this potentially harmful medication.

There is strict monitoring for pregnancy during these treatments. Any female about to take Accutane must first take one, and in some cases two, pregnancy tests to ensure there is no possibility of a birth before going on this drug.

If a female patient is or might become sexually active during the course of treatment, she is required to use two different forms of birth control at least one month prior to treatment, throughout the entire course of treatment, and then for at least one month following the discontinuation of Accutane treatment. Regardless of sexual activity, female patients must take birth control pills for the duration of treatment. There are even strict policies that require a negative pregnancy test before a female patient can pick up her next month's supply of Accutane at the pharmacy.

A formal consent form must be signed before initiating treatment with this drug. It mentions the obvious and most notable potential for severe birth defects and the patient's agreement to take birth control for the duration of treatment. It also goes into great detail about depression and the possible signs of a depressive mental state while on Accutane.

Depression and Accutane. When you take anything orally, the substance enters the bloodstream and is introduced to all the cells it comes in contact with. Whether it is a medication or vitamin pill, it affects your body chemistry. And this includes brain chemistry. Depression, which occurs due to altered chemicals in the brain, is one of the side effects that can be caused by taking Accutane. If you choose to take Accutane, I caution you to pay close attention to your emotional life. If you think you may be experiencing medication-induced depression (depression brought on by the use of this oral medication), *call your doctor!*

The following are the symptoms listed on the Informed Consent/Patient Agreement form that must be filled out by every patient about to undergo Accutane treatments. It instructs you to immediately tell your doctor if you start to *feel sad or have crying spells; lose interest in your usual activities; have changes in your normal activities; become more irritable; lose your appetite; become unusually tired; have trouble concentrating; withdraw socially; or start having suicidal thoughts.* This is an instance where you are trying to fix a problem (acne), and you may accidentally create another, more undesirable problem (depression).

Obviously Accutane does not cause depression in every patient. But without knowing the possibility of it occurring, you may not be watching out for the signs of depression. I recommend talking with your doctor about this aspect of Accutane specifically so you can be clear about what to watch out for and what to do should you start feeling emotional changes. I realize you want clear skin, but don't make your body (and mind) pay the price. Knowledge is power; know what all the roadblocks are and keep your eyes open.

What does Accutane do? Accutane causes your sebaceous or oil glands to shrink. This naturally causes a reduction in the amount of oil the glands are able to produce. Smaller oil glands, less oil production. Problem solved, right?

Hardly. This brings me onto my soapbox—well, *one* of my soapboxes, anyway. Shrinking the oil glands, resulting in less oil production, sounds good on the surface. And the 'surface' is exactly as far as this treatment really goes. Like other so-called cures for acne, Accutane treats the symptom, not the actual cause of the problem. Symptom: too much sebaceous activity. Solution: stop sebaceous activity through drug interaction. And in the meantime, you cause a host of events to occur. Yes, the drug causes a physiological action in your body (shrinking glands), but it does nothing to address *why* the glands are overactive in the first place.

I believe without a shadow of doubt that you are what you eat. Therefore, the following, contained in a handout from the drug company that produces Accutane, leaves me shaking my head. It says, "Acne is *not caused* by a poor diet." How can it possibly be true that if you eat a diet filled with fast-food hamburgers, French fries and sugar-laden sodas, all of which I consider to be part of a poor diet, you won't run the risk of your entire elimination system (which includes your skin) being affected? Diet is not always the sole cause of problems, and certainly not with acne in particular, but to suggest that how you are nourishing your body doesn't *affect* your body, inside and out, is absurd to me.

For some people, oil production can, will, and does increase after a given time following Accutane treatments. The oil glands probably don't produce the same amount of oil after treatment, but some people still have skin problems after using this drug. It is not necessarily a once-and-for-all treatment. This is especially true if your lifestyle habits (namely diet) have not been altered since taking Accutane. (See **Jennifer's story** later in this section.) Granted, other factors may be present, like a hormone imbalance or genetics, but diet cannot be ruled out as a major contributor to your breakouts.

Is Accutane good for acne? The answer to this question is not as straightforward as you may think. Accutane has helped hundreds and thousands of people with acne. Some people can go through one round of the drug and be cured. Others find little or no relief. There are also what I call serial Accutane users; people who continue to go back to this medication after its effects have worn off.

In defense of Accutane (or any other treatment for problem skin), if you do not take away the *cause* of problem skin, then Accutane or any other treatment is compromised as to its efficacy. If you keep bumping into a door, you can treat the bruises with ointments to help them fade, but unless you determine that bumping into the door is causing the bruises in the first place, you can see how ineffective any treatment might be.

Do some investigation and try to find out the source of your problem skin. This can take time and definitely requires patience. You may not have either of these to spare. But if you decide to go on Accutane treatments, or any medication, please be well-versed in the side effects and take whatever precautions recommended by the drug company. That information will be found on the long list of contraindications and drug interactions provided with all prescription medications.

Although Accutane is supposed to be prescribed for stage IV, nodular acne—the most severe cases—I have found that many of my clients who didn't have such severe cases were readily given a prescription. Later in this section there is a reader comment and question that addresses this very concern. From the experiences of my clients coming in and relating their stories to me, I have also found many people have been on Accutane more than a few times, without even having major problems with their skin.

Are there alternatives to Accutane? I was discussing Accutane with a client who was concerned about her skin. She didn't have a lot of problems, but was experiencing ongoing breakouts. Her diet wasn't great—she is in college and is subject to peer pressure—and most notably, almost all of her friends are taking Accutane. Convincing someone to go the opposite way of everyone around them (especially their friends) is next to impossible, especially at that malleable age.

Since a woman has to use the birth control pill in order to take Accutane, I thought perhaps she could try going on the Pill only and see if it might help her skin. Please read this: I am in NO WAY advocating going on birth control pills. But since she wasn't currently taking it and would be required to in order to take Accutane, why not see if the Pill alone might help her skin? Perhaps it's the lesser of two evils, even though I am certainly not a proponent of taking birth control pills in order to clear up skin problems.

> My [teenage] daughter has had problem skin for several years. She has been treated by a local dermatologist with antibiotics and has been using special cleansers, but nothing is working. Now he wants to put her on Accutane, and after reading about the side effects of this medication, I'm really opposed to it.

The first question I would ask this woman is "how is your daughter's diet?" What is bad in her diet? Other than raging hormones, chronic skin problems can surface due to poor dietary habits. My guess, especially since she is a teenager, is that she eats a lot of sweets. If you are sensitive to sugar and you continue to consume it, you will probably end up with (chronic) problems.

Diet may have little to do with her skin problems. She may be predisposed genetically to having teenage acne. This is always a possibility. But in all of my years in practice, I find that even when there's a genetic predisposition, diet plays a key role in problem and acne skin—whether it is happening to a teenager or an adult.

I agree with this mother's hesitation about putting her child on Accutane, especially because of all the possible side effects. Since she hasn't responded favorably to previous attempts to clear her skin up, it indicates to me that she is probably continuing to feed the problem, which might be centered around sugar.

Accutane may indeed help this young lady's skin to finally and totally clear up. But before subjecting your body's health to this or any drug, wouldn't it be worth it to try a new dietary plan and see what effects changing food has on the state of your skin? You may end up saving your skin and avoiding all the potential side effects of taking Accutane.

I've been on Accutane for four months now and my skin has totally cleared up. This is my second time on it for the same thing. Thankfully, I found a liberal doctor who would prescribe it for me because I don't have a "severe" acne problem. It's actually a rash I get all over my forehead and temples and on my chest and upper back too. Now I can use whatever shampoo, conditioner, or styling product I like without getting any reaction, but I'm afraid that will stop when I go off the drug.

My skin looks somewhat dry and dull-looking from the Accutane treatments. It also seems really sensitive to products. When I use heavy creams or even creamy cleansers to combat the dryness, they just make me break out. Is there a heavier cream I can use that won't clog my pores? I'm really worried that when I go off the medication, the rash will come back like it did the last time I went off Accutane.

I am using this email as a doubly bad example of Accutane abuse. Not only did she go on several rounds of this medication, but apparently she doesn't even have true acne.

Thankfully, I found a liberal doctor who would prescribe [Accutane] for me because I don't have a "severe" acne problem. I wonder how many people could have written the very same thing. Prescribing Accutane is serious business. I am worried and disappointed about this "liberal" doctor. Need I explain? I'm sure it's frustrating having to find products that won't cause reactions, but the potential problems caused by using Accutane far outweigh this annoyance.

I'm afraid [my ability to freely use products] will stop when I go off the drug. This is why it is crucial to find out what is causing your skin problems, be it sensitivities to ingredients or foods or other factors. Until you eliminate the *cause* of the problem, you won't stop creating the symptom. It really *is* as simple as that.

My skin looks somewhat dry and dull-looking from the Accutane treatments. When I use heavy creams or even creamy cleansers to combat it, they just make me break out. Here is a perfect example of why I want to educate you about the difference between dry and dehydrated skin. Although this truly is a special case and perhaps this young lady's skin really isn't producing much oil now that she has taken Accutane, using heavy creams aren't the solution. Is her skin truly dry or just dehydrated from the use of Accutane? (See **Dehydrated Skin.**)

Is there a heavier cream I can use that won't clog my pores? No! Heavy creams will clog your pores if you don't need all the oil they contain. Only true-dry, oil-deficient skin can use heavy creams with relatively no problems. If a cream is breaking you out—especially if it is a "heavy" cream—it is not appropriate for your skin.

I'm really worried that when I go off the medication, the rash will come back like it did the last time I went off Accutane. First of all, we haven't established that this person even has acne. It sounds like a rash, even though Accutane helped eliminate it—temporarily.

But still, she clearly illustrates a concern I have about taking Accutane. Why is she having skin problems in the first place? Whatever the source of her problem, she probably has not eliminated it from her life. As long as she continues to introduce products that are irritating her skin, she will continue to have the rash and the problem skin she describes. Eliminating the root cause (whether it's a rash or acne) will help to control or eliminate the problem skin.

Are you willing to take a strong drug, but unwilling to change your lifestyle habits? If you are unwilling to change your ways, I hate to think you will rely on Accutane (which can and does have side effects) to do all the work for you. In the long run, I think your body loses.

Jennifer's story. Jennifer came to me years ago for a facial and has been a loyal, monthly client ever since. She is a lovely, conscientious woman in her late 20s. By her own admission, Jennifer is overweight. She doesn't drink alcohol or smoke cigarettes, but she does have a wicked sweet tooth; something she has "no control" over.

Throughout our years together, I have seen Jennifer's skin go through many ups and downs. She has attempted to lose weight many times, unable to find a way to drop the unwanted pounds. The same holds true for her attempt at eliminating sugar from her diet. Jennifer's skin is now and has always been broken out—sometimes severely. She truly has an acneic condition—comedones, milia, pustules, and cysts. I am not saying that sugar is the sole reason for her skin problems, but sugar is a top factor in how her skin appears and how her skin is indeed functioning, or rather dysfunctioning.

After trying all the different routes to "curing" her acne and without changing her lifestyle habits and dietary choices, Jennifer decided to take the leap into Accutane. Because her acne had become so severe, I actually was in agreement and thought this would make an interesting case study.

Jennifer's skin improved on Accutane—temporarily. It was definitely helping with the large cysts under her skin as well as helping to stop new cysts from developing. If new problem areas did come, they were smaller and less noticeable. Both Jennifer and I were encouraged with her progress and she surely thought her skin problems were over.

Jennifer's treatment course ended, and eventually so did her clear skin. Within a six-month period, her skin was right back where it started, and Jennifer was depressed. And no doubt her emotions were also fueling her food intake. She was gaining weight along with her skin breaking out again.

Talk and counsel her as I did, I couldn't get Jennifer to stop eating sugar and other foods even though she knew they were huge contributors to her skin problems. It's true that you can lead a horse to water, but you can't make her drink. Jennifer went on to take several rounds of Accutane. All helped for a period of time, but then her problems would always return.

My point in sharing Jennifer's story with you is to illustrate how denial and reliance on drugs and medications will not necessarily get you clear skin. Maintaining awareness and making conscious choices are always the best ways to achieve a goal. And if your goal is clear skin and you have an acneic condition, before taking medications, ask yourself what you may be doing to contribute to your circumstances. Acne is happening for a reason. It is up to you to decide how you are contributing to your problem skin.

Last of all, it's interesting to me that in all the literature I have read about Accutane, the consequences to the liver are barely touched on. I think more attention should be paid to the liver and the potential damage Accutane can cause. As you have read, only about 15% of patients develop liver problems, and those problems are usually curable and temporary. But do patients really understand what their liver will go through while taking this drug?

I will leave you with this question: Why do you have acne? After reading this book, I hope you will have more answers to this pivotal question.

Acidophilus

What is acidophilus? Acidophilus, or technically *lactobacillus acidophilus*, is the friendly bacteria found in your intestines. These health providers are always present in varying numbers, helping to defend their territory against pathogens and invaders.

There is a balance of friendly and unfriendly bacteria in the colon. This balance is so vital to the health and vitality of your colon that making sure you have enough friendly bacteria is of great importance. This is especially true if you are or have been taking antibiotics. As you will read, antibiotics take a toll on friendly bacteria. In essence, taking acidophilus helps to balance. It helps restore a healthy intestinal environment so jobs like digestion and elimination go smoothly day in, day out.

Acidophilus and antibiotics. Antibiotics, as we all know, are important tools for our health. And just like many things in life, they can also have adverse effects, especially if overused or abused. In some cases colitis, which is essentially inflammation of the bowel, has been linked with taking antibiotics.

For anyone currently taking antibiotics or even if you have just recently been on a round of antibiotics, I highly recommend taking acidophilus. Why? To reinstate and ensure a healthy balance of good bacteria in your colon, which was probably destroyed or in some way altered by the use of antibiotics.

The following is reproduced with permission of The McGraw-Hill Companies (1999). It comes from a wonderful little booklet found in most health food stores or online bookstores called *The Friendly Bacteria: How Lactobacilli and Bifidobacteria Can Transform Your Health*, by William H. Lee, R.Ph., Ph.D.

Antibiotics: The Destructive Lifesavers

Antibiotic drugs have a valued and necessary place in therapy, and have been focally instrumental in saving immense numbers of lives. They are an effective emergency measure, destroying disease-producing bacteria in a manner which seemed miraculous to those who first experienced and observed their action. Many diseases, such as pneumonia, which had been at best life-threatening, became routinely curable.

But antibiotic means, literally, "against life." When the "life" that is destroyed is that of harmful micro-organisms, all well and good. Antibiotics are not selective, though, and, like aerial bombing, are not geared to spare the friendly organisms which inhabit the same space as the hostile ones. After a course of antibiotic treatment, the intestinal flora are severely diminished, the good along with the bad.

At the least, this is likely to cause some digestive upset, anything from diarrhea and flatulence [gas] to severe constipation. As a routine precaution, many people have now learned to add yogurt [plain, not flavored with sugar added] to their diets—making sure that it has live cultures and is not pasteurized—after such treatment, or to take a guaranteed high-potency supplement of acidophilus or bifidobacteria.

An upset stomach* is not the worst result of the destruction of your population of friendly bacteria. In their absence, other organisms normally present and innocuous can seize the opportunity offered and expand their numbers explosively and dangerously.

One of the most prevalent and troublesome—and sometimes deadly—of these organisms is the yeast Candida albicans.

*As I tell my clients, usually when they are talking about their stomach, as in a stomach ache or upset stomach, they could mean their small intestine or transverse colon. Why do I say this? Because when I ask them to point to the place they are talking about, they point to the area around the belly button, which is where these organs are located. The stomach is much further up and to the left.

Although antibiotics are taken to restore our body's health, they also create a threat to the bacterium in the intestines that are designed to support health. Antibiotics have a place in the world of medicine and treatment, but their overuse is common and can cause real problems. Treating problem skin with antibiotics is a good example of this. I have come across hundreds of people who have been on antibiotics for their skin *for years!* This *cannot* be a good thing! After reading the previous excerpt from the acidophilus booklet, I hope you begin to understand that long-term use of antibiotics—for whatever reason—can be a real threat to your body's balanced state of health.

What and when to take acidophilus. There are approximately 11 trillion bacteria in residence in your intestines. Eleven *trillion!* That's about 3½ pounds of bacteria—the good kind. I mention this not only because it is an amazing fact, but also because some clients have expressed concern over taking acidophilus, which can (and should) contain up to a billion live bacteria in a single dose. When you compare these numbers, a billion vs. 11 trillion, it doesn't seem so daunting.

After talking with several health care professionals, they all agree you want to take acidophilus that requires refrigeration. These supplements usually come in capsule form, although powdered acidophilus is available. There are several brand names, so I recommend talking to a qualified person who works in the herb and supplement section of your health food store. They will (or should) be well-versed in what the store offers and what the best source of acidophilus is for you. Be sure the product has been refrigerated at the store.

Directions vary on when to take acidophilus, but generally it is recommended to take one to three capsules 20 to 60 minutes after eating.

I started taking acidophilus after I was on antibiotics. Now that I've stopped the antibiotics, should I keep taking acidophilus?

I would continue taking acidophilus because it is just so important for colon health. Perhaps after a few months off antibiotics and taking acidophilus you could stop, but I would give your colon plenty of time to regroup and regain a healthy balance after antibiotic use. There isn't any reason that I know of to stop taking acidophilus. It will do you no harm to continue using it, whether or not you are currently taking antibiotics.

Acne

I have broken up all the material regarding problem skin into different segments. After reading this piece, be sure to check out **Breakouts**, **Problem Skin**, as well as any other sections related to problems you are experiencing.

Treating acne or any constant skin care problem is a twofold process. If you do one step but forsake the other step, it's doubtful you'll see long-term results. As I read skin care books and articles in magazines and even listen to skin care experts on TV, I am always amazed that the treatments for problem skin usually recommend doing only one thing: treating the breakout. The question in my mind is always "What is causing the breakout in the first place?"

Here is one analogy. You are driving your car down a street with nails all over the place. You drive, and lo and behold, you get a flat tire. You fix the flat tire and keep driving down the same road. Later, you get another flat, and you fix it. What you don't realize is until you get off the road with all the nails in it, you will continue to get flat tires. Translate this to your skin. You may not even realize you are doing things that are contributing to your problem skin.

Until you become more aware, you will probably continue to have problems—even if you're using topical (or oral) medications. You must go to the root to find the cure. And even then there are no guarantees. But causal treatment (treating from the cause or root) will surely help you get a better hold on why you are breaking out. If you alter your behavior in order to stop contributing to your breakouts, hopefully then you will have clearer skin. You may not be able to afford to eat so much (or any) sugar—or whatever it is you may have in your diet that is a major contributor. But you have a choice. You can choose to continue to be frustrated with your blemishes or decide to do something about them, which usually includes discontinuing items currently found in your diet.

I have dry, scaly patches on my cheeks, but my dermatologist said I have acne. He gave me a topical ointment plus oral antibiotics. Is my skin dry or is it acne? It's all so confusing! Help! Plus an aesthetician said I have a little rosacea on my cheeks. I'm so sensitive and have spent so much money at the dermatologist and having different treatments...what should I do? What is my skin type?

I love this person's remarks. She exemplifies the confusion so many people face when it comes to their skin. A doctor said this, and I am taking a prescription medication, but with little or no results. I don't understand my skin. Sometimes clients even say "My skin is confused." Your skin isn't confused; it is simply reacting to its environment (internally *and* externally). Your skin, in fact, knows exactly what to do—and is doing exactly what it needs to do. It is the consumer who gets confused, and for good reason. I will break down her comments to see if I can make better sense of what is going on with her skin.

I have dry, scaly patches on my cheeks, but my dermatologist said I have acne. Dry and scaly skin does not equal acne. If your skin feels dry and looks scaly, you probably need to exfoliate. True scaliness could mean your skin is having an allergic reaction or perhaps an intolerance to a product, especially a new product. Dry and scaly skin could be eczema—a condition explained under **Dermatitis**. Dry and scaly could also be your skin's reaction to harsh and drying products you may be using to decrease oiliness or problem skin. Remember: your skin is reacting to something when it becomes dry and scaly. Look to your skin care habits and the products you are using, even extreme weather conditions, to find out what may be causing these reactions.

He gave me a topical ointment plus oral antibiotics. A topical product for acne may help with breakouts, but it also may be causing the dry and scaly condition of your skin to continue or even get worse. Many times dermatologists prescribe creams and ointments that are meant to dry things out. This, as you know (or will find out), is *not* how I would go about treating an acne or problem skin condition. If your skin seems drier and more scaly or red and irritated after the prescribed treatment products, don't use them! Monitor your skin and let it be your guide, but do contact your doctor about any reactions.

Regarding antibiotics, taking *anything* orally affects your entire body. Constant or repeated use of oral antibiotics can cause several problems. First, it can create a healthy environment for unhealthy bacteria to flourish in your large intestines. Your colon is set up with a particular balance of both good and bad bacteria; antibiotics kill both the bad *and* the good bacteria. Second, your immune system can weaken from constant use of antibiotics. If and when you really do need to produce antibodies to fight off bacteria, your system is less able to do so, which makes you vulnerable to getting sick. Antibiotics—long term—set up imbalance. (See **Acidophilus/ Acidophilus and antibiotics.**)

Is my skin dry or is it acne? It's all so confusing! Plus an aesthetician said I have a little rosacea on my cheeks. I have found acne and rosacea to be the most misdiagnosed conditions or at least the two most overused words to describe skin problems. You may very well have rosacea, although the description of your skin didn't necessarily indicate that. I would suggest reading about rosacea so you can see if the symptoms match your skin's condition. The treatment for rosacea is miles apart from acne treatment. Perhaps you truly do have acne or even rosacea, but you may just have problem skin that has been adversely affected by the actual treatment of your problems. Now *that* is confusing. You may simply have problem/dehydrated skin.

I'm so sensitive and have spent so much money at the dermatologist and having different treatments...what should I do? What is my skin type? If you take away all the treatments and medications that could be causing problems, it might be easier to determine your true skin type. Your skin's *condition* is what you need to treat first and foremost. It is the immediate need, secondary to skin type. Once your skin has normalized, you can better determine what products would be effective for your actual type of skin or skin type.

It's difficult to treat skin conditions yourself if you don't know what is going on. That is the purpose of my writing—to help you determine for yourself what the problems are and how to go about solving them. I want to give you the knowledge and the tools to help you help yourself. If you have acne and cannot get rid of it by changing your lifestyle habits (or because you refuse to), then absolutely, go see your doctor. Medications may indeed help you, but in this person's case, it didn't help her and seemed to cause her skin more problems.

Can you provide any referrals for products that treat severe acne?

Severe acne will not be totally eradicated by using products, even with an exceptional treatment product. True acne is a sign of an internal imbalance that needs to be attended to more than just topically. However, treatment products that employ essential oils, which are antiseptic and antibacterial, are perfect for helping to calm down infected skin. Again, nothing used topically is going to fix a problem that stems from the inside, but these types of products can definitely help.

How long does it take to clear up problem skin?

There is no definitive answer to that question. It is totally individual and depends on numerous factors. "*Why* is my skin not clear?" would be a good first question to ask yourself. If you continue to do things that contribute to poor-quality skin, then your skin may never clear up. Improper cleansing, sleeping with makeup on, using products that are drying, eating sugar or junk food, disregarding constipation, and not drinking enough water are just some of the factors that help to create unhealthy-looking, unclear skin.

Then there is the genetic component that cannot be overlooked. You can have all the unhealthy habits in the world and still (perhaps) get away with it due to inheriting miraculous genes for good skin. On the other hand, the opposite can also be true. You can do all the "right" things to support internal and external health, and having clear skin still may be a struggle if you have a genetic makeup that predisposes you to having problem skin.

So my answer to the question "How long does it take to clear up problem skin?" is: *Good question!*

What are you willing to do to improve the balance of health inside *and* out? Dr. Phil (McGraw) has a wonderful life philosophy that says you are either contributing to or contaminating situations in your life.

Although he is not talking about skin care specifically, it can apply to any and every area of your life—including your diet and how you are taking care of your skin. Ask yourself these questions: How are you contributing to or contaminating your skin? Your body? Your health? I bet the answers you come up with will not only be interesting, but will help you understand how you could be causing your skin problems. And also (here's the good news), how you can be the creator of healthy skin.

Actinic Keratosis

What is actinic keratosis? Actinic keratosis, sometimes called *solar keratosis*, is basically a premalignant lesion of the skin caused by excess exposure to sunlight. *Keratosis* means an over-accumulation of keratin or skin. These skin growths start out as flat and sometimes scaly places that can later develop into a scaly surface that resembles a wart. Although these are precancerous growths, around 10% of actinic keratoses become skin cancers called squamous cell carcinomas. These precancerous growths tend to form on lighter skin that receives sun exposure.

My story. It was time for my annual checkup at the dermatologist, so I went in to get a full body check of my moles. I looked over my body the night before my appointment so I would be familiar with my moles and I could ask about questionable places.

As I sat in the exam room, I took a marker I brought in with me (specifically for this purpose) and marked an "X" next to all the moles I had questions about. This may seem strange to you, but to me this is serious business, and I wanted to have all moles checked and didn't want to forget any I thought were questionable. Normally you will be given a cloth gown to wear for your examination. Since I had a few moles up and around my breasts and near my armpits, I decided to wear my roller blading shorts and a workout-type bra, clothing more conducive for the doctor to examine those hard-to-reach areas.

The Physician's Assistant, Gabriel, came in and the exam began. As we went through each section of my body, I asked questions about marked *and* unmarked moles so I could get some perspective on places that were OK versus moles that were suspicious. Gabriel came upon a place of concern on the outside of my left leg about five inches above my ankle bone. I had marked an "X" there because this mole looked questionable to me. This mole was small and relatively insignificant, and I believe that most people wouldn't have even considered it to be questionable.

The dermatologist concurred with Gabriel's findings, and it was decided a biopsy was in order. The area was numbed with a shot. Then Gabriel used a scraping instrument to take a scoop of skin off. I was glad the mole wasn't on my face since this procedure takes off a fair amount of skin. A bandage was put over the spot, and I was on my way.

A few days later, Gabriel called with the biopsy's results: actinic keratosis. He said it wasn't cancer, and wasn't actually considered precancerous, although if left unattended, over time it certainly could have become a cancerous growth (squamous cell carcinoma). I was amazed. It wasn't in a very obvious area on my body and was such an unassuming little spot of pigmentation. It did have somewhat irregular borders and had dark brown dots mixed with the normal brown color of a regular mole. The dermatologist said this was the biggest clue— the dark brown shade within the normal mole color.

This tiny spot turned out to be potentially problematic. Technically, it wasn't yet a precancerous mole, but it was unusual enough for the dermatologist to be concerned. The fact it was so small leads me to discard one of the common beliefs about cancerous growths: that they usually appear to be at least the size of a pencil eraser.

My mole was only ¼ that size. Granted, it wasn't cancerous, but if I was only looking for pencil-eraser sized moles, I would have passed this one by.

Since I have been involved in outdoor sports in recent years, I knew my body had been getting a lot of sun exposure even though I always wear waterproof sun protection. During my teenage years and early adulthood, I hadn't spent any measurable time in the sun. However, I had received several bad sunburns as a kid, and actually had sunpoisoning during a frivolous adventure in Florida one summer when I was 16. But compared to most people, my suntime had been short. That's why I was so surprised at the diagnosis.

Anytime I go to the dermatologist for whatever reason, I have them do a thorough check of my entire body—head to toe, front and back—to see if there are any moles that need attention. I highly recommend you do the same as well. Even if you aren't going in for sun damage, have them check your moles. And if you have spent anytime in the sun, go in *now* for a baseline if you haven't already; then you will have a point of reference for the next checkup. If you have any hint of a question about a mole on your body, don't second-guess yourself—do go see your dermatologist!

Acupuncture

New clients who come in for facials or return clients who may have a major skin change are asked a series of questions geared to help me determine areas in their lives that may be contributing to their skin problems. I am looking for dietary habits with the number one offender being sugar. However, sometimes a client has major skin eruptions, but clearly follows a strict and clean diet, free from sugar and other toxic foods. If my client is female, I ask if she is having normal (for her) periods along with other questions that might lead me to believe she has some imbalances hormonally. If it is a male client, he could also be experiencing some hormonal fluctuations that might be factors in skin problems.

When it comes to hormonal matters, this is where my expertise ends, and I send them to a specialist. And my specialist of choice is an acupuncturist. Unlike some medical doctors, a doctor of acupuncture has a unique and wholistic view of the human body and how it functions. Acupuncture and its medicinal attributes have been practiced, as far as recorded history tells us, for well over 2,000 years. How can I ignore the potential benefits of something that has survived this long? I can't! And I welcome you to explore this ancient healing technique, not only to help balance your skin problems, but also to ensure the health of your entire body—on a regular basis.

I get acupuncture as a matter of course once a month. I do this not because I have health issues or problem skin, but as a *preventative* measure to ensure my body stays in a balanced state. Anyone who knows me well can attest to this: I don't get sick. I do many preventative things to support my body's wellness, and receiving a monthly acupuncture treatment is one of my insurance policies.

When I initially started receiving regular treatments, I noticed a normalizing of my monthly cycle. The duration of my periods was shorter, cramping was less severe, and I just felt more in balance. I can directly relate these changes to my acupuncture treatments. In fact, my acupuncturist said it is optimal to get the treatment just before my period starts, so each month I schedule it just before I am expecting to menstruate.

Why should you get acupuncture? Speaking as an aesthetician, I would send someone to an acupuncturist if he or she is having skin problems that I cannot identify as having a dietary base. I realize some of my clients don't admit to all the bad things they may be eating, but there are some people for whom diet is not the issue with their skin.

Many women have irregular menstrual cycles. This not only can affect their skin, but it is simply not good for a healthy, balanced body. So even if skin is not a problem, if a female client comes in who I know has menstrual problems, I will recommend acupuncture.

Speaking as an acupuncture client, I think everyone should get acupuncture. It helps to balance and maintain health. Who couldn't benefit from that? I realize there is a stigma in the West concerning services like acupuncture. If the fear of needles doesn't stop you, then perhaps the intangible nature of the healing power of acupuncture will. I assure you, as you can read later in this section, the needles are not an issue in the slightest. In most cases you won't even know when they are being used—really! I have a client who I sent to get treatment. She was so apprehensive—mostly because of the needles. Once she was on the treatment table for a few minutes, she asked the doctor when he was going to start working on her. He chuckled and told her to look down where he was standing. She had several acupuncture needles already going to work, and she didn't feel a thing as he administered them. By the way, this was years ago, and this client continues to get regular acupuncture treatments today.

What is acupuncture and how does it help skin problems?
The following is an explanation of what acupuncture is, what it does, and how it can help you. This section was written by my friend and licensed acupuncturist, Sharon Kraus, D.O.M.

> *When some people think of acupuncture, they cannot get past the word "needle." For them it conjures the image of thick hypodermics and the pain of an injection or perhaps some comedic Hollywood image of a person with 400 needles stuck into every square inch of his or her body. Well, this could not be further from the truth!*

Imagine instead walking into a serene setting, complete with soft music and gentle lighting. You are arriving at the end of a hectic day of meetings and frantic work deadlines. Your shoulders are so tense that they practically touch your ears. Your head aches and is heavy, and your stomach is slightly queasy from the greasy lunch you grabbed on the run. Imagine entering this tranquil space after your long and stressful day. You change into loose-fitting clothing and lie down on a soft massage table. Your acupuncturist enters the room and begins a series of gentle diagnostic procedures such as feeling your pulse, looking at your tongue, and palpating certain areas of your body such as your arms and legs, belly or back. You will have a chance to tell your acupuncture practitioner what's been on your mind and your concerns about your body. In addition to paying attention to what you say, he or she will be noticing the sound of your voice, the color and tone of your skin, and your general state of well-being. All of this goes into the diagnosis of your condition and the course of your treatment.

As the treatment begins, he or she may gently insert fine filaments (aka needles)—about the width and diameter of a hair—into specific points on your body. These points are chosen for their location on what is called an acupuncture meridian. Although sometimes there is a sensation of pressure, tingling, or the occasional pinch when the needles are inserted, it truly should be a comfortable process. As you lie on the table, you begin to feel your shoulders relax and the pressure begins to drain from your head. The queasiness in your stomach begins to subside as you float into a state of heavy relaxation. When the hour is up, you leave feeling renewed and perhaps a little sleepy. Or, if you lacked energy before, you might feel like going home and cleaning your house or tackling a project. You might just notice that you feel back in harmony with your world again.

Obviously the above is an idealized view of an acupuncture experience. Your acupuncturist may run a noisy, busy clinic with five tables, each separated by a cloth. But if you have a qualified acupuncturist, the setting is not the main issue. Once the treatment begins, it is likely that your body will relax and go into a slightly altered state of relaxation and healing. It is important, however, to find an acupuncturist who is licensed either statewide or nationally, and whom you can relate to. There are many styles of acupuncture, so I encourage you to try a few different people until you find the person who is right for you.

What is acupuncture and how does it work? Acupuncture is a system that balances the flow of bioelectrical energy in the body. We are conductive beings, composed largely of water, and the functioning of our very cells is regulated by the flow of positive and negative ions. Although modern science still cannot explain it, the ancient Chinese, probably about 3,000 years ago, began mapping the electrical flows of energy in our bodies through a series of channels called acupuncture meridians. These channels invigorate the organs and the tissue, the flow of the blood, as well as the free-flowing expression of emotions. In that culture there was an understanding that the health of an individual depended on the harmonious interrelationship between all of one's parts.

Over the centuries, this body of information grew and has continued to be refined throughout China, Japan, and other Asian cultures until present times. Now we see the vast tradition of Oriental medicine, which is a primary system of health care for millions of people, interfacing with modern medicine and Western science. More and more we see Oriental medicine being looked to here in the West to address the "gray" areas for which Western medicine has no clear answer, such as hormonal imbalance, fatigue, fibromyalgia, insomnia, chronic pain, arthritis, menstrual discomfort, and even infertility. The fact is, Oriental medicine can address any condition because it's not treating the symptom, but the underlying imbalance. Regardless of the other therapies you might be receiving, acupuncture can be a very helpful addition.

In relation to skin care, most of us know that our skin is a major organ of elimination. In Oriental medicine, the skin is associated with the lungs and large intestine, otherwise known as the "metal" element. As you may also know, a buildup of toxicity in the body can lead to problem skin. If toxins can't be properly eliminated through the bowel, they are likely to be expelled through the sinuses and the skin. Obviously the liver and the kidneys play an important role in the detoxification process as well. Keeping the metal element balanced with all of the other elements and their related organ systems through the use of acupuncture and herbs is one way to assist in the detoxification and maintenance of healthier skin.

Hormonal changes can cause breakouts and sometimes deep, scarring acne. Although hormones were an unknown entity 2,000 years ago in ancient China, there was an understanding that supporting a free flow in all the acupuncture meridians eased stress in the body, allowed for better assimilation of food and elimination of waste, normalized sleep, and improved the regulation of all the body's cycles. In fact, acupuncture and Chinese herbs are known to be particularly helpful in regulating menstrual cycles and menstrual discomfort, as well as easing symptoms associated with menopause.

In the clinic, I have found that improving the flow of the lymph fluid in the upper part of the body with acupuncture, especially when there is a lot of upper body tension, helps to clear up acne. I have also discovered that many women with hormonal imbalances have either blood stagnation or weak "qi" (diminished energy flow) in the lower abdomen, often accompanied by tight upper *bodies—stiff neck and shoulders. We sometimes diagnose this as weak kidney or spleen qi, with liver qi or blood stagnation that can lead to "damp heat" conditions such as hormonal acne.*

Let me translate! What this actually means is that a weakness in the body leads to stagnation of fluids, sometimes referred to as "dampness" in Oriental medicine. Many things can lead to this type of weakness or "qi deficiency," but it's important because in some cases the resulting accumulation of fluids can lead to a heat buildup in the body. Toxicity due to sluggish functioning of other organ systems such as the liver and large intestine can also lead to localized heat accumulations. In fact, heat buildup can be generated through repressed or expressed emotions like anger or overexcitement, as well as through elements of diet. Foods such as alcohol, coffee, greasy and spicy foods, excessive intake of "the whites" (i.e., refined sugar and flour), or foods to which one may be allergic can also lead to heat or damp conditions. Truly, the term damp heat *can encompass all sorts of inflammatory, viral and bacterial conditions, including acne or herpes, as mentioned before.*

Skin problems can have many different etiologies, but the beauty of Oriental medicine is that we examine the cause in each individual and balance the body accordingly. Acupuncture is becoming increasingly popular in the West as our society begins to realize the importance not just of healing a single part but of considering the whole. This concept is inherent in Oriental medicine. We can no longer afford to focus on just one part at the expense of all others, whether it be in relationship to our bodies and our skin, to our planet, or to the whole of humanity.

What should you look for in an acupuncturist? I think whenever you are looking for a therapist, finding someone who speaks your language is important. I don't mean your language as in English or Spanish. I mean finding a doctor who you can relate to and who can relate to you—someone you are comfortable with. If you don't have a good feeling about your therapist or they relate to you in some way that makes you feel uncomfortable, this can compromise the efficacy of your treatments.

I always recommend making an initial phone call to the person you are thinking about going to. This way you can ask some basic questions and also get a feel for who this person is and how he or she might treat your problems. Obviously the information you receive over the phone will be limited, but still you can gain some insight into your prospective therapist by calling first.

Where can you find acupuncture? Getting referrals is always a good place to start. Ask around and see if you can find someone in your circle of friends who gets acupuncture or knows someone who does and who is satisfied with his or her specialist. If you see a D.O. (Doctor of Osteopathy), many times they are in the know about "alternative" treatments such as acupuncture. In the **Resources** section is information on finding an acupuncturist in your area.

How often should you get acupuncture? This question is best answered by your acupuncturist. For years I have gotten monthly acupuncture treatments. I do this for the benefit of prevention, not because I have specific needs. My need is to keep my body in balance and to do as many things possible to ensure this state of health. Acupuncture is one of my favorite ways of staying well. And acupuncture is something I *highly* recommend.

Melanie's story. Melanie has been a client of mine for years. I have always enjoyed our health and diet discussions during her monthly visits. She is an avid reader about diet and how it affects the body. She is a fit, thirty-something mother of three wonderful boys.

Melanie has always had some problems with breakouts—generally around her mouth and chin area. Through the years, I have cautioned her to keep her cell phone away from her face. She is on the phone all day long and as I will explain (see **Breakout**), resting the phone on your face can and will cause problems—eventually if not immediately.

Melanie has pared down the amount of sugar in her diet, yet her problems persist. Something else you need to know about Melanie: she has never had a normal menstrual cycle. This is a very important key to this story. As with so many bodily functions, menstruation is a clue to a woman's health. If you are not menstruating, or your cycle is abnormal, it is your body warning you that something is out of balance.

Because of her monthly irregularities, I have—for years—encouraged Melanie to start getting regular acupuncture treatments. This is exactly the kind of imbalance that I believe acupuncture is so proficient at helping to normalize. When the hormones are out of whack, it can and does throw off so many of our body's normal cycles. This keeps us from being in a balanced state of health.

I moved from Dallas to Chicago to open another skin care salon. When I would return for my quarterly trips to Dallas, Melanie was always on my schedule. This past visit (after not seeing her for over 5 months), I was pleased to see her skin had made an obvious improvement. Melanie told me that she finally committed to experimenting with acupuncture and had been going regularly for the past year. Well, not so regularly as you will find out.

She started to go and saw improvements in her skin and also in her menstrual cycle; things did seem to be changing for the better. But then life took over, and Melanie was unable to keep her regular appointments with her acupuncturist. Over the past summer, she hardly went for treatment and finally fell off the wagon completely.

What she noticed was surprising to her, but is what convinced her to start up again. Melanie noticed, once she wasn't getting acupuncture treatments, that her period was becoming nonexistent again and her skin problems were also returning. She hadn't given much credence to the whole alternative treatment course she had begun months earlier. But now, the evidence of how beneficial the treatments had been was in.

Melanie once again began getting regular acupuncture treatments, but this time she was more dedicated to not missing any appointments and going as prescribed by her acupuncturist. She saw and felt undeniable results after this second go-round with acupuncture. Melanie insists it is acupuncture alone that has regulated her menstrual cycle and therefore, finally, helped to clear up her persistent skin problems.

Aestheticians

I am interested in going to school to be an aesthetician. I am a little confused about some of the programs that are out there. I read your book, and I really liked the information I got out of it. I have even managed to give up sugar! The schools that I've researched have a lot of programs where you learn how to hook people up to batteries and dump chemicals on them, and I am pretty turned off by that. Can you give me some good ideas about what to look for in a program or better yet a good school in my area?

I'm glad you found some good information in my book. As far as schools go, I have no idea about the school programs in your particular location. It sounds like you've done some research, and that is what you'll need to do; find out where the schools are in your area, what their programs are, and which one sounds like the best fit. Because of the state of skin care these days, you may just have to contend with being taught things you may not agree with, but you'll certainly have control over what you do and use in your practice once you have graduated.

I learned very little in skin care school. My real learning came as I was working with clients and doing a lot of self-study. I studied things that meant something to me. And that is what I recommend whether you love the school you are attending or not. Experience is always going to be your greatest teacher. And until you have been working with skin for several years, you will just be learning and taking in information.

I have heard from a lot of people who want to become aestheticians and from aestheticians already in practice. I graduated in the mid-'80s, so my school experience may be a bit dated compared to the education available today in skin care schools throughout the country. But regardless where or when you went to school and how much you learned, continuing education (whether through self-study or classes) is a must. As you grow your practice and have clients who have come to you regularly for years and years, you will learn a lot about how skin changes and what the best treatments are.

Good luck to any of you who may already be working in skin care and for aspiring aestheticians just beginning your career. Go forth, study, and do good work.

You made a comment in your book that people should not go to an aesthetician who is just starting out. I think that is an unfair statement. I know I have put a great many hours not only in my state requirements, but also in my research, education and technique. I know I will learn more each day, not only in the next couple of years but hopefully for the rest of my career. I also believe, because this is so exciting and new for me, I will be giving my clients 110%. It seems that this profession, as with any, can have a burnout effect. I have had several facials by seasoned aestheticians who didn't seem to enjoy what they were doing. I really enjoyed the rest of your book and will use it as a tool in helping my clients. It is wonderful reading.

I appreciate this reader's comments. I believe the line I use in the book is "A novice aesthetician is not what you are looking for" when it comes to getting a facial. Someone who has stood the test of time—in any profession—will tend to be more qualified. However, the burnout comment can also apply. Due to the minimal amount of time it takes to become an aesthetician in most states, it can be a very easy career choice for some who may be unqualified, and that is where my comment stems from. I am quite sure many of you have put in a lot of hard work to become licensed in skin care, and I commend you for your commitment.

There are always exceptions to the rules and people with exceptional talent: aestheticians who will be heads above the rest in terms of qualifications as well as just an inherent understanding of the skin. However, having been one of these exceptions myself, I still know from my own experience that in the first few years as an aesthetician I simply wasn't able to help people on the level I can now.

Everyone has to start somewhere. My goal with my writing is to give readers the best information I can, knowing that ultimately they will be the decision-makers. Going to a novice anything wouldn't be my first choice; however, there may be benefits that will supersede a client's need for expertise. Trial and error along with getting personal referrals will be the determining factors in finding a good facial and aesthetician.

Why did you become an aesthetician?

Since I was young, I have always had a fascination with the human body. Perhaps because I grew up as a ballet dancer, I had a unique view into how the body functions under unusual circumstances, since dancing is quite an athletic event, and ballet in particular puts you in touch with your body—like it or not!

After 20 years of ballet, I wanted to switch careers and become a massage therapist. But I was offered a position as an aesthetician at a friend's salon, and she was kind enough to put me through skin care school. I jumped at the chance since my interests were not only in massage, but skin care as well.

Of course, straight out of school I knew nothing compared to what I know now, but I did my best. Through struggling to learn more and more about the body and skin in particular, I achieved my current level of expertise.

Eventually, by the way, I did graduate from massage school. I worked for several years both in skin care and massage, but I discovered that helping people with their skin in the context of a facial was the best application for my talents. After several years in practice, I stopped renewing my massage license in favor of being an aesthetician only. I guess I felt "jack of all trades, master of none" might apply if I didn't concentrate my efforts.

Being an aesthetician and now writing about skin care has brought me much joy. I am lucky to say I truly love what I do. For me, this is my life path; the work I was put here to do. It truly is my number one passion.

As a licensed aesthetician who no longer works in the industry, skin care is really more of a hobby that I enjoy reading and talking about. Your book is a must-have for aestheticians, who could definitely benefit from your experience, and for the consumer whose dermatologist and aesthetician isn't helping! Thanks for the fabulous tips in your book and for making my skin just that much more beautiful!

Alcohol in Products

Why is alcohol [in products] bad for my skin?

Alcohol, the bad kind, basically dries everything on the surface of your skin. In theory, this may sound appropriate, especially if you have an oilier skin type. But in practice, stripping away all the oil from your skin can cause your oil glands to produce more oil to compensate for the loss. Add to that the moisture (water) evaporation alcohol causes, and you could be causing the very things you are trying to avoid. Namely, oily skin that feels dry and looks flaky.

Some of my skin care products contain alcohol, mostly cetyl and cetearyl alcohol. Does this mean I can't use them?

I hear from people who are worried that alcohol is an ingredient in a product they are using. There are many alcohols that are OK as ingredients, as well as many that are not good. I had a woman call me who had read my book and was worried because she saw that Cetaphil® cleanser contained alcohol. This particular product has cetyl alcohol (an emulsifier) and stearyl alcohol (a waxy filler); these are both acceptable kinds of alcohol.

This is important: *Not all alcohol is bad.* To clarify the difference, here is a list of many of the alcohols, good and bad, that are used in skin care products. Some of them are seldom used, but many are very common. Bad alcohols are marked with a "B" before their names; if they are good or acceptable types of alcohol, they are marked with a "G." This list was compiled from Ruth Winter's *A Consumer's Dictionary of Cosmetic Ingredients, What's in Your Cosmetics?* by Aubrey Hampton, and *Milady's Skin Care and Cosmetic Ingredients Dictionary* by Natalia Michalun. Permissions listed on copyright page.

G/B—*abietyl alcohol; abietic acid; sylvic acid.* A texturizer for soaps derived from pine rosin. May cause allergic reactions.

G—*acetylated lanolin alcohol.* An emulsifier, emollient, and skin softening agent.

B—*alcohol; ethyl alcohol; ethanol.* Although this alcohol has antiseptic and degreasing abilities, don't use it! It is drying, absorbing the water on the surface of your skin.

G—*batyl alcohol.* A stabilizer that is derived from glycerin.

G—*behenyl alcohol.* A thickener, emulsifier, and stabilizer; increases viscosity.

B—*benzyl alcohol.* Derived from pure alcohol.

B—*butyl alcohol.* Sometimes listed as *n-butyl alcohol.* This is in the same league as other bad alcohols like ethyl and isopropyl.

G—*caprylic alcohol.* Occurs naturally in many essential oils (lavender, lemon, lime). A surfactant, or wetting agent.

G—*cetearyl alcohol.* A mixture of cetyl and stearyl alcohols, it is an emollient, thickener, and emulsifying wax.

G—*cetyl alcohol.* An emollient, emulsifier, and thickener.

B—*cinnamic alcohol.* A common allergen used as a fragrance ingredient.

G—*coconut alcohol.* Sometimes called *coconut fatty alcohol*; an emollient and lathering agent.

G—*decyl alcohol.* Derived from coconut oil or synthetically; it is an emollient, emulsifier, and antifoam agent.

B—*denatured alcohol.* See *methanol.*

B—*ethanol or ethyl alcohol.* Known as *rubbing alcohol,* it is a topical antiseptic, astringent, anti-bacterial. Avoid this alcohol!

B—*isopropyl alcohol.* Another rubbing alcohol. Made from propylene, which is a petroleum derivative. It is antibacterial, but is the bad kind of alcohol.

G—*lanolin alcohol.* An emulsifier and emollient.

G—*lauryl alcohol.* Used primarily in perfumes, this coconut oil derivative is used as a stabilizer, a skin conditioner, and for its sudsing abilities. May contribute to clogging the pores (comedogenic).

B—*methanol; methyl alcohol; wood alcohol.* This is basically denatured alcohol—the bad kind. It is flammable and toxic.

G—*myristyl alcohol; myristyl betaine; myristyloctadecanol.* An emollient, emulsifier, and foaming agent.

G/B—*oleyl alcohol.* An emollient and antifoam agent; it may be irritating to the skin.

B—*propyl alcohol.* Comes from crude oil; has a drying effect on skin.

B—*rubbing alcohol.* This is just another name for isopropyl alcohol and ethanol, which are the bad kinds of alcohol. Irritating and poisonous if ingested.

G—*stearyl alcohol.* Derived from sperm whale oil or synthetically produced from stearic acid; a lubricant.

B—*wood alcohol* (see *methanol*).

To reiterate, the most commonly used "bad" alcohols are ethyl, isopropyl, and SD alcohol. These are used quite frequently in products for problem or oily skin. No matter where they are used, you want to avoid these three plus any of the other alcohols listed above as "bad."

Allergic Reactions to Products

How do I know if I'm having an allergic reaction to a new product? And what should I do if I'm having a reaction?

If your skin changes for the worse after starting a new product, you may be having an allergic reaction. Or you could just be intolerant to one or more ingredients in one or more of the new products. Contrary to what you might have heard, a product should not cause breakouts when you first start using it. One client said she was told to give a new product three weeks for her skin to adapt. Even though she was breaking out from using this product, that was acceptable as far as the salesperson was concerned.

If your skin reacts adversely upon first using a new product, stop using it! In order to perform a controlled study and get some definite answers for yourself, I recommend taking the 72-Hour Test (see below). This seems to be a good experiment to find out what products are causing the reactions.

But first, I want to differentiate between initial reactions to a new product and developing an intolerance to a product over time. The following test is to help you figure out what product or products that you just began using might have caused any skin reaction you experienced. If you develop a skin condition such as eczema (discussed later in this section) or some other intolerance to a product you have successfully used in the past and just now are reacting to, try the 72-Hour Test. But this test is most helpful to narrow down possible culprits that have caused an immediate skin reaction.

Many times allergic reactions like a dermatitis can occur because something is compromising your immune system. And a product that you have used without any problems for a long time may suddenly give you problems. Stress is a known culprit when it comes to skin reactions and allergies. So if you are in a stressful state and are having problems with products you normally have no reactions to, I think you have to look to your state of inner health before completely discarding your skin care regime.

You may have to find other products in the interim that you can use without reaction, but you may not have to give up your old products altogether. Once the stress in your life has subsided, you may want to dig up these formerly OK products and give them another try. They may cause no reaction, and then again, you may have to forgo using them if you do indeed react. In this case, as well as with new products that may have caused reactions, take the following test to determine whether or not you can use a particular product.

The 72-Hour Test. Let's say you just purchased a whole line of skin care products (or even just a single product), and after using them for a few days, you notice redness or skin sensitivity you didn't have before. First, stop using all the new products and go back to what you had been using. You want your skin back to normal before proceeding with the test.

Once your skin has calmed down, take one product, let's say the new cleanser, and use it for three days (72 hours) along with your other old products (toner, moisturizer, eye cream). If your skin is OK, use a second new product for three days (your old cleanser and now the new toner, for instance). If at any point you introduce a product and have a reaction, at least you'll know which product is the trouble-maker. Keep in mind, you may only have a reaction to one or two of the products—not the whole line. So by doing the 72-Hour Test, you can find out which products you can use and which ones you can't. This process takes time, but if you want to find an answer to what is causing the reaction, it's worth the time.

If all goes well and you don't react to the individual products, it may have been too much for your skin to try out so many products at one time. Sometimes this happens, but most likely if you had a reaction the first time you used it, you will find at least one product causes a reaction when doing the test. If every product causes a reaction, there may be a common ingredient in the line that may prohibit you from using any of it.

If you are reacting to a product three or more weeks after using it, I doubt it is really the product breaking you out. Usually your body (skin) will react within a short period of time after trying a new product—instantly or within a few days. This is not an absolute, but it's doubtful it will take your skin three weeks to realize it is intolerant to particular ingredients. The breakout could be due to something new in your daily routine, severe weather changes, or stress—something current in your life. Don't automatically blame a product for causing problems when it could be something unrelated. Take the 72-Hour Test and see what you come up with.

With all that said, over time you can develop intolerances to certain products or ingredients, just like with foods. You may have been able to eat certain foods in the past that today you are intolerant to. Sometimes this can happen with skin care products as well. It all boils down to ingredients and your skin and how the two are suited to each other. If you feel like you have become intolerant to a certain product (or even the entire line of products) simply stop using them, go back to products that in the past didn't cause problems, and then take the 72-Hour Test.

Regardless of what is causing the problem, having a reaction is undesirable. If you have just purchased new products you can't use, try to return them. Companies have varying return policies (something you might want to consider before purchasing). Make sure you are aware of the likelihood of getting your money back (or not).

I'm 23 years old and have very sensitive skin. Any product I use wears out its welcome after three months. About three weeks ago I began waking up with lines on the bridge of my nose. Two weeks ago I noticed lines forming under my eyes, and this week the skin under my eyes looks dry (but isn't) and is full of lines and wrinkles. It even seems a little loose. What is happening? My skin was smooth with tiny, barely visible lines three weeks ago; now it's as if it has aged 10 years overnight! Why would this happen, and will my skin ever go back to the way it was before? Could this be an allergic reaction?

Based on your symptoms, I would say this is a classic allergic reaction. Crepey skin, especially when you find wrinkles overnight, is definitely a symptom of an intolerance to something used, and is probably a dermatitis called eczema. The eyes are so sensitive, and many times an allergic reaction to a new skin care product will occur near the eyes, even if the offending product was used on the entire face.

Depending on the severity of the reaction, you may need to see your dermatologist and get a prescription cream to help calm your skin down. First you could try a topical cortisone cream (found at any drug or grocery store) and see if this helps. You must, however, read the directions and be very careful about how close to your eyes you apply the cream. The doctor will be able to prescribe a higher strength steroid cream if the over the counter type isn't effective enough.

Look at the ingredients of the offending product and see if you can find anything you know you are allergic to. Sometimes just fragrance in products can cause reactions like the kind mentioned above. Your skin, once calmed down, should resume its natural, normal state. How long this will take varies with the individual. But surely within a week or perhaps a bit longer, you will have your old skin back.

Recently I went to purchase some new products—an experience that turned out to be a living nightmare! First, I got my skin analyzed and was told that I have normal, combination skin. I purchased a papaya exfoliant, clay mask, and a moisturizing mask for dehydrated skin.

After several weeks of exfoliating and masking, to my horror I woke up one day with welts all over my face, redness, burning, and itching. My eyes were almost swollen shut! I have never reacted like this to anything before. Needless to say, I am mortified that my skin may have been permanently ruined.

My doctor has prescribed methylprednisolone (cortisone) for six days. It has brought the swelling down a bit, but I still have redness and itchiness, not to mention that my skin feels very taut and dry—appearing to have wrinkled up (I didn't have any wrinkles before this!!!!).

Everything I have tried on my face to alleviate the burning and itching has not worked, except for petroleum jelly, which soothed it considerably. I am worried and don't know what to do next. I am thinking of going to an allergist.

Would you have any advice for me? Is my skin ruined forever?
Please respond as soon as possible because I desperately need your
expert advice. I am afraid of the cortisone I am taking, but feel I
have no choice since my symptoms are severe. I am desperate!

Your reactions sound like a dermatitis, probably eczema: red, itchy skin that feels like it is burning, along with severe dryness and crinkling. A topical cortisone cream will probably relieve the symptoms, but that doesn't tell you why you had the reaction in the first place. If you are game, you could also take the 72-Hour Test to help narrow down which product caused the problems. It may have been all of the products, but maybe not. Of course, you may not be willing to develop those reactions in order to figure out which products you can or cannot use. In that case, an allergist will probably be able to figure it out for you. There may be common allergens contained in one or all of those products that the specialist can tell you about. If you are going to do the 72-Hour Test, I highly recommend you wait until your skin has completely recovered and even wait a few more weeks to be sure you aren't still in reaction mode.

This client told me that after about a week of severe redness, itching, swelling, and pain her skin did finally calm down. She made an appointment to see an allergist, but wasn't able to get in to see someone for almost four months.

I have noticed that certain hair products seem to irritate my skin.
Do you recommend a certain type of conditioner? I have really long
hair so I have to use lots of product in it every day. I try to keep
it off my face, but I noticed recently that a new conditioner I was
trying has aggravated my face. Any recommendations?

One recommendation is to really rinse the conditioner out of your hair before you leave the shower. I realize you are using it to soften and probably detangle your hair, but just the excess product left on your hair might be a big contributor to your problems.

If you are using something that you know is aggravating your skin, of course stop using it. If you can, go back to products that didn't bother your skin, even though they might not be as effective for your hair. It may be a trade-off; you'll have to decide which you'd rather have, clear skin or more manageable hair.

Allergies & Skin

Allergies (airborne) can equal dark circles, puffiness under your eyes, and possibly eczema or another dermatitis, to say nothing about sneezing, wheezing, and generally feeling miserable. When your body is dealing with invading allergens, it cannot possibly keep up with everything, and your immune system becomes compromised.

If you have allergies, you may be taking medication to suppress the symptoms. Most over the counter products have decongestant ingredients that can dry out your system. Allergy medications can also wreak havoc on your skin. I recommend adding hydrating elixirs to your moisturizers and exfoliating as often as possible to help keep your skin feeling hydrated and looking flake-free.

To help your body function under the stress of allergies, be sure to get all the proper nutrients on a daily basis and try to avoid drinking alcohol and eating sugar. Both of these can stress your immune system as well as cause inflammation, which is exactly what your sinuses don't need. Dairy products, namely milk and cheese, are mucous forming, so avoid these if possible while you are experiencing allergies.

When the pressure gets to be too much and my sinuses feel painful, I will do a little bit of acupressure on the areas. All this means is that I apply pressure to points on my sinus cavity, which really does help to temporarily relieve some of the pain. I usually start with the area where my brow bone slopes down to the nose. Next I work on all the bones surrounding the eyes, and then around my cheek bones, and even my middle forehead area. If you have allergies and your sinuses are congested, you will feel where you need to apply pressure. I usually press as hard as I can and stay with that pressure for at least 10 seconds for each area. (Don't forget to breathe!) You can experiment and see what works for you, but using this technique can really help to relieve some of the pain and tension in your sinuses. It can work for headaches as well.

Aloe Vera

Aloe vera is a plant that is known for its healing abilities. Today, it can be found as an ingredient in many skin care products, both for the face as well as the body. Personally, I have had many success stories where aloe came to my skin's rescue, and I have many friends and clients who have discovered the miraculous healing abilities of this desert plant.

However, as with most things in life, not everything works for everybody, and such is the case with aloe. Along with all the success stories about how aloe saved people's skin, I have heard from some people who had reactions to it as well. If you are unsure if you are allergic, read through this section as well as **Allergic Reactions to Products** to gather more information. As great as aloe vera is, you might react to it.

Aloe and sunburn. Probably the best known treatment for sunburn is aloe vera. If this is news to you, next time you have a severe or even just a slight sunburn, be sure to have aloe vera gel handy to help treat your damaged skin.

Aloe is almost entirely made up of water along with proteins. Since sunburned skin has essentially had all the water sucked out of it, replenishing this vital hydrating liquid is all-important. Aloe vera gel will not only soothe the pain and swelling of a sunburn, it will also speed healing of your sun-damaged skin. Since sunburns do happen, always have aloe vera gel (95% or higher) in your medicine cabinet for those times when the sun has gotten the better of you.

One of my own aloe stories. Years ago, while under tremendous stress, I started developing a stomach ulcer. After reading about the healing power of aloe vera, I started drinking aloe juice (not to be confused with the gel) daily and the ulcer went away—very quickly. Granted, I also changed some unhealthy aspects of my diet and worked on relaxing more during the day, but I believe the highest percentage of healing came from the aloe juice.

In the **Canker Sores** section, I talk about swishing salt water in your mouth several times a day to help with these mouth irritations. Although stomach ulcers and mouth ulcers aren't the same thing, there is a similarity, and therefore aloe juice can make an effective treatment for both.

I was told by a pharmacist that aloe worked well to clear up acne because it was natural and oil-free. So I would put aloe on periodically, thinking it would soothe my face. I would usually break out soon afterwards. I never connected the breakout to the aloe because I was only using it off and on.

I have read the ingredients in my body lotions and many have aloe in them. It seems to be fine on my body, but as far as my face goes I will not use something that has any aloe—I can't afford to aggravate my face.

I am including stories of how aloe didn't work to let you know it is not uncommon to have an intolerance to this product. Unfortunate as that may be, if you find you get irritated after using aloe vera, stop using it. Regarding this email, although aloe vera is a great product and I'm sure its benefits would be good for almost any skin condition, it wouldn't be the first thing I'd reach for to treat problem skin, including acne.

The following comes from my neighbor Teressa who called me up one day after putting aloe gel on her face. She had a bad burning reaction that left her skin bright red. In the following email, she is updating me on her aloe investigation.

> *After my face calmed down from using aloe gel, I purchased a brand new bottle of Lily of the Desert®. I opened it up, put it on my face, and the same thing happened again—it burned and made my skin red and irritated. I know aloe is supposed to be good for me, but I guess I'm allergic to it.*

Yes, Teressa, you are one of many people I have encountered who just have an intolerance to aloe. You might want to be careful in the future and watch your skin's reaction if you use products that have aloe in the ingredient list. You may not be able to use it straight on your skin, while still being able to use products with aloe in them. Because the percentage of aloe will be low if it is in a product, compared to the nearly 100% strength you have been using, you may be able to tolerate it.

Lily of the Desert is actually a good choice for a high-strength aloe vera gel. After Teressa's email, I went out and purchased this brand and was happy to see it was 99% aloe. It is inexpensive and can be found in most health food stores. Lily of the Desert isn't the only brand available, but it certainly is a good choice—as long as you don't have allergies to aloe.

"Anti-Aging"

I'm always amazed when I hear the term *anti-aging*. It makes aging sound like a bad thing. Yet this term is used every day in conversations and advertisements for products (not just skin care products). You name it—people view aging negatively.

A client telephoned and asked me what anti-aging products I thought she should use. I told her the best recommendation I could give her for anti-aging was to step away from the mirror. The phone went silent, and I think I caught her off guard, but I was actually halfway serious. It is only because we see our reflections in the mirror that we know what we look like. The less you look in the mirror, you will see less of your so-called flaws.

I promise I don't say these things to trivialize your thoughts and fears about getting older. I say them in order to give a voice to the other side of the story. We are constantly inundated with anti-aging-this, look-younger-that, and I'm quite sure that will not be changing soon. But *I* can change—and so can you. You don't have to give in to the theory that as you age you have to look younger than you are. Strive to look your best, of course, but getting rid of age is not only impossible, it takes up a lot of energy. Personally, I barely have enough energy to get me through a normal day. If I chose to spend a good deal of time worrying about how young or how old I look, I wouldn't have time to simply have a good day.

I'm just advocating paying attention to the other side of aging: the *anti*-anti-aging side. Take the best care of yourself you can and do whatever you feel is appropriate for you to look your best. And give yourself a break at the same time. Remember, what you put your attention to is what you will attract into your life. Put your attention toward being healthy and at peace—no matter what your age. To me these things far surpass erasing any wrinkles I might be accumulating.

Antibiotics & Skin

Sara's story. My client Sara has been on tetracycline for at least two years for problem skin. However, after talking with her, I found that her skin problems are very intermittent and occasional. Once her dermatologist suggested Accutane, but Sara's problems weren't severe, and from what she knew about that medication, she thought Accutane sounded like overkill. She went on to tell me she had a hysterectomy at 27 years of age due to complications with her ovaries, and since then she has had over eight surgeries for endometriosis. This information shows something is inherently out of whack with Sara's body. Most likely she has a hormone imbalance, which can adversely affect the skin.

She called me wanting help with occasional breakouts that came in the form of deep cysts about once a week. We discussed diet, and she didn't have too much sugar in her diet although she did admit to her one bad habit: Diet Coke®. She drinks about 6-8 per day. These may not be causing her skin troubles directly, but they surely aren't helping her overall health. Diet or not, carbonated beverages—especially consumed in excess—can be harmful to the delicate balance in our bodies.

As an example of why being on antibiotics can affect you adversely, recently Sara burned her arm, causing a fair-sized wound. She went swimming, as she usually does for exercise, and wound up with a large infection at the sight of the burn. She called a doctor friend of hers who proceeded to tell her he couldn't believe she had been on antibiotics and still developed an infection. The body gets used to anything, and it can get used to antibiotics if they are used for an extended period of time. That is one reason I am so against long-term antibiotic use for problem skin. It is only treating, temporarily at best, the symptom and doing nothing to protect or enhance the body's immune system—something you need if you get sick, or in Sara's case, sustain an injury.

She told me sometimes she doesn't take the antibiotics and nothing bad happens with her skin. Maybe she could stop altogether and see if her skin problems persist. I can tell you this much: her problems will persist if she doesn't locate and isolate the offending party (which could be a hormone imbalance, diet, stress, lifestyle habits) and eliminate or in some other way alter it to end the skin reaction.

Long-term use of antibiotics for skin problems is a slippery slope. My personal experience with antibiotics is limited since I haven't taken them for many years, but in the past whenever I would take antibiotics, my skin would break out. I wouldn't get a huge breakout, but I'd always get one or two really deep, red papules; the kind of blemish that doesn't have a head and cannot be extracted. It is also the kind of spot that tends to take a long time to go away. I think this is because my body was trying to throw off the toxic effect of the medication.

In the short term, antibiotics can be helpful and useful. It is their long-term use and abuse that I disagree with, as in Sara's case and many other stories I have heard from clients over the years. Take notice of how long you have been taking antibiotics for your skin and consider finding alternative ways to ensure clear skin. This includes putting on your investigator's hat and trying to discern what the cause of the breakouts is in the first place. (See **Acidophilus/Acidophilus and antibiotics**.) As a side note, I suggested Sara go to an acupuncturist to see if that would make some headway with her hormonal concerns.

A teenager's story. Linda's son, Michael, has had problem skin his whole teenage life. He has been on tetracycline (a commonly prescribed antibiotic) for years and now, at age 19, his skin is a mess. The antibiotics have long since stopped working and his dermatologist is suggesting Accutane. His mother is, to say the least, disappointed and unsure of what to do.

Linda told me Michael eats a diet rich in poor-quality foods. She insists he doesn't drink sodas and juice at home. Teenagers and soda pop pretty much go hand in hand, so if his friends are drinking sodas, he probably is too. Although she makes her own house as sugarfree as possible, the world is a huge candy store just waiting for teenagers to come and partake.

I told Linda that her son can go on and stay on drugs his whole life, but until he stops feeding the problem—literally—the skin troubles will continue. Due to his age, his hormones may still be surging and will settle down with time, but in the meantime it would be great if he could learn to change his eating habits.

The special challenge with teens is not only are their hormones kicking in, but they don't usually eat a balanced diet. Even some adults have a hard time understanding that what they are eating may be affecting their bodies, their health, and their skin. And in my experience, I find most teens haven't made that connection yet either.

One positive thing about Michael is he is coming to his mom and expressing disgust with his skin. That's actually a good sign because it means he will be open (to some degree) to changing his ways and listening to helpful advice. Here is a fact that has repeated itself to me over and over again: If people see improvement after making a change (like cutting back or quitting sugar), they are more prone to continuing to change. If no improvement is seen (like after buying expensive but ineffective products, for instance), then they are less likely to keep changing.

The point to this story is to say that taking antibiotics won't necessarily clear up your skin. It may be a temporary fix, but unless you change your eating habits (or just grow out of the teenage hormonal years), antibiotics aren't a cure-all. And they can actually affect your body's immune system by weakening it. Start at the source and see what positive changes you can make that will surely result in positive changes in your skin's health—and of course for the health of your entire body.

Antioxidants

What are antioxidants and should I take them for my skin?

Anything you swallow (pills included) will get into your bloodstream and affect your entire body. Although antioxidants can help your skin look its best, they are important and beneficial to much more than just your skin. I mention this because the mindset of taking supplements to affect one thing is akin to exercising to spot reduce a certain body part. It just can't be done. Exercise will affect your whole body; antioxidants will too.

Antioxidants help rid the body of free radicals; free radicals contribute to the destruction of healthy cells. If you are eating a balanced diet with a high fruit and vegetable content, you are probably getting lots of antioxidants. But diets are not so balanced for many people. I'm not a big believer in taking pills, especially using supplements as a way of substituting for a poor diet. However, due to our modern lifestyles and busy schedules, supplementing is not only inevitable, but probably necessary.

Free radicals. Free radicals are running rampant in our bodies due to the polluted world we live in. Pollution from the outside can and does create pollution inside our bodies. We can easily cause imbalance inside by making poor nutritional choices as well as sustaining emotional stress. Luckily there are many avenues you can take to help keep free radical damage to a minimum.

Surely you are asking, "What is a free radical? " Normally functioning molecules have two or three electrons; free radicals are missing one electron, making that molecule unstable. So they hunt for an electron they can take from a neighboring molecule. Free radicals aren't particular—they attack the nearest stable molecule in order to create stability for themselves. So free radicals are constantly searching to complete themselves with their missing half. Once the free radical finds its "mate," it sets up a domino effect of scavenging. The molecule it took the electron from becomes unstable and has to steal another molecule's electron. Each free radical that finds an electron in turn makes the molecule it stole from a free radical. It is an endless cycle of search and swipe, and so the vicious cycle continues.

Free radicals are necessary in certain amounts to promote circulation and other vital functions of the body. Smog, cigarette smoke, and poor food choices are some of the major causes of an overabundance of free radicals in our bodies. When they get out of hand, it's time to bring in the heavy artillery. This is where antioxidants come into play. If you want to take care of your skin, you want to be sure your body has a good supply of these free radical-destroying nutrients.

Antioxidants. If free radicals cause damage in the body, antioxidants are their worst enemy. Antioxidants basically help to stop the domino effect of free radical scavenging and restore the normal, whole functioning of the cell both inside and out. In supplement form, there are many antioxidants to choose from. If you only take one, vitamin C for instance, you will still derive benefits that outweigh no supplementing at all, but used in combination, antioxidants form a stronger bond and thus a more potent effect.

Alpha lipoic acid and protective are synonymous. A powerful antioxidant, alpha lipoic acid has the ability to actually help regenerate other antioxidants that have been wounded in the process of ridding the body of free radicals. Alpha lipoic acid can also be very helpful in regulating blood sugar levels. This is something that diabetics and people who suffer from hypo- or hyperglycemia may want to know about. I am interested in alpha lipoic acid not only for its antioxidant abilities but also for its benefits with inflammation; both of these factors have an effect on the health of your cells. And as with many of the supplements available in the anti-aging range, anything that increases the health of your body will naturally be reflected in healthier-looking skin.

Alpha lipoic acid in supplement form is fairly expensive. As an ingredient in skin care products, alpha lipoic acid is outrageously expensive. Even if these products did work wonders for your lines and wrinkles, unless you are well-off financially, you will never be able to afford to keep up this habit. You'll just have to age with the rest of us and find less expensive ways to keep your skin looking clear, healthy, and if you must, young. I'm still not convinced putting alpha lipoic acid, vitamin C, or any other anti-aging miracle ingredients topically on your skin is truly effective against aging. I prefer to eat my vitamins, whether in food or with supplements.

There is no RDA (recommended daily allowance) for alpha lipoic acid; recommendations vary from 10mg to 600mg daily. Doses over 100mg might have the effect of lowering blood sugar levels in some individuals, even non-diabetics. I am prone to hypoglycemia so I closely monitored how I felt when I first started experimenting with alpha lipoic acid. When I took 100-200mg per day, I had no adverse reaction in regard to my blood sugar levels.

Note: Alpha lipoic acid should not be confused with alpha-linolenic acid (ALA), an omega-3 essential fatty acid. They are both beneficial for different reasons. (See **Essential Fatty Acids.**)

Also known as *ubiquinone*, **Coenzyme Q10** (more commonly called CoQ10) has shown signs of rejuvenating brain cells in laboratory animals. There is no conclusive evidence yet to show there is an appreciable difference in the human brain, but tests are underway to bring new information to the forefront. What is known is CoQ10 is a powerful antioxidant. It has been shown to help boost the power of vitamin E in the fatty part of cells. This is the part that can sustain the worst free radical damage. These fatty cells are concentrated in the brain, so taking CoQ10 may help to protect the all-important brain. There is no established dosage for Coenzyme Q10.

Grape seed extract enjoyed a bit of popularity a few years ago, but has since slipped behind so many of the up and coming antioxidants. Grape seed extract, however, is an excellent source of a complex of antioxidants called OPCs (oligomeric proanthocyanidin complexes). You can take capsules ranging anywhere from 250-1000mg daily. It is the OPCs in red wine that is thought to be good for certain health issues. Grape seed extract is the best all around source for OPCs, so don't drink wine as your only source for this complex of antioxidants!

If **vitamin C** isn't the best-known antioxidant, surely it is the best-known vitamin. It started when we were kids, hearing how vitamin C helps to keep the common cold away. In fact *Vitamin C and the Common Cold* is the title of a wonderful book written by Dr. Linus Pauling. Among many other contributions (both social and scientific), Linus Pauling is perhaps best known by the general public for his research and advocacy of high-dosing vitamin C. This investigative pioneer began ground-breaking research into the value and disease-fighting ability of vitamin C, and lived to the ripe age of 93 (1901-1994). He truly was an example of his research and work in nutritional studies.

Now we know that vitamin C is one of the most powerful antioxidants. It is helpful with brain function as well as repairing free radical damage. One of the more interesting benefits of vitamin C is its ability to improve the quality as well as the quantity of brain transmissions. Translation: it helps your brain function optimally.

Vitamin C helps with many other bodily functions. It helps in the production of collagen, which is the supporting structure of your skin. It is the collagen and elastin fibers that break down through sun exposure and the natural aging process, creating lines and wrinkles on our faces as well as flaccid or sagging skin. This antioxidant also helps with bruising as well as the healing of wounds and burns.

Vitamin C is water-soluble and not manufactured by the body. Therefore, we have to get this antioxidant through our food and/or supplementation. Vitamin C is found in numerous foods you are probably already eating. Because most of this vitamin leaves through the urine, you might consider taking it in supplement form as well.

Taking anywhere from 500 to 1000 milligrams daily is thought to be sufficient to help protect the brain. Even in large doses, vitamin C doesn't seem to be toxic. Of course, too much of anything is not a good thing. You will know if you've taken too much vitamin C because you'll get loose bowels or possibly diarrhea. Some people even use high-dosing of vitamin C in order to clean out their colon. If you experience diarrhea, whether you are inducing this type of evacuation or because you are sick, you must also increase your water intake to compensate for the loss of water through these eliminations.

Vitamin E, sometimes known by the name *tocopherol*, is an important vitamin if you are interested in your brain having maximum help to ward off free radical invasion. This antioxidant works on the fatty parts of the cells that comprise the brain. Research is increasing to see if vitamin E can help fend off such debilitating brain diseases as Alzheimer's and Parkinson's.

You want to take *natural* vitamin E. How do you know if it's natural? It will always have a "d" in front of the chemical name, such as d-alpha tocopherol. *Tocotrienols* are another form of vitamin E, and can be found alone or in the mixed tocopherol supplements. The mixed vitamin E supplements might contain d-alpha as well as d-beta, d-delta, and d-gamma tocopherols. The mixed forms of vitamin E are said to be the best for brain protection. In most of the literature I've read, it says taking 400 IUs (international units) of vitamin E is sufficient; taking more, especially over 800 IUs, can get you into trouble. Most notably, it has blood thinning abilities at these higher doses. I would stick with the lower 400 IUs per day, unless instructed otherwise by your health care practitioner.

The antioxidants you just read about are the most powerful, but certainly not the only ones available. Other antioxidants include bilberry, an herb; cysteine, an amino acid; ginkgo biloba, an herb; glutathione, a protein; green tea; melatonin, a hormone; selenium, an enzyme; superoxide dismutase, an enzyme; vitamin A as well as beta carotene; and zinc, a mineral.

Food sources containing antioxidants are numerous. Many fruits and vegetables have high antioxidant contents, as well as some fish like salmon, which is my all-time favorite. I encourage you to try to incorporate as many antioxidants as you can into your life and your diet for optimal health of your entire body, including your skin.

Ashy Skin

African-Americans sometimes find their skin to be "ashy." I really think it is just flaky, dry skin that appears to look like ashes due to the dark color of the skin and the lighter color of the flakes. In the winter months, for instance, my legs become very dry and flaky and if not for my light-colored skin, I would probably say my skin looked ashy. But regardless of the semantics, the problem is dry, flaky skin, no matter whose skin it is occurring on.

> *I have ash on my legs, and it doesn't look good. I have to go to the beach this summer. Is there anything I can do to even out my skin tone, and what's the best and least harmful way to get rid of this ashy look?*

Simply making sure you always have moisturizer on your body's skin can go a long way to helping the dry condition. This means that after every bath and shower you need to apply a good moisturizing cream or lotion—or even an oil—to give the skin extra hydration. The use of alpha hydroxy acids (AHAs) might be applicable here. AHAs help to passively exfoliate dead skin cells, leaving a smoother, less flaky surface. I don't recommend AHAs for the face in most cases; it can create problems with the delicate capillaries. But for the legs, these acids may indeed give you the smooth texture you are looking for.

Gently exfoliating this ashy skin is also of importance. Although AHAs do help to passively remove dead skin, you need to also actively get the dry, flaky skin off. Using a body scrub or even exfoliation gloves can get the job done. I don't recommend loofahs; they're too harsh on the skin, plus they are hard to keep clean and bacteria-free. Terry cloth towels and washcloths are also not recommended here. Getting too aggressive with "rubbing" the skin off can actually cause the skin to thicken—something you don't want to happen. Stick with scrubs and good moisturizers to help keep the ashy skin away.

Avobenzone

Avobenzone or Parsol 1789 is one of the few truly effective sunscreen ingredients. The other two are titanium dioxide and zinc oxide. All three are considered physical blocks.

Avobenzone, unlike many other sunscreens, helps to block out UVA radiation from the sun. This is important—you want to use sunscreens that are classified as *full spectrum*, which means they are able to protect you against both UVA and UVB sun rays.

On one of the talk shows I was a guest on, there was also a dermatologist there giving information about sun-related skin damage. He went on and on about the benefits of this relatively new sunscreen ingredient, Parsol 1789.

So when you are shopping for the best ingredients to have in your sunscreen, look for the name Avobenzone or Parsol 1789. Of course nothing except the great indoors is going to keep you from receiving sun exposure, thus sun damage. But wearing a product with this or any of the other physical sunscreen ingredients mentioned above will give you the best coverage you can find—short of an umbrella or inside a building.

Azelaic Acid

Azelex® is the name for a prescription topical antibiotic cream containing azelaic acid that is used for acne. It is said to be less irritating than other topical blemish medications derived from vitamin A like Retin-A, which can cause a lot of redness and flaking.

Azelex contains 20% azelaic acid, which comes from wheat and grain. It helps to decrease inflammation and is an antimicrobial, which means it kills bacteria. Azelaic acid's antibacterial abilities are similar to essential oils, and I happen to be a fan of essential oils. They are easy to find, inexpensive, and do not require a doctor's prescription. I also think essential oils work better than most topical medications used to diminish blemishes.

One of the more interesting benefits listed for azelaic acid and specifically Azelex is its reported ability to lessen pigmentation. It doesn't have a bleaching action, but helps to disrupt the melanocytes' activity, inhibiting melanin production wherever the product is applied. This theory is not absolute, but it might be one way to help lessen hyperpigmentation. Some topical medications, however, can have the opposite effect, causing photo or sun sensitivity, which actually increases pigmentation. It just goes to show you nothing works for everybody. Rosacea is another skin condition this antibiotic cream is reported to be beneficial for.

All of my writing is experience-based—either personal or from my clients' experiences. To date, I haven't had enough clients using this acne treatment to give you anything other than the facts available on this product's label.

Age is just a number. Old is a state of mind.

– Carolyn Ash

Back Breakout

In a popular beauty book, the author recommends using dishwashing detergent followed by benzoyl peroxide for back breakouts. Now, I am only one person, but I have a fair amount of common sense. I can see how the author thinks if detergent gets the grease off her dishes surely it would be an acceptable product to use on human skin. Because as we all know, skin and porcelain and/or glass are virtually the same thing, right?

OK, I'll stop being sarcastic and just tell it like it is. Using dish washing detergent on your skin is the most ridiculous thing I have ever heard of! I did a TV show where I had degreasing detergent on the table of what *not* to use on problem skin. I once knew a client who put dishwashing detergent on her blemishes in an attempt to dry them out. She thought, perhaps as the above mentioned author does, that a degreasing agent would degrease her skin. But the results for my client were irritation coupled with severe peeling on and around the blemishes. I can't imagine what would happen to the skin on your back if you applied dishwashing detergent even just one time, and then followed it with another known skin irritant: benzoyl peroxide.

This author goes on to recommend applying the dishwashing detergent not with your hands but with a bath brush. You have not only set up the potential for irritation using a product never intended for human skin, but to add insult to injury you are going to ensure severe irritation by using a brush to massage in the product! Is she crazy? No, just very ill-informed. She is not an aesthetician or even a person who has had any experience (from what her bio reads) with skin on a real, up close and personal level. The kind of advice in that book is the kind of advice I recommend avoiding at all costs. Those suggestions might look good in a magazine or flash advertising, but to actually be recommending this for readers who have problem skin on their backs (or faces, or wherever) is preposterous. I can only hope that if you choose to read books like that one, you will also use your common sense. How much sense does it make to use dishwashing detergent (meant for dishes and glassware) on your delicate skin? If your answer is, "It kind of makes sense," then I will just tell you straight up: don't do it! Dishes are dishes, but human skin is a living organ that needs special care.

With that said, you came to this section to get help with back breakout. Because we are dealing with skin, its location is less relevant than you may think. As long as you are producing infected blemishes, you want to essentially treat them the same no matter where they appear on your body.

I get a lot of breakout on my back. It is practically impossible for me to reach this area. What can I do to help the problem, and why does my back break out in the first place?

When it comes to treating the skin on your back, it can be challenging. But there are ways you can get to that skin, even if you have to employ another person in the process. The answer to why you are breaking out there is the same as if you were having breakouts on your face. Internally something is out of balance, and in my opinion, diet is most likely at the root of the problem.

Watch your sugar intake. See the **Sugar** section to find out more about how this common ingredient can cause a lot of problems with skin—namely breakouts. **Water** is one of the best things for your body. If you aren't currently drinking enough (or any) water each day, start now to drink more water, which helps to rid toxins from your body. If you **sweat** a lot, are you able to rinse it off your back? Or does the sweat just sit there on your skin for long periods of time? This can be a source of irritation and potential breakout, especially if you are sweating during workouts. Rinse the sweat off your entire body before it has a chance to dry on the skin.

If you can afford it, get a **back facial** at a salon or spa. Call first to be sure they offer this service and if you have the time, go by the establishment and see where you will be receiving the treatment before you even make an appointment. Why? Some facial chairs just don't translate into good tables for back facials. You want a versatile chair that will ensure your comfort during the process. The salon may have you lie on a massage table, which is fine. Ask them to prop up your feet if that makes you feel more comfortable. They probably have a bolster to put under the tops of your ankles for this very purpose.

Ask a friend for help. If there is someone in your life you trust to do a good job, ask them to give you a back facial. You could get a back facial as often as you can find someone to give one to you. Just like any treatment for blemishes on your face, the more kind attention you give problem skin, the better it is for helping the healing process.

After taking a shower to get yourself cleaned off, lay a towel or two down on the floor and lie face down. Have your helper use a mild scrub mixed with water on your back. If you have large red and pus-filled blemishes, a scrub is not a good idea. It is important to exfoliate back there, but you certainly don't want to break open the spots and possibly spread the bacteria to other places on your skin. Other than scrubs, a gel-peel (like a gommage) or another type of non-abrasive peel, like a papaya enzyme peel, would be preferable. If you don't have access to an exfoliant or if it would be inappropriate to use one, just skip to the next step.

After the scrub (or other exfoliator) is removed, apply a clay mask. Usually back breakouts are in the upper region, near the shoulders. If your entire back is broken out, you will probably go through a lot of mask, but it is very helpful to get it on the spots. If you don't have enough mask to go over the entire area, be sure to dot clay liberally on all the blemishes individually—even if they cover your whole back.

If possible, spread the clay over the entire area as mentioned above. Ideally you want to keep the mask moist. This way you won't dry out the outer skin. You can either spray the mask with toner or filtered water. Or, if you are so inclined, your assistant can take tissues and soak them in either toner or water and place them on your skin as a compress where the clay has been applied.

Leave the mask for 15 minutes or so. Then you can either shower to remove the clay or your helper can remove it with a warm (not hot) washcloth. Just be sure not to rub hard or scrub with the washcloth. After the mask is cleaned off, I suggest spraying one last application of toner on the area and massaging it in. If you have any medications or special products you are using for the blemishes, apply those last. Geranium oil (see section) would be a good choice to help treat the individual spots.

I have one last recommendation: Don't let your helper pick at your blemishes unless he or she knows how to extract properly. I have heard countless stories of partners who actually relish popping their mate's spots. I suppose it is just a natural maternal instinct that we have. But if done incorrectly, this process can cause more harm than good. However, some places may need to be extracted. See **Extractions** to read up on how to do it for the best results.

Please understand, facials, whether for your back or your face, will not eliminate your skin problems completely. Your breakout originates from a systemic imbalance, and treating the symptom (breakout) topically will only go so far. Treating the problem from the outside can and will help it on many levels, but I want to be sure you are also taking steps to figure out the real cause of the problems. Without figuring out the cause of the imbalance along with action taken toward healthier lifestyle habits, no amount of facials, back or otherwise, will fix the problem at hand.

Basal Cell Carcinoma

Basal cell carcinoma is a very common form of skin cancer that you need to know about. Over 800,000 people are diagnosed with basal cell carcinoma annually, and that number is only going to increase as the years go by. Basal cell carcinomas occur in the basal cell layer of the skin and are primarily caused by sun exposure.

There are many different looks to basal cell cancers; sometimes they may just look like regular moles on the skin. They don't have clear-cut identifying markers, like, for instance a melanoma. Unlike this deadly form of skin cancer (melanoma), basal cell carcinomas rarely spread to other parts of the body. The most common area for this type of skin cancer to surface is the face, ears, even the scalp. They also can appear on the upper part of the back and chest. Sometimes the spots can bleed, and as you will read, left untreated basal cell carcinomas can become disfiguring.

I am including two stories of basal cell cancers and their removal. Hopefully some of you will read these stories and decide that you need to go have an unusual spot or mole looked at by your dermatologist. Don't have a skin doctor? See the **Resources** section at the back of the book to get some ideas on finding one in your area. I hope these stories are helpful. The key is to listen to your intuition and don't wait to get things checked out.

David's story. My friend David is now sporting a fairly large scar on his left cheek. Although at first he struggled to come to terms with this new facial characteristic, he now sees it as a gift and a reminder of how lucky he truly is. Here's his story.

It was the summer of 1999. David, like many men, had a small blemish on his left cheek. And, like many men, David decided to do what he always does—try to pop it. The place bled a little bit and seemed to scab over; this went on for several days. He thought perhaps there was a hair caught inside the pore because as soon as the place seemed like it was going away, it would get irritated and red again. Eventually the spot did go away, although a small red bump was left on his cheek.

Every so often when David was shaving, the small red bump would bleed due to the razor hitting it. This went on for a month or two. Then the place scaled over, and he thought finally it was starting to heal. What David didn't know is that many times when dry, scaly skin grows over a spot (especially one that has bled in the past), it is a sign that something is wrong with that tissue.

During the winter, David started noticing tiny spots of blood on his pillowcase. Perplexed at first, he finally realized the blood droplets were coming from his little red bump. Soon after that he was out to dinner with a radiologist friend who saw the place on David's left cheek and thought he should get it checked out.

This next part of David's story is similar to many of the tales I hear. Although he knew something was wrong, and even after a doctor said it looked funny, David still did not get his red bump checked out—not for another four or five months. (This is *so* typical.)

Finally in June of 2000 David decided he needed to have the strange place (that never went away 100%) on his left cheek checked out by a dermatologist. The impetus for action was because the spot had started to grow and was now almost the size of a pencil eraser. David finally gave in to the possibility something might be up. (Denial is very common when it comes to getting tested for possible problems with our health.)

He made an appointment with a dermatologist. She came into the room, sat down next to David and immediately said she didn't like the way the place looked. Without hesitation she ordered a biopsy. She was so sure it was going to be a problem that she insisted David schedule himself for surgery just in case the test results came back positive for cancer. When it comes to skin cancer, timing is everything. (Note: Basal cell cancers are not as serious as melanomas, but they still grow and spread and time is a factor nonetheless.) So he scheduled surgery and waited for the test results, which came back positive for basal cell carcinoma.

David went to the clinic where the surgery would take place. He would have Mohs' surgery, a newer procedure that is used to remove cancerous cells. When David walked through the door, he said it looked like a M.A.S.H. unit; people everywhere were bandaged in the different places they were having skin cancers removed. There were young and old alike in the waiting room. David, at 41 years old, was in the middle age range, not the older range. After looking around at all these people in varying stages of skin cancer and treatment, he got scared and almost walked out.

Hearing he had skin cancer didn't really faze David. He knew it was treatable and figured the doctor would cut it out of his face, the skin would heal, and that would be that. It wasn't until he was being prepped for surgery that his demeanor took a sharp turn. David said the moment he knew this was serious was when his doctor drew on his face with a marker. Not only did she circle the actual cancerous lesion, but she drew a line 2$^{1}/_{4}$" north and south and another line an inch-wide left and right. (If you haven't ever had surgery, drawing on the skin at the place of incision is a common practice.) Once he saw all the lines drawn on his face, he realized the area affected was much bigger that he ever expected or realized.

David felt a sense of panic. Was he going to be wearing a big huge scar after all was said and done? He asked the doctor, and she said that because of the Mohs' surgery, it would be a flat scar, and she would take great care to make the lines go with the natural lines of his face, namely his laugh lines coming down his cheek. She would do the best cosmetic job possible while at the same time being sure to get all the cancer out.

After the procedure, David was talking with the attendant. Since David's face was already bandaged up, he couldn't tell the size of the surface area affected. The attendant offered to show him some of the still photographs taken at every stage of the Mohs' surgery. When David saw the final shot and how much tissue had actually been taken out of his face in order to reach and extract all of the cancer, David was blown away. He was speechless and in a state of shock at the size of the opening in his face.

It took three passes to get all of the cancer. Twenty-two stitches inside and out. David thought it would be a few stitches and no big deal. What he learned is when it comes to skin cancer, it is anything but "no big deal." He also wished he had asked more questions. He truly had no idea it was going to take almost two dozen stitches to patch his poor face back together. But how do you know what questions to ask when you're going through something you have never gone through before?

Something David learned after the surgery was that the cancer got so deep, it came very close to one of his salivary glands. If the cancer had gotten down that far, David would have needed radiation as well as the surgery. Radiation? David was feeling luckier by the minute.

Once the bandages came off and David could see the reality of the large scar he now had on his face, he said it really bothered him at first. Then, after the tissue around the scar had healed and he had gotten used to his new appearance, it didn't bother him much at all. I think any change in our appearance takes time to get used to. But in David's case, he chooses to see his scar as a reminder of how lucky he is—he dodged a bullet with his salivary gland. And he truly sees the scar as a blessing rather than a curse. A blessing because the alternative he could have faced would have been so much worse.

David has become somewhat of an activist for skin cancer. He even says he can spot a basal cell a mile away and doesn't hesitate to go up to people, even strangers, and tell them to get checked by a dermatologist.

The moral of the story for David was he knew there was something wrong, but didn't do anything about it. And the irony was that originally he was worried about having a zit on his face (in the very beginning), and now he has a noticeable scar. David learned a valuable lesson about listening to that inner voice and following through.

David now "butters up" (his way of saying he slathers on the sunscreen) before he goes out. He is in the construction business, so he does spend a considerable amount of time outside—necessarily. He also goes to his dermatologist whenever he sees a spot that looks unusual or that doesn't perform the way a normal blemish (or mole) does.

In closing, David wanted me to tell you this simple thought, "If it doesn't heal, something's wrong." Thank you, David, for sharing your story with us!

Carol's story. Since my friend Carol had a basal cell carcinoma removed from her face and she had a story to tell, I asked her to write about her experience. Her story, especially her hesitation going to the dermatologist (sound familiar?), is a common one and is an important point in her message. Here is some of what Carol wrote:

> I put off going to the dermatologist, but probably only for 6-7 months* because [the mole] looked like a freckle, so friendly and benign. You, however, advised me to go get it checked out, especially because it was new.
>
> A doctor-friend wanted me to have an ophthalmological surgeon do the biopsy and removal because it was so close to my eye. The eye surgeon was certain beforehand that it wasn't cancer, but while I was out and still under the knife, the pathology report came back—basal cell carcinoma.
>
> So out it came with more tissue than expected and a skin graft to boot. All because you really urged me to have it looked at. Most likely if I'd gone sooner it would have been smaller and not as big a deal.

*Six to seven months can be a long time for cancer to grow.

Because I see Carol's skin on a semi-regular basis (she gets facials on a quarterly basis, sometimes more often), I have had the advantage of becoming familiar with her skin and am able to notice changes from time to time. Because I am not superhuman, I do write down changes or abnormalities I see on a chart I have for each and every client, something every aesthetician should do without question.

I had marked down what I thought was a place on Carol's face (near her eye) with unusual tissue formation. So the next time she came in (3 months later), I knew it wasn't a blemish. Spots don't take three months to heal, and this place looked the same as it did, no changes. That is unusual. Plus the tissue looked strange to me.

Even though I encouraged Carol to see her dermatologist, she did what many people routinely do—she didn't do anything. Just like David, Carol let many months pass before she decided to take the plunge and have her moles checked. I think it is part of human nature to avoid something we don't want to know about, such as the possibility of cancer. I hope you will bypass this perhaps natural inclination if you indeed find a funny-looking mole—no matter where it is located on your body—and have it checked out.

It is common for me to send my clients to the dermatologist to have a mole checked. Nine times out of ten, they come back with a clean bill of health. But as I tell them, I would rather be safe than sorry. And in the case of skin cancer, this should be your anthem. And anytime you have had a cancerous lesion removed, you should (if not instructed by your doctor) get a checkup at least every six months to a year. I advise the shorter time frame because once you have one place removed, I believe there will inevitably be more to come. And the more time you have spent in the sun (over your lifetime, not just recently), the higher the chances of problems cropping up.

I recommend going to your dermatologist for a baseline mole check. The baseline gives the doctor a marker of what your moles look like now, so if in the future they change, it may be easier to detect potential problem areas.

I hope these stories have helped you understand the importance of getting funny looking moles or places on your face (or anywhere) you have questions about checked by your dermatologist. Just remember: Don't wait, don't hesitate, get your moles checked today!

The Basics 1-2-3

Back to The Basics. Skin care is not rocket science. How our skin functions and how to take care of it is pretty basic. If you look back at history, the successful diets, exercise programs, and skin care regimes all reflect this concept of simplicity. Jack LaLane's workout programs, dating back to the 50s, are chockfull of simple tips and advice. Most of the diet programs today are simply taking us back to an "old" way of eating; making sure we get our fruits, vegetables, not too much refined food and adequate protein. That's pretty simple, right? And so, too, I am striving to get all of you to adhere to a simple program for your skin. Cleansing, toning, and moisturizing every day plus weekly exfoliation and masking along with monthly facials if possible. What's complicated about that?

I am 45 years old and have been blessed with extraordinary clear skin. Except for it being very sensitive to fragrance, I never have a problem. Everyone has always commented on how flawless and young my skin looks. I purchased your book because I thought that someday my "luck" would run out and I wanted to prepare to maintain the healthy glow and clarity of my skin.

The main thing I would stress is this: Don't ruin a good thing! If it ain't broke, don't fix it! And certainly, don't go changing to try to please anybody! I think if we don't have problems and we have idle time, maybe we start focusing on problems that don't exist. If you have flawless, no-problem skin, congratulations! You are the envy of most people in the world. You probably are blessed with good genes and perhaps common sense as well. Because you don't have problems, you don't require a lot from your products—at least not as much as a person with problem skin does.

The daily routine for everyone is The Basics 1-2-3: Cleansing, toning, and moisturizing. Eye cream and sunscreen are included in your basic daily habits. Don't forget to stay out of direct sunlight, even though you are wearing sunscreen. Drinking water, eating a healthy, balanced diet, and not too much of the bad stuff or anything in excess (even the good things) will go a long way to keeping you looking and feeling your best.

It's really very basic—like life. And don't we really know in our hearts what works and what is just a fantasy? Common sense, to me, is the ability to discern the difference between the two. Left at the cosmetic counter unarmed, you may make costly mistakes, which can lead you down the path of skin care confusion. If that happens, take out this book, and look through *Timeless Skin*, and remind yourself that taking care of your face is a simple procedure. Fall back on your Basics 1-2-3 program plus The Extras (see section). Remember that you are in control of your daily skin care routine. Even taxed with a newborn or a hectic work schedule, surely you can find two or three *minutes* a day to do your morning and evening routine. It doesn't have to take longer than that to take basic care of your skin.

For a very detailed look at The Basics, refer to Chapter One of *Timeless Skin*.

Bath & Body

Is it OK to use body lotions that contain petroleum? I know in your book you say the molecule is very large so moisturizers with petroleum derivatives like mineral oil don't penetrate very well. Do you opt for the natural, health food store body lotions?

I don't recommend using petroleum products on the face—or at least for skin that is normal or oily. These cheaper ingredients (like petroleum or mineral oil) have a large molecular structure, and the creams they are in tend to sit on the surface of the skin. For anything other than true-dry skin, this can cause congestion and possibly breakout.

When it comes to my body, I tend to use less expensive products than I do on my face. I actually use a health food store brand body moisturizer that is under $5 for 12 ounces. (It doesn't happen to contain petroleum.) It's certainly not the highest quality product available, but it's inexpensive. I take lots of baths—especially in the winter—and every time I get out of the tub, I slather my entire body (except for my face and neck) with this moisturizer. Therefore I go through a lot of product in a short time. There are other inexpensive brands like Lubriderm® or Vaseline Intensive Care®, and these do have petroleum derivatives in them. I wouldn't use these products on my face, but my body's skin is different and does very well with these cheaper creams. You may, however, prefer to use more expensive products on your body. Regardless of the price, I am not against using mineral oil or other petroleum derivatives on the body.

For an inexpensive **bubble bath**, I use bath gel in place of the more expensive bubble bath products. Bath gels contain ingredients that will foam up just like a bubble bath product but for a fraction of the cost. My health food store sells its own brand of bath and shower gel for under $2 for a 12 ounce bottle. I may get six to eight bubble baths with this, compared to many bubble bath products that cost ten times as much.

I never use bubble bath products that are alkaline—and neither should you. Here is another good use for your pH test papers. Many bubble bath products have alkaline ingredients in them; these ingredients help produce the foaming action, similar to bar soap. Some of these ingredients include *sodium laureth-13 carboxylate* and *disodium laureth sulfosuccinate*. If your bath water becomes alkaline, this not only will cause your body's skin to get dry and flaky (just like your facial skin will with alkaline soap), but women have the added worry of developing urinary tract infections from sitting in an alkaline bubble bath.

I can remember as a kid loving my Mr. Bubble® bubble bath. Even now when I see the box at the store, it triggers happy memories for me. But I also remember having chronic bladder infections, no doubt caused at least in part from my wonderful Mr. Bubble. I tested Mr. Bubble and a few other commonly found bubble bath products. The results were as I expected: they all turned the litmus papers dark purple. In other words, the test showed they were alkaline.

The above mentioned shower gel I use as bubble bath is acidic. I checked the label, and it has few ingredients (that's a good sign) and although it contains sodium laureth sulfate, which is a very common soap-like ingredient derived from coconut, it did not contain either of the alkaline ingredients listed above. Test your bath products to ensure the skin over your entire body is being pampered with the proper products. Then draw a bath and relax!

Aveeno® has two bath products for dry skin. One is called "Daily Moisturizing Bath with 43% Natural Colloidal Oatmeal." (*Colloidal* means crushed.) It is meant to help give soothing relief for dry, itchy skin. It is fragrance free. The second product is "Soothing Bath

Treatment with 100% Natural Colloidal Oatmeal" (there are no other ingredients). It helps relieve itchy, irritated skin due to poison ivy, poison oak, poison sumac rashes, insect bites, eczema, prickly heat, chicken pox, hives, and sunburn. Both products are powders and come in individual packets or envelopes. The average cost is close to one dollar per bath, and eight packets come in each box.

In the winter I use these products a lot. The oatmeal really helps to moisturize the skin, thus taking the itch of dry, winter skin away. Be sure to clean the tub after the water has drained out. These as well as most bath products leave a slippery substance in the tub, so be careful!

Exfoliation gloves make an excellent choice for getting rid of the dead skin on your body. You simply slip the gloves on, apply a bath gel, and go over all parts of your body. These gloves are easily rinsed out and can make exfoliating not only easy but fun as well. Be sure not to rub too hard, lest you cause skin irritation. And do be sure to thoroughly rinse the gloves before hanging them on the towel rack to dry, or throw them in the washing machine.

Adding **essential oils** to your bath can have a wonderful effect not only on your body but on your psyche as well. Lavender is relaxing; birch and juniper are both good for soothing aching muscles; and any of the mints (wintergreen, peppermint, spearmint) are invigorating and energizing. Usually, 10-15 drops of assorted oils is what you would add to your bath water.

Note: Essential oils are lighter than water, so they may float on the surface of your bath water. When you are soaking in the tub, wherever your skin meets the water you may get a concentration of essential oils. I recommend once you have stepped into the tub to then splash the water around, helping to disperse the oils. If you are using strong oils like birch or peppermint, you really need to use this splashing technique or you may end up causing skin irritation. I usually add the drops as I'm filling the tub. This seems to disperse the oils. Even using 15 drops of peppermint hasn't irritated my skin.

Why is it beneficial to soak in Epson salts? Is there anything else that is good to put in my bath that is relaxing and will help sore muscles?

Epson salts are high in magnesium. This mineral is a well-known muscle relaxer. Adding these mineral salts to your bath can really help relieve sore, aching muscles. Even if you are just tired after a long day, soaking in a hot (not too hot) salt bath can help to revive your body and relax your mind.

Many companies make mineral salt bath products. Many of them are predominately Epson salts along with other ingredients. You can get plain Epson salt very inexpensively at the grocery or drug store, then add some essential oils to your bath. This will give you the benefits of the salts and the essential oils, which are therapeutic and wonderfully aromatic, without spending a lot of money.

Dry hands. I have come to a place in my life where I cannot stand to have dry, scaly hands anymore! Getting through a Chicago winter is really challenging unless you have a plan. My hands are in water a lot because of my profession; during each facial I wash my hands or utensils 3 or 4 times. When I'm home, the last thing I want to do is compound my already dry hands with more hard water. So I have succumbed to wearing rubber gloves. I wear them to do the dishes, I wear them to clean the house, I wear rubber gloves whenever I want to keep water—especially hot water—off my hands.

At first, I felt silly and confined. But I bought gloves that really fit my hands, and therefore my dexterity is improved over when I was wearing more oversized gloves. I can feel through the gloves, and my hands don't suffer with exposure to water or cleaning supplies. Putting a little talc, like baby powder, inside the gloves will help your hands get in and out of them easier.

Wearing rubber gloves may sound like an obvious solution, but I have asked many people who have problems with dry hands, and most of them have not yet discovered the benefits of wearing rubber gloves. I noticed an immediate difference in the level of dryness of my hands once I started to use gloves. I didn't have to apply lotion as frequently, and my skin just felt better in general. I don't do special hand treatments, like paraffin or warm oil with gloves. These would be wonderful, but I just don't have the time or inclination to do any more than I have to to have smooth-feeling skin on my hands.

> *I had my ovaries removed 3 months ago and my skin on my entire body is so dry, it's driving me crazy. I can literally scrape the dead skin off! I am on estrogen medication, and when I asked my doctor what I could do, he said the dry skin is part of "the change" and that maybe in 6 months or so it will get better. I live in Florida, so dry skin shouldn't be such a problem in my life. Is there anything I can do to keep my skin from itching and get rid of all this dry skin?*

This is a common problem for women who are going through peri-menopause. To add to that, this client also had her estrogen-producing ovaries removed, so her skin just doesn't have much of a chance to lubricate itself. Although, as the doctor said, there may not be any cures for the dry skin, I do believe there are things you can do to help the dryness from driving you crazy.

I asked this client if she had ever used body oils. Her answer was no. I asked if she had olive oil in her kitchen, she said yes. I told her to pour out about ¼ cup of the oil into a container she could take into her shower with her. After she had done everything in the shower and was about to leave, I instructed her to keep the shower water running and take some of the oil and start spreading it over her body. Start with the legs, but don't put oil on the bottoms of your feet! Otherwise you might slip and fall in the tub. Apply the oil in a medium layer to your entire body, back, front, up and down. Massage the oil in to the skin, then let the water rinse any oil off that will come off. Once you are out of the shower, don't rub with your towel, but pat dry. This way the oil will have a better chance of staying on your skin. You can apply an oil after you have gotten out of the shower or bathtub. But don't dry your skin off first; apply any oil to wet skin, massage in and let it have time to soak in. I wouldn't dress immediately—or I wouldn't dress up. Bed or house clothes won't matter as much if any oil residue gets on them.

You may not be going through menopause, but perhaps you live in a cold and/or dry environment. The same oil application can help you too. During winter here in Chicago, if the cold air doesn't get you, the heat inside the buildings will! Using oil on truly dried out skin is the most effective way to get rid of that dry feeling.

Beards

My husband has a full beard. I was wondering what he needs to do, if anything, to keep the skin underneath healthy. Is it better for the skin to be covered with hair or clean-shaven?

My husband's skin underneath his beard is beginning to itch, and it's driving him (and me) crazy! What is causing this, and how can he remedy it?

Deciding to have facial hair or not is purely personal preference. And although having a beard may seem easier on your skin than being clean-shaven, the skin underneath does go through its own hardship. The hair inhibits some of the skin's natural exfoliation, whether it be from shaving or just having that skin rubbed or touched throughout the day. Since the hair is in essence shielding any activity in the covered area, this skin needs **exfoliation**. It will keep the skin from itching and flaking as sometimes happens underneath a beard.

Since exfoliating underneath facial hair really cannot be done through conventional means (scrubs and gommage), this is a good application for **AHAs**. Fruit acids help to exfoliate just by lying on top of the skin. After you have done your morning or evening routine (assuming you have a skin care routine), take some AHA cream or gel and try to get it onto the skin under your beard by massaging it in with your fingertips. What you don't want to do is pile on a bunch of moisturizer just because it contains AHAs, so be careful how much you use. Towel off any excess.

Using a **facial brush** can help to exfoliate the area under your beard. You want to be careful not to irritate the skin by using the brush too aggressively. And you always want to thoroughly wash the facial brush after every use. See **Facial Brushes** for more details.

Glycerin (see section) is another option for getting needed moisture to the skin underneath your beard. Pure glycerin is a runny liquid that can be massaged into the area with the excess blotted off the hair. This should not cause any adverse effects, yet can really help to keep that skin soft and moisturized.

Finally, if you are experiencing severe problems underneath your beard, it may be time to **shave it** and see exactly what is going on. If you choose to shave, **getting a facial** before you regrow your beard would be an excellent idea. Getting that skin in good shape before the hair covers it up will help, even if temporarily. If the skin doesn't respond to exfoliating and moisturizing, you may want to **visit your dermatologist** and see if there is something more serious going on.

Benzoyl Peroxide

In one of the many skin care books in my library, the author states he is "appalled to see so-called beauty experts claiming that salicylic acid and benzoyl peroxide don't work against acne." I may be one of the "so-called beauty experts" this author is speaking of. It's not that I think benzoyl peroxide (BP) doesn't work against acne, but I do think it is harmful compared to the other types of treatments that I espouse. I'm sure BP does work against acne and for clearing up skin in some cases. But how it does this is what I am opposed to.

In over two decades of working on people's skin I have found alternate ways to improve problem skin that aren't irritating or caustic. Those alternate ways are what I believe are the most beneficial in the long run for my clients and anyone interested in clearing up problem skin. My way is about a whole body approach, not simply putting a drying product or an antibiotic treatment on a blemish to help dry it up. My point in sharing what I know is to inform you of alternatives to the prevalent (and in my opinion many times ineffective) treatments readily available for problem and acne skin. Your own personal experience is going to be the proof in the pudding. Try benzoyl peroxide and see if you like its effect. If not, you will find alternative treatments for problem skin throughout this book and *Timeless Skin*.

Benzoyl peroxide products are relatively inexpensive, and they are very easy to find. Sold over the counter (OTC), they usually come in three strengths: 2.5%, 5%, and 10%. Although the lower 2.5% strength is available, from the OTC products I researched, most have the higher percentages of benzoyl peroxide in them. It is also available by prescription, but you can bet that in prescription form the benzoyl peroxide is strong enough to blast a pimple out of the water—so watch out! Because benzoyl peroxide is also a known irritant, I don't recommend using it in these higher strengths. If you're going to use BP, go for the lower 2.5% versions.

What is benzoyl peroxide and what does it do? Other than being a bleaching agent for certain foods, it is defined as a drying agent in cosmetics, toxic if inhaled, as well as a possible skin irritant. Benzoyl peroxide is said to have antimicrobial qualities and helps to loosen debris lodged in the pores. It releases oxygen into the infected area, which helps prevent bacteria proliferation.

Some people see good results when first using BP, but after a while their skin becomes dry and flaky, and because they have been treating the symptom only (the breakout) and not looking at what the cause might be, their skin problems continue.

Why should I use benzoyl peroxide? I don't necessarily think you should use BP products. In my experience and in the tales told by my clients, all it really does is dry out the area and the surrounding skin. This sometimes leads to irritation and generally doesn't help to clear the blemish. It may appear to be clearing the problem because the skin feels drier and tighter after using BP. The infection may seem to go away, but long-term, BP isn't as effective as you may initially think it is. The best way to know if it will work for you is to try it and see. Something that works for me or my clients may not work for you or vice versa. Nothing is absolute, in life or in the skin care world. And skin is as individual as personalities are, so experiment for yourself if you are unsure of the results you are reading about.

A note of caution: Those of you with darker skin tones, especially black skin, need to use BP with caution. The higher concentrations (5% and 10%) can cause an increase in inflammation due to the peroxide's irritation, which may and probably will cause hyperpigmentation—dark spots.

Where do I find benzoyl peroxide? BP products are everywhere acne or problem skin medications are sold over the counter. Benzoyl peroxide can also be prescribed by your dermatologist.

My dermatologist recommends that I use Benza-Clin® for my occasional breakouts. Can I continue to use this product along with my regular skin care products or is it really necessary?

I'm not going to tell this client to stop using something a doctor prescribed for her skin. However, Benza-Clin is a prescription benzoyl peroxide product, which means it probably has a high BP content, and benzoyl peroxide is very drying. For occasional breakouts or *any* breakout, I recommend using geranium or an alternate essential oil. They are antibacterial (like BP), but they won't dry out the surface skin like BP can and will. I think, however, she should try her skin care products with the medication and see how it goes. As you are learning, drying out the skin does little or nothing to get rid of infected blemishes. If this reader feels she needs to use the prescription medication and she can use it without adverse (drying) reactions, then that is her prerogative. If not, there are definitely alternatives that don't dry out the skin but help with the infection and the breakout as a whole.

As a general rule, I do not like benzoyl peroxide or the types of products this ingredient comes in. If BP works at all, it also causes adverse side effects, namely dry, flaky skin. Read through the sections on skin troubles as well as **Geranium** and **Clay Masks** to see other ways to treat blemishes. Also, my thoughts on helping to stop breakouts from occurring in the first place can be found in many parts of this book.

HOT TIP: Because it is a peroxide, not unlike hair color, benzoyl peroxide can bleach your clothing—so be careful where you are using it.

Biking & Skin

I ride a bike every weekend and sometimes on weekdays if I have time. How can I keep my skin (especially my face) protected from all the sun I know I am getting?

If you are an ardent cyclist out on your bike for many hours each week, or even just a weekend warrior, you'll have a tough job protecting your skin from the sun. Like any activity that keeps you in the sunlight for extended periods of time, cycling is going to create an environment for sun damage to occur—there are no two ways around it. Sun exposure and sun damage are one and the same.

Many years ago, while in my 20s, I was an avid cyclist. I even got a license to race. My biking schedule consisted of sitting in the saddle at least 10 miles a day and well over 70 miles on the weekends. I cycled in the cold, the heat of Texas summer, wind, rain—you name it; I was on my bike. When it came time to protect my face, I kept running across a problem: how to do it.

Cycling caps, in case you've never seen one, have a bill only a few inches long—probably ¼ the length of a baseball cap's bill. I always assumed they were just for show; certainly they were not meant to keep sun off the face. Since these caps offer almost no protection from the sun, I wore a baseball cap under my helmet. I got teased by all the guys I rode with because of it, but I didn't care. Protecting my face was more important to me than making a fashion statement.

One problem with wearing baseball caps while riding a bike is you might have some problems with obstruction of vision. Different bikes have different handle bars. Some keep your posture more upright than others. Regardless of my position on the bike, I know that even when I wore the baseball cap under my helmet, I still got a lot of sun.

As you may already know, baseball caps and visors offer very little in the way of protecting your face from full-on sun exposure. The only parts of your face that are shielded from the sun are your forehead and a little bit of your nose; the lower half and both sides of your face are totally and continually exposed to UV rays. Take that information and add to it a 30, 60, or even a 90-minute bike ride and you can see how easily you will accumulate a lot of sun exposure while riding your bike. This kind of exposure is really no different than driving in a convertible, lying on the beach, playing golf, etc. The position of your body will be different with each activity, and the clothing—or lack of it—is certainly a factor, but exposure is exposure. As I will say over and over again, the sun does not make any distinction about the kind of activity you are engaged in versus how much UV light will be absorbed into your skin.

Obviously, the number one course of action is to wear sunscreen. You always want to have **waterproof sunscreen** all over your face, neck, tops and backs of ears, hands, body—every nook and cranny that will be exposed to the sun while you are out enjoying your bike ride. Make sure to get sunscreen up under your clothes where they meet your skin. While exercising, clothing can ride up and slide around, so be sure to protect those areas of skin just at the edge of your clothes.

You might consider wearing a pure **zinc product** (at least on your nose and mouth) that will offer a physical block from UV light while on a long bike ride. True zinc oxide is pure white and does not absorb into your skin. You may look silly in someone's eyes, but better that than having part of your nose cut off in order to get all the cancer cells out of your face. (If you doubt my seriousness, just ask your dermatologist about the potential disfiguring results of long-term overexposure coupled with waiting too long to have cancerous lesions removed. It can be an eye-opening experience, to say the very least.) If you are prone to chloasma (dark patches of pigmentation) you may want to spread some zinc on those places to keep them from getting darker.

Wearing a **baseball cap** under your helmet will help. You can also tie a **bandana** around your head, fully covering your forehead at least. This will also help to absorb sweat, preventing it from dripping into your eyes while you are cycling.

Dehydration can also be a factor when you are exercising outside for extended periods of time. If you become dehydrated, your skin will be more susceptible to burning. To state the obvious, drinking a lot of water is crucial in this or any exercising scenario. You can easily carry large amounts of water with you in the form of a **Camelbak® water pack**. These came out just as I was ending the cycling phase of my life; they are a wonderful invention, and you probably should have one handy for long (or even short) excursions. You fill it up with water and strap it onto your back. There is a feeding tube that attaches to the water pack, enabling you to drink water with little effort while you are riding. Your bike will also have one or two cages to put water bottles in. Fill these up and use them too. While exercising, you can't have too much water to drink.

For a little extra boost, I always liked to keep a few packets of **Emergen-C®*** with me during a long ride. I would open a packet, suck on the powder, and immediately feel refreshed. The sourness of the vitamin C would make my mouth water, helping with dry mouth. Chewable vitamin C tablets are another possibility. They will also help to keep your mouth from getting dry while at the same time getting vitamin C into your system. I also keep these chewables handy at home.

Depending on where you began your ride, you might still be a car ride away from a nice hot shower. If you are not riding your bike directly home, you may want to have extra water in the car so you can at least **thoroughly rinse off** your face before arriving home. This way you will avoid letting all that sweat, dirt, and debris just sit on your skin causing the potential for irritation and possibly breakout.

I would also recommend slathering your sun-soaked body with **aloe vera gel** following your shower. Aloe will help replace the water lost on the surface of your skin, along with providing amino acids to help your sundrenched cells replenish themselves.

The bottom line when trying to protect your skin while cycling is being extra diligent and knowing you are getting some amount of exposure no matter how protected you may be or feel. There is only so much you can do; then you have to live your life, enjoy yourself, and in this case, ride your bike.

There isn't really an ironclad, foolproof answer to the question of how to protect your face while bicycling. But wearing a baseball cap and/or bandana, using a waterproof sunscreen and possibly zinc oxide, and drinking lots of water are all important factors in helping to protect your skin while on your bike.

*Emergen-C is a powder vitamin C supplement that can be found at most health food stores.

Blackheads

I don't know exactly what blackheads are. The pores on the sides of my nose are dark. I'm assuming these are blackheads. What should I do to keep them from getting worse?

Basically, blackheads (also termed *comedos* or *comedones*) are clogged pores. The pore, which is a tiny opening on the surface of the skin, can collect skin cells, excreted oil, as well as debris in the air. This mixture can oxidize, causing it to turn a dark color. That is probably what you are seeing on the sides of your nose.

The best thing to do is to make sure you are cleaning your skin properly on a daily basis and if possible, using a clay mask once or twice a week. Clay has a deep cleansing effect, helping to unclog the pores, which is just what you need to use on blackheads.

Much to my surprise (and disgust!) my husband informed me that I have a bunch of blackheads in my ears. And when I put my finger there, it feels very oily. Help! What can I do to get rid of these unsightly blackheads?

You are not alone in your concerns. Whenever I give a client a facial, I always check inside his or her ears to make sure they are staying clean and blackhead-free. Our ears are sometimes a forgotten place in regard to our skin care routines. But just like other parts of our bodies, our ears have active oil glands and pores that, if left uncleansed for a period of time, will accumulate oil and debris that can create blackheads.

It is a lot harder to get rid of blackheads inside your ears than it is to help prevent them in the first place. If you already have congestion there, first you want to get into the habit of cleaning your ears—something that you have undoubtedly not done for most or all of your life.

I use the same cleanser for my ears as I do for my face. I take a little bit and put the cleanser on the tips of my fingers and stick them right in my ears. Not down the ear canal, just in that pocket that's like the cup part of the ear. I just massage the cleanser in a little bit—not for very long—and rinse when I rinse my face. I actually only do this in the shower, but you can certainly do it at your sink if you prefer. The shower is just easier for me because I can get the shower spray right above my ear and really get the residue of the cleanser all out before getting out of the shower. This should be a daily habit, especially if you are having blackhead problems.

If you are trying to get rid of existing blackheads, you will want to take a more active approach. My first suggestion would be to take your clay mask, and after thoroughly cleansing the area, gently put some mask in the cup of your ear or wherever the blackheads are. Let it dry for 10-15 minutes and remove carefully with warm water, or in the shower. I say carefully because you really don't want cleansers or clay or anything to go down your ear canal. Ears are very delicate organs, and although I am suggesting you clean the area, I am also imploring you to be very careful and not let anything actually go inside your ears. When rinsing, the best thing to do is to tilt your head with the ear you're cleaning pointed down to the ground so that gravity will take care of the rest. Then with your finger, make sure all the product gets out of the ear cup. Tilting like this will ensure nothing drips or seeps inside of your ear.

If you have a bad blackhead problem, you may want to use the clay for several consecutive days, eventually backing off to 1-3 times per week. When the problem goes away, be sure to continue to cleanse the ears daily in the shower and use the mask when you feel it's necessary, maybe once a week for maintenance.

Can I get the blackheads inside my ears extracted by a facialist?

I have extracted some enlarged plugs in the ears of my clients, but this is extremely hard to do. It has to be done with Q-tips® because fingers are too big to fit inside an ear. And truthfully, I rarely get the entire blackhead extracted—the area is so confined and hard to maneuver in. This wouldn't be a job for someone you don't know or who you don't have a great deal of confidence in. But if you have a skilled aesthetician, she may indeed be able to make some headway extracting your ear blackheads. In my experience, I have found that only part of the plug actually comes out during the extraction process. But getting the process started usually helps to clear the blackheads eventually. Plus, you will now be paying more attention to this area.

I treat the inside ear with an essential oil solution (for me, this is the toner I use), and when I put the clay mask on my client's face, I put some in the ear, too. Make sure the aesthetician doesn't forget to remove the clay from your ears before you leave the facial chair. People might begin to talk!

Maybe you don't know if you have blackheads inside your ears. Ask your aesthetician during your next facial (if she doesn't volunteer the information), or simply ask a trusted friend. Ask someone with a gentle spirit who won't throw out an answer that hurts once it's heard. Remember, no one except your significant other is looking that closely at your ears. And perhaps he or she doesn't even notice your ear's insides. So don't get all fanatical about how the insides of your ears look! Just keep your ears clean and worry about more important things.

What can I do about blackheads around my lips? I recently had a facial and the technician removed them (it hurt!). What, if anything, can I do to prevent them?

I recommend having these blackheads removed professionally during a facial. The area around the lip line is very sensitive, as you found out, and if these places are not extracted properly (you try too hard or extract incorrectly), the tissue can swell and potentially cause infection.

If you decide to extract these blackheads yourself, follow the rules of extraction and proceed with caution. In other words, go slowly. The tissue of the lip is less flexible than your facial skin. These blackheads are usually located right on the edge of the lip tissue and the facial skin. So the blackhead, even if it is small, will have a harder time dislodging from this area. Always have your fingers wrapped in tissue (Kleenex®) and don't skip putting a dot of clay mask on each place you have extracted. And don't wear lipstick immediately after extraction! If you have to extract, do it at night before you go to bed. This way the places have all night long to recuperate.

Note that wherever you extract on your lips, it will probably swell more so than when you extract places on your face. This is due to the difference in the tissue. The swelling will recede, especially with the application of clay.

Botox®

Botox is a very popular anti-aging treatment. It is one of the least harmful procedures, but alas, it is also temporary. Only your inner core belief about life and the aging process is something that can hold its shape unchanged over time.

Botox isn't technically wrinkle removal; consider it wrinkle postponement. Botox doesn't truly erase wrinkles; it paralyzes the muscles at the site of injection, prohibiting movement during expressions. Once the toxin is absorbed and removed from the muscle, your ability to express will return, and so will the wrinkles.

Some of you will obviously choose Botox. But where does it really get you in the end? And do we know about the possible long-term detrimental effects of using this toxin over and over again in particular muscles of the face? The answer is no—at this point there are no long-term studies on botulism's effect long-term. Botox was approved for use in the facial area by the FDA in 2002.

Mental Botox. What I'm introducing is a way to begin being consciously aware of how you are creating your lines and wrinkles through your repetitive and unconscious facial expressions. If you decide to get Botox injections, it will prohibit facial movements but will do nothing to teach you to control your unconscious expressions. Once the Botox wears off, you will be right back where you started, albeit a few months further away from deepening the lines.

I'm beginning to form lines between my brows. The only reason these lines are forming is from crunching up my face from squinting in the bright sun or when I'm worried or upset. Nevertheless it is something I am creating (the wrinkle); nothing else is causing it. Mental Botox is this: I have simply, over time, learned to direct my conscious awareness to my facial expressions. Sometimes I don't realize I am making wrinkle-producing expressions immediately, but now when I do become aware that I am, I relax that part of my face so the line will cease to increase. Sometimes I put my finger up there and massage the skin a little bit to help the muscles relax. Because I am getting older and because skin changes as we age, these lines will end up forming on some level even with this Mental Botox application. However, I can certainly delay their coming and decrease their depth by learning to relax those muscles. This way I am in control of my destiny, and I don't have to pay hundreds of dollars for a Botox injection. And Mental Botox can be used for the rest of my life. It also enables me to make expressions, which are something that is a part of everyday communication.

I believe you can consciously direct yourself away from bad behaviors and habits as well as into new and improved habits. For example, I have not only used this self-programing for when I'm wrinkling my face, but also for when I am grinding my teeth. I now wake myself up when I am grinding my teeth, whereas before I would just wake up in the morning with a jaw ache from grinding all night. I simply told myself to become consciously aware of the grinding and to wake up when it was happening. Although it may sound impossible, it actually works. It's just a matter of determination, setting a goal, and prioritizing its achievement.

They say we only use a very small percentage of our brain's capacity. You have the resources within you to make changes, large and small, within your own life and body. Why not give Mental Botox a try? You have nothing to lose and maybe better body awareness to gain.

I had a bit of Botox around my eyes two weeks ago. I've been very afraid of that treatment but caved in. I have to say, it has made quite a difference. I just pray that it is safe! What are your thoughts on Botox?

I have said that if I had to get an anti-aging procedure (emphasis on *had* to), I would most likely choose Botox. To me, it seems the least invasive as well as the least problematic. And the results are temporary, so if it doesn't do what you want it to do, you aren't stuck with the results. But for now I will continue to go along using my mind to help me with aging. Yes, I mean using Mental Botox, but more so I mean I will continue to work on developing a healthy attitude of acceptance vs. resistance to the most natural process in our lives and our bodies— the aging process.

Breakout

What causes breakout?

That is the $64,000 question! There are numerous things that cause breakouts and reasons why breakouts occur. The short list is **hormonal fluctuations** (including **puberty**, a woman's **monthly menstrual cycle, pregnancy** and **breast feeding, menopause, hormone imbalances** that can occur in either sex), **diet, sweating, stress, a genetic predisposition, allergies** and **intolerances** to either products or environment. So the answer basically is life in general!

What is causing your breakout? I am going to help you answer this question, and so together we can try to figure out what is causing your problem skin. You may not find out the answers immediately, but the following questions and their answers will at least begin to give you a better picture of the possible causes of your breakout. At my salons, by utilizing this list of questions when interviewing clients about their problem skin, we can begin to narrow down potential culprits and help find some answers that have proved helpful in determining what is causing breakout.

To start with, I always like to find out some background on your skin's condition. In other words, **how would you describe your problems?** Are you plagued with only blackheads, or do you have whiteheads instead, or both? If you have whiteheads, is there any redness in the area, or are they simply bumps under skin that look white or yellowish? If there is redness, they are technically small pustules. The redness indicates infection, and that means there is bacterial contamination. A true whitehead is just sebum (oil) trapped beneath several layers of dead skin (albeit thin, see-through skin). What about cysts? Do you experience small to large bumps under the skin that don't form a clear pus-filled head? Are they just red and often painful bumps? And then there are the breakouts that are what most people mean when they say "breakout." These are pustules that are small, medium, or large bumps that are not only red but have a clear and defined puss-filled head as well.

Next, I would ask **where is the breakout located?** Is it always contained within a certain area, or does it migrate—changing places and not usually coming back in the same place all the time? If it is in one or two places always, is it on both sides of the face or usually only one side? What about size? Is the breakout usually limited to small spots, or do they always appear as big places on your face?

If you continue to get breakout in the same place on your face, it may be due to contact with something. Telephones and cell phones, equipment like sports helmets or pads, even pillows you sleep on can cause a sort of contact breakout. (See Q & A later in this section.) If the places are symmetrical on both sides of your face, this is usually a sign of hormonal breakout.

My questioning the size of the breakout is really just to let me know how deep your blemishes are. Almost always, the bigger the spot, the deeper the infection. Or, if we are talking about blackheads, if they are large, this indicates the pores have been clogged for a long time. Large blackheads don't generally form quickly. The same is true with whiteheads. They enlarge over time, so the bigger they are, the longer they have been forming.

Now I want to find out **what are you using on your skin?** I will tell you about some things that I think you shouldn't use on your skin, and you can determine whether or not you are possibly contributing to your problems by using one or several of the following.

Breakout contributors: Products with alcohol. Not all alcohol is bad; it is primarily SD, ethyl, and isopropyl (rubbing) alcohol that are not good to use on your skin. Alcohol merely puts out the fire, so to speak, but does nothing to douse the origination of the flame. It causes dry skin to form in and around the affected pore, which can cause problems of its own. Although drying something up seems to be effective, it is simply a temporary fix and is not part of a real solution for ending your breakouts. (See **Alcohol in Products**.)

Witch hazel contains roughly 15% ethyl alcohol. So although it is not pure alcohol, it still contains some bad alcohol nonetheless. Witch hazel is said to increase "microcirculation," which I interpret as stimulating blood circulation due to the irritating effects of the alcohol contained in this common ingredient. Since it does contain alcohol, I think witch hazel should be avoided, especially as a main ingredient in a product. (See **Witch Hazel**.)

Benzoyl peroxide (see section) is a popular ingredient in many problem skin products. Go to any grocery or drug store and there are numerous "oxy" products lining the shelves, waiting for unsuspecting customers to take them home—only to find they usually don't work. Benzoyl peroxide is antibacterial, which is good. But it is also a skin irritant and can cause dryness, sensitivity, and irritation, which is bad. You want to soothe and heal your blemishes, not irradiate them by using a nuclear bomb!

Fragrance as a skin care ingredient can cause problems with many people's skin. Even fragrance worn as perfume can cause allergic reactions in a large percentage of the population. *Fragrance* is an ambiguous term. It is similar to *natural flavoring* in foods. What is the fragrance made of? I have seen many decent, natural face products that employ fragrance in their formulations. This can ruin an otherwise good product. Fragrance can also cause big problems with your skin. Allergy to fragrance is one of the most common reasons someone cannot use a particular skin care product. Watch out for this ingredient.

Soap is a skin care no-no as far as I'm concerned. There just isn't any good reason for using it—on your face. Soap, by its very nature, has ingredients in it that help hold its shape and keep it hard—ingredients the skin on your face really doesn't benefit from. Soaps are generally alkaline vs. being pH balanced; alkalinity is bad; pH balanced is what you want. If you are currently using soap, try switching to a liquid soap or face wash. Sometimes these, too, will be alkaline, so testing with pH papers is always the best way to find the right cleanser for you. (See **pH**.) Because alkalinity strips all the oil and water off your face, your oil glands may overproduce to compensate for the loss, which can cause oiliness, dehydration, as well as breakouts.

Although not an ingredient in skin care products, the trace mineral **iodine** is known to cause breakout in some people. And I happen to be one of those people sensitive to this vital mineral. I know this because in the past I have taken kelp tablets, high in iodine, and every time I do my skin starts to break out. One time I experimented to see if it was indeed the kelp that was disturbing my skin. I stopped taking the kelp, let my skin clear up completely, then once again starting taking kelp tablets while not changing anything else in either my diet or my skin care routine. Sure enough, my skin started reacting by breaking out. Therefore taking kelp tablets as an easy way to get iodine is just not for me. Although important for a healthy-functioning thyroid, iodine is easy to get through foods, namely fish, seaweeds (high in kelp), and iodized table salt.

Other contributing factors: Anything in excess. This can mean too much of something in your diet, but it can also mean too much exercise, too much stress, and of course too much soda, caffeine, alcohol, or cigarettes. Just look at your day-to-day routines and see where you hit the excess meter. This way you may discover something that is contributing to your breakout in your everyday life.

As you have learned (I *hope*), **sugar and sugary foods** are huge contributors to problem skin. So if you are eating excessive amounts of sugar (I consider excessive to be eating some form of sugar every day), you probably have breakout. And if you don't, you may have regular headaches. And if you don't have either, believe me, something is going on in your body to counteract all the toxic, sugary foods, and it's not a positive effect.

Exercise as we all know is an important part of daily (or at least three times weekly) life. But like any other good thing, too much of it can turn against you. Wanting to be in shape and keeping your body fit and healthy is obviously a good thing. But I'm sure you know someone (is it you?) who just cannot get off the exercise treadmill. I mean that metaphorically, but I suppose it could be taken literally too. For some, exercise has turned into an unhealthy addiction, and unfortunately your skin may be paying the price for those extreme efforts.

You may be wondering how this affects your skin. First, if you exercise—at all—you have to get more water than the daily recommended eight glasses a day we all grew up hearing about. Your body is throwing off sweat in order to keep your inner core body temperature down, since you are heating it up by increasing circulation and raising your body's heat index. Without drinking water all throughout the day and even while exercising, your smart and creative body will simply take the water it needs from wherever it can get it—namely your blood (which is 60-70 percent water) and your organs. Your skin is an organ—the largest one—so why not take water from it?

Not drinking enough water and dehydration go hand in hand. Dehydration can take the form of dehydrated skin on the outside as well as dehydration inside your body. And you don't want your insides to become dehydrated. That is why the eight 8-oz. glasses theory is drilled into us from such an early age. It is absolutely necessary. If you exercise excessively I seriously doubt you could get enough water in your system to compensate for the loss. Think about it and adjust your water intake accordingly.

Too much coffee, sodas, iced tea, candy, sugar in your coffee, and artificial sweeteners. All of these and more can contribute to your skin problems. Do I need to go over why drinking too many sodas may be contributing to your skin care woes? If you drink regular, sugary, caffeinated sodas you are shoveling 10-15 teaspoons of sugar into your body with each and every soda pop, to say nothing of the caffeine your poor adrenal glands have to contend with. Sugar is lethal for many reasons and is a common denominator I have found to cause breakouts in a high percentage of my clients. (See **Sugar**, *please!*)

Even drinking **fruit juice** can cause some people to break out. Store-bought juice is a concentrate of sugar with some vitamins added. And although the sugar is fructose (fruit sugar), this kind of juice will have added sugar if it's from concentrate. People down glass upon glass of juice thinking it is a healthy drink. I have many clients who come in for facials with breakout and after finding out about their diets, I discover they are drinking juice every day or on some kind of regular basis—even just a small amount. Remember, when you drink juice, you are getting a lot of carbohydrates from sugar and also a lot of calories. I heard someone say they don't like to drink their meals—meaning they want to eat foods with high nutrient contents rather than a glass of sugary juice. See **Juicing** to find an alternative to drinking conventional juice.

Stress plays a huge role in skin care problems. Stress breaks down your immune system, leaving your body ill-equipped to function optimally. This includes its ability to excrete toxic waste and eliminate properly. Many times when the body is under a lot of stress, one of the unfortunate symptoms is breakout.

If you have **a genetic predisposition** to have oily, problem, or acne skin, there is little you can do to stop this driving force fueled by your ancestry. However, keeping all other areas in check (diet, stress, lifestyle habits, skin care routine) can and will contribute to keeping your skin clear and breakout-free.

Sleeping with your makeup on is another no-no in the skin care realm. My dictum is if you brush your teeth at night, you should also wash your face. (I suppose this saying would backfire if you don't brush your teeth before going to bed.) But I think you understand my point here. See **Cleansers & Cleansing** for more detailed information.

Birth control pills can, in many cases, cause breakouts. Some women find help with their problem skin while on the Pill; others find their skin becomes worse or starts breaking out when they didn't have any problems prior to taking these hormones. Going off the Pill can cause problems too. Hormones are what cause breakouts. Since the Pill contains hormones, it makes sense that this seemingly "harmless" form of birth control can and in many cases does cause problems.

I'm 27 years old, and I have very oily skin. In the past, I've had minimal breakouts, usually around my period, but overall pretty good skin. I've always had a good regime; your 3-step program plus exfoliating and using a mask at least once a week. But for the past 6-8 months I've developed a lot more breakouts, blemishes, zits, blackheads, whiteheads, and so forth. I swear I've developed acne, which I've never had. And now I have spots from the bigger zits. I don't know what to do anymore. I do see my aesthetician every few months or so. I should go every month, but you know how pricey that can get. I know more or less what is adding to my problem: I got off birth control pills about six months ago (I was on them for about two years), I just went back to school, and I work a lot of hours at my job. So my stress level is definitely high right now. I welcome any suggestions you might have. Too bad your salons are so far away from me!

This emailer exemplifies how stress can cause dramatic effects in your body, which affects your skin. She has a lot of stress from work and school, plus the added stress of going off hormone medication (the Pill). Six months ago she got off the Pill; six months ago her skin became problematic. I tell my clients that it can take six months to a year or more for your body to readjust after going off the Pill. For some it may be a longer or shorter timeframe, and for others going off the Pill may not affect their skin at all. Patience is an important practice to exercise.

Have you recently gone off birth control pills and are now experiencing breakout? Did you just begin taking the Pill and find you have problem skin? You must question all things, including stress, as either contributing to your skin's condition or helping it to clear. (The spots she is referring to are probably due to post-inflammatory hyperpigmentation. See that section for more information.)

As I will continue to say, the breakouts are there for a reason, or reasons. I like to look at problem skin as your body sending you a message, a signal that something needs to change in order for the skin to clear up. Hopefully you can identify the cause or causes of your problem skin so you can have a little more control over it. In this case, ignorance is not bliss; knowledge is power. Be honest with yourself and with how you are contributing to the breakouts. Whether it's through diet, poor skin care habits, or something else, own up to your part of the process and take some steps to help your body free itself of the toxins it is expelling through your skin. And remember:

Treat the system, not just the symptom.

I have this red, rashy breakout around my mouth. But it's only on one side. What is causing this?

Believe it or not, I see this quite often. Whenever there is breakout on one side of the face, it's time to ask yourself a few questions. First, do you talk on the phone a lot? If so, on which side of your face do you hold the phone? And further, do you let the phone rest on your face?

Telephones get dirty quickly. Even if you are the only person using a particular phone, oil and debris collect on the receiver, and especially if you rest the phone on your face, this will easily get transferred to your skin. Sometimes the oil will cause breakouts, and sometimes constant handling of the phone can cause contact dermatitis, a skin inflammation that is caused by contact with offending materials. Cell phones are contributors to irritations on the skin. They are almost always resting on your face and therefore can create problems, especially if you talk on a cell telephone throughout the day.

Step one in solving your problem is to keep the phone off your face. This won't be easy, but without stopping contact, I'm afraid your problem will continue. Second, clean your phone. One of my clients was experiencing contact dermatitis caused by her cell phone. I recommended she keep baby wipes handy to clean her phone with. You'll be amazed at how much junk gets piled up after just one day of using the telephone. Next, keep your hands off your face. Constantly feeling the breakout with your fingers will just encourage it to stay there. For the time being, don't use an abrasive scrub on this area, but do use a clay mask to help encourage any congestion to vacate the premises. Keeping the area clean, which includes keeping the phone off your face, is your best bet for helping the problem go away.

If the phone doesn't seem to be the culprit, what is your body position when you sleep? Do you lie on your right or left side, on your back, or even face down? I have found some people can get a small amount of breakout if they sleep on their side. It is the side that is crushed against the pillow all night long that suffers. Changing how you position your body to sleep may be a huge leap, but if you are sure this is what is causing your breakouts, the true solution is to change your habits.

The only explanation I have come up with for this type of break-out is that lying on your face all night inhibits elimination. If you have always slept on your side and just now think this is causing some skin problems, perhaps it is simply new laundry soap.

To help with the breakout around your mouth, no matter the cause, use clay mask on the area at night. Be sure to let the clay dry before you get into bed, otherwise the clay will stick to your pillow-case instead of your skin. Do this for several consecutive nights and see if it clears the problem. (I can hear you saying, "But you said to always keep the clay mask moist on my face." Yes, that is true when you are applying clay to your entire face. You don't want that much surface area to become dried out. However, when dotting the clay mask on small spots or blemishes then going to bed, you have no choice but to let the clay dry. Because you are only applying the mask on tiny spots, this shouldn't cause your skin to become excessively dry.)

I am 27 years old and have fair to medium skin tone. I have combination skin; oily in the t-zone with frequent breakouts on the chin, around my nose, and between the cheek and mouth area, especially around my cycle or when I'm under stress. I have mild breakouts, but they never seem to cease.

I have tried numerous products along with making visits to dermatologists and even switching to a birth control pill that claims to help with acne breakouts. I am guilty of picking at those annoying little bumps and using alcohol. I have also used topical products such as benzoyl peroxide and products that contain salicylic acid.

My skin seems to have become less oily this year, but it still keeps breaking out! Since reading your book I have stopped wearing foundation, except to cover blemishes. I have stopped going to the tanning salon, started to drink lots more water, have been trying to limit the amount of sugar I consume in my diet, and have become better regimented about cleaning my face twice a day.

In addition, I am concerned about all of the various products and medications that I have used, and cost is important to me at this time. I would like to continue to make skin care a top priority.

I am including this email because I want to break it down and see if I can clear up some important points as well as give you some solutions to your problem skin.

I am 27 years old and have fair to medium skin tone. I have combination skin; oily in the t-zone with frequent breakouts on the chin, around my nose, and between the cheek and mouth area, especially around my cycle or when I'm under stress. This is a pretty standard description that I hear. She has light to medium skin color, normal to oily skin, with occasional breakouts during or around her period and usually under stress as well.

I have mild breakouts, but they never seem to cease. That the breakouts are never-ceasing says to me that there is something she is doing (ingesting or using) that is continually feeding the breakouts, as mild as they might be.

I have tried numerous products along with making visits to dermatologists and even switching to a birth control pill that claims to help with acne breakouts. Ortho Tri-Cyclen® is the birth control pill that is advertised to help with acne. For some women this pill (or any birth control pill) may help with breakouts, and for others it can cause problem skin.

I am guilty of picking at those annoying little bumps and using alcohol. I have also used topical products such as benzoyl peroxide and products that contain salicylic acid. Picking, especially if done incorrectly, is not a good thing. Alcohol will not help the problem in the long run—or really even in the short term. Benzoyl peroxide and salicylic acid aren't the best things to use on blemishes and can be too harsh—depending on what kind of products they are in.

My skin seems to have become less oily this year, but it still keeps breaking out! Since reading your book I have stopped wearing foundation, except to cover blemishes. I have stopped going to the tanning salon, started to drink lots more water, have been trying to limit the amount of sugar I consume in my diet, and have become better regimented about cleaning my face twice a day. It sounds like she didn't have a very good or consistent routine, both in her skin care program and also in her diet and lifestyle habits. She made a few common mistakes. She used "acne control" products that are so prevalent out in the marketplace, along with not drinking very much water, eating a lot of sugary foods, and not being consistent with washing her face on a daily basis. And then there was the tanning salon. If you listen to the owners or people who work at these establishments, you will think this form of UV exposure is the safest thing in the world. Because of her acceptance of the safety of tanning beds, I am going to question what else she may be doing that is contributing to her skin problems that she also may think is OK. All in all, if she just does the "right" things and cuts out all the other stuff she has been doing, my guess is her skin will reflect this better care, which up until now it had not been receiving.

In addition, I am concerned about all of the various products and medications that I have used and cost is important to me at this time.

I would like to continue to make skin care a top priority. I agree on all counts. There are so many products to choose from out on the market, along with prescriptions available from doctors. I encourage you to become a responsible consumer; know what you are taking and its effects on your skin *and* body. If you find products that work for you, money may become secondary. If you can stick with something that makes a difference, you will save money by not needing to experiment anymore. I think making skin care a top priority is a great choice. It sounds like change from the past is what she needs in order to have clearer skin in the future.

> *I've recently been experiencing small bumps on my forehead and the occasional painful zit on my cheek or chin. What is causing this, and what can I use? Also, is it a good idea to use two different brands of skin care products?*

To answer your last question first, as long as all the products individually don't cause problems with your skin, I doubt combining them is a bad idea. It is a myth that mixing different product lines together is bad. It's just not true.

Regarding your breakouts, do you eat much sugar? Milk? Cheese? Anything you are eating in excess (or even on a daily basis) can cause bumps and blemishes. Whenever your skin is breaking out, you can usually look at what you are putting in your mouth to find at least one reason it has become problematic. Stress and environment are also contributing factors for some people, but in my experience foods and drinks are the major contributors if you are experiencing regular breakouts. See **Clay Masks** and **Geranium** for ideas to treat the problem areas.

> *I am 26 years old and just this summer I started to break out really badly on my forehead and temples. They are fairly big places and are in clusters way underneath the skin. What should I use?*

117

My first question for this young lady would be: what changed in your life over the summer or just before that time? Because her troubles began in the summer, it might be something as simple as sweating. Perhaps during the summer she was outside more than in the past and wasn't as diligent about keeping her skin sweat-free. There may have been other contributing factors that led to her breakout, such as dietary factors that I have already spoken about.

In the meantime, she needs to be sure her Basics 1-2-3 program is in place, as well as using pH-proper products. Doing The Extras (exfoliating and clay mask) is important, and also making sure to rinse the sweat off her skin if she is exercising or sweating on a hot summer's day. Breakout doesn't just happen, it happens as a result of some cause, no matter what that might be. So her job is to find out what could be the cause and then she can help to stop the breakout in its tracks.

Case study: Stephanie

Stephanie moved from San Francisco to Dallas in August. She moved from the sea to a land-locked city where there is a lot of air pollution and humidity. There is not a lot of air circulation in Dallas (certainly not the kind of ocean breeze that the West Coast receives) helping to keep the city air cleaner. Not only was her physical environment different, but emotionally she was going through withdrawals, having left the Northern California coast for a city far from the ocean.

Stephanie was starting a new life in all ways. It is said that the five life events that cause the most stress are marriage or divorce, giving birth, death of a loved one, starting a new job, and moving to a new city. I'd like to add to the list being laid off or fired and going through a chronic illness—either your own or a loved one's. Whatever the cause, stress creates all kinds of changes in your body (and mind), so stress cannot be dismissed as being a major factor in problem skin.

When Stephanie showed up at one of my seminars, her skin was a mess. She had widespread breakout in the form of pustules (pimples) and papules (hard cysts under the skin) as well as blackheads and dehydration. According to Stephanie, in California her skin was perfect; she rarely had breakouts and never experienced the kind of skin problems that she had now.

Because of the blemishes, Stephanie was doing something that is very common with people experiencing breakout. It is also something that, unfortunately, usually causes more problems. She was putting all kinds of drying agents on her face, from Clearasil® to oxy products, in hopes of getting rid of the spots. She was even using products for dry skin because the other things were drying her skin out. Her thinking was common: treat the breakout topically with products on the market for problem skin. And in essence, she had the right idea. But specifically, she was using the wrong products.

When stress is the biggest factor in a new breakout, until your body adjusts or until the stress is eliminated (which sometimes never happens), the breakouts will probably continue. Breakouts caused by diet are a lot easier to solve than the stress-induced kind. You simply eliminate the cause (certain aggravating foods), and the breakout will diminish in time. If only it were this simple to eliminate stress! And breakouts due to environment are also a big challenge to fix. So Stephanie was facing two of the more difficult types of breakouts to get rid of: stress-induced and environmental.

Clearing up breakouts that are caused by moving to a new city with different water, weather, and air quality will usually come with time. Your body will eventually adjust and hopefully the breakouts will cease or at least diminish. The same is true for stress breakouts. As soon as your body can adjust and when the stress (hopefully) ends or evens out, your skin should adjust back to being normal. How long the body will take to adjust is the big question. When it comes to patience with ourselves and especially our bodies, many times we fail.

Unfortunately, we are usually impatient when it comes to allowing our bodies time to adjust to adverse conditions, like illness or injury, moving, or dealing with new and bigger than normal stress. Read the **Relaxation** section to get some ideas on how to bring a peaceful energy into your life on a regular basis, whether or not you have problem skin or stress.

The program I put Stephanie on consisted of moisturizer for problem skin (*not* dry skin), gommaging and clay masking every other day for the first week or two, then 1-2 times each week thereafter. I told her to drink lots of water, take stress reduction classes like yoga or Pilates, cut out sugar (but allow some indulgences), and get facials if she could afford them.

Once Stephanie started using products meant to clear problems in a healing vs. drying way, her skin responded favorably and eventually normalized. And although her skin did clear up, I don't think Stephanie will ever get used to living away from the ocean.

Case study: Donna

Donna has blackheads on her nose and rarely gets whiteheads. She experiences most of her breakouts in the hollows of her cheeks. She complains of oily eyelids. Other than her normal daily routine, she uses a peel-off mask now and then.

For breakfast, she has oatmeal or cereal, and sometimes a bagel and eggs. On a normal work day, she has fast food for lunch. The sugar she knows she eats comes in the form of muffins, which is just like cake in terms of sugar content—no matter how healthy they may appear to be. Donna says she is "very constipated."

Donna used Proactiv for three months; then she said it stopped working. This is something a lot of people have told me. But I will say this: No matter what regime you are using product-wise, if you don't change your eating habits, there is no guarantee your skin troubles will exit your life.

Donna's case is actually easy to help. She wasn't really aware of how much sugar she was getting just by eating cereal and muffins, which are loaded with sugar, let alone other sugary foods she did know about. Fast food is not good for either her skin or her colon. Without eating at least as much good food as bad food in her diet, she shouldn't expect constipation and problem skin to be out of the ordinary.

Diet is key here. Preparation is going to be Donna's challenge as well as her saving grace. The reason we eat fast food is convenience. If she were to be very organized and prepare lunch for herself, which would also include healthy snacks for her work week, she would be able to eliminate a lot of her problem foods. Getting away from all the sugar is a little harder. Sugar is physically addicting and an acquired craving not so readily dismissed by the body.

I would recommend Donna immediately start taking both chlorophyll and acidophilus. Chlorophyll (see section), if taken regularly, can really help with constipation and elimination. Because of the buildup of old debris in her colon, there is no doubt an unhealthy amount of bad bacteria growing there as well. Taking acidophilus will help to restore a healthy balance of good and bad bacteria. (See **Acidophilus**.)

Above all else, water is essential to Donna's skin care program. I can't stress this enough: *Drink more water!* For Donna, it will help with her constipation, it will help with her skin, and it will indeed help every cell in her body function better. Without adequate amounts of water, our entire body's health is compromised.

I believe with conscientious design, Donna's skin problems can be a thing of the past. She has to be willing to let go of old patterns of eating and accept some new lifestyle changes. If clear skin really is a priority for her, Donna will make these all-important changes.

Case study: Paige

Paige suddenly noticed her skin breaking out, and she couldn't figure out why. Nothing had changed in her diet, and her stress levels were unchanged as well. After further investigation, asking Paige about anything that might be new or different in any area of her life, she finally came up with the answer to her skin care problems.

Earlier she found out she had an ovarian cyst. Rather than operate, her treatment consisted of a shot that would stop her periods for perhaps an entire year, which would reduce and hopefully eliminate the cyst. Her skin was breaking out because her body's hormonal balance was out of whack. Not having a menstrual cycle is a big deal! Women menstruate for a purpose, so not having this release can wreak havoc with your skin.

Paige had to basically wait out the year and contend with her new skin problems. Like with pregnancy, there wasn't a lot she could do because of the course of her medical treatment. She continued to get her monthly facials and did a lot of at-home extra care for her blemishes. I recommended acupuncture to help Paige's body adjust and get her back in balance, as well as previously mentioned helpers for her actual breakouts. Eventually her skin cleared, and I am happy to report her cyst disappeared.

I keep saying the breakouts you are experiencing are there for a reason. In other words, you are not breaking out for no apparent reason; it just may not be apparent to you—yet. Ask yourself questions to help determine the cause of the "sudden" breakouts. What has changed in your life recently or at the time your skin problems started appearing? Look at what you are eating to see if there is a correlation to the break-outs you are experiencing. Usually you can figure out the cause of the problems by going back in time to when the breakouts began and what was going on in your life at that time. For more information on breakouts, turn to the sections on **Acne** and **Problem Skin** if you haven't already. Between these three sections, hopefully you will have a better understanding of what might be causing your breakouts as well as how to go about clearing up your skin.

Bruises

What causes bruising?

It's pretty basic, really. When a hard object delivers a blow to the body or you fall down on a hard surface, something's got to give. The harder the trauma, the deeper the bruise, and the longer it will take the tissue to return to normal.

An area of your body that contains a lot of adipose or fat tissue (your buttocks, for example) will sustain a blow with less visible damage than your forearm, for instance, which doesn't have a lot of body fat to cushion against a strike. Without that blanket of fat to protect the blood network underneath the skin, your capillaries don't stand a chance and will break due to the trauma. This causes blood to leak out of the vessels and into the surrounding skin, making for discoloration of the affected area.

A bruise, sometimes called a contusion or hematoma, will usually start off looking like a dull or not-so-dull red or purple color under the skin, and finally it fades into more green or yellowish hues. Depending on how hard the impact was, the blood will eventually be reabsorbed into the blood stream, and the skin will go back to its normal color. Using bruises as one example, we once again are able to see and experience the amazing, miraculous healing abilities of our bodies.

If you have thin skin you will be more susceptible to bruising. A woman's skin is generally thinner than a man's, so women tend to bruise easier than men do. An older person's skin will be thinner with less fat, collagen and elastin fibers, which thin out over the years. With less to cushion the skin, an older person tends to collect bruises very easily. If you are deficient in vitamin C, you will tend to bruise fairly easily. Vitamin C, and bioflavinoids specifically, help to keep the capillary walls strong. If you have spent a lifetime in the sun, this too could make you more susceptible to bruising. Why? Sun damages the capillaries as well as altering collagen and elastin, which are the supporting structures of your skin. Without this wall of protection, bruising comes easier.

Is there anything I can put on a bruise to make it heal and go away faster?

Arnica, or *arnica montana*, is a daisy-like flower that has anti-inflammatory actions and has been found to help alleviate the edema (swelling) and blood clots that occur due to a blunt trauma, like bumping into something. Arnica is able to help lessen this blood congestion due to its ability to stimulate white blood cell activity. Arnica ointments and creams can be purchased at most health food stores. Use as directed. Arnica should never be used on open sores or broken skin, only on bruises, sprains, and swelling. Unlike other herbal medications, arnica should not be taken internally. (There are arnica pills that can be taken for shock after an accident, but these are homeopathic and are the only way to ingest arnica.)

C

Camping & Skin

When I go camping with my husband, we backpack and therefore I don't have much room to bring my cosmetics with me. Do you have any "bare minimum" suggestions for products I can take camping that wouldn't take up too much room in my pack?

Through the years I have had many clients and friends ask me how to go about taking care of their skin while under unusual circumstances. One friend was on her way to Washington state to summit Mount Rainier, while several clients have gone on no-frills safaris in the wilds of Africa. Whether you are scaling a mountain, on safari, or you're just a weekend camper, you will want to take only the essentials to save room yet save your face at the same time.

When I go camping, it is usually the no-frills kind. No bathrooms, no water other than a (very) cold stream near the campsite, and sometimes not even that. If there is no stream, I am left with water from a canteen to brush my teeth and wash my face. Needless to say, this limits my routine to the bare bones. And admittedly, although I always do my morning routine, the evening routine doesn't always get accomplished. After sitting around the campfire in the deep darkness of night, sometimes just climbing into the tent to go to sleep is my top priority.

I'm telling you this to say don't worry about skipping your routine if your circumstances dictate it. I don't go camping very often, and I certainly take exceptional care of my skin every day of my life otherwise. So if you find yourself unable (or maybe just unwilling) to do all the right things, don't worry about it. Just know that you will have some catching up to do once you get home, and your skin may show the signs of improper care, which may include congestion (more blackheads than you normally have) and flakiness from lack of exfoliation. My skin usually goes through a minor breakout during a camping trip, but frankly I'm more focused on the environmental beauty I am surrounded by and not on how I look. Fortunately, there are no mirrors out in the woods, so out of sight, out of mind!

If possible, get a facial after your trip. This will ensure that your neglected skin will get all the attention it needs. If you can get a facial before you go, do—before to prepare, after to repair. A good clay mask done right after returning from a camping trip will do wonders to immediately perk up your skin as well as clean out your pores.

Travel companions. The first order of business is getting any products you plan to take with you in travel sizes. If these smaller versions aren't available, make your own. You can find small plastic containers at almost any drug or grocery store. If your products are housed in glass or metal, they probably need to remain in containers made out of those materials, rather than plastic.

If the product you use offers sample sizes, get hold of some (you may have to purchase them, or sometimes they are given away) and take these with you instead of your travel-size products. Saving space is always the name of the game. If you end up bringing samples, be sure to take a few self-sealing plastic bags with you to use as "trash cans" for your used sample containers. When you go camping, especially backpacking, you always take out whatever you bring in, and this includes trash.

The following are the most important ingredients in your **basic travel kit:**

- Cleanser (To cleanse day and night.)
- Sunscreen (Used amply and frequently.)
- Moisturizer (Used at night, and even under your sunscreen if you need the extra moisture, and as your eye cream if you can't take a separate product.)
- Lip balm (Your lips will thank you for this one!)
- Toner in a spray bottle (If room allows.)

Keeping your skin clean and protected from the sun are the top two concerns to focus on. With that said, you have the added challenge of limited space in your pack and limited time to stick to a routine. The following suggestions are based on special, limited circumstances and are in no way recommendations for normal, daily skin care at home. When I have gone camping, if I was able to brush my teeth morning and night, it was an accomplishment!

The first ingredient in your camping travel kit is a **non-alkaline cleanser**. If water is limited, I recommend a change from how you are cleansing at home. First, spend a few more seconds applying the cleanser to your face. Next, only if water is limited, wipe the cleanser off with a towel; then rinse with water from your canteen or, if available, a stream. If stream water is your only option, you won't want to splash too much of that ice cold water on your face. It's damaging to your capillaries. Toweling or wiping off cleanser is not a practice I recommend if you are at home—there you want to splash-rinse with water. But in these limited circumstances, this wiping off procedure will require less water in order to get the cleanser off your face.

In the morning, after you have removed the cleanser as thoroughly as possible and rinsed with water, pour on the **sunscreen**! And be sure to take some with you when you go hiking. Sunscreens work on a temporary basis only, and one application in the morning *will not last* throughout the day. It should be waterproof (or water-resistant) so you won't sweat it off. Please, don't go on any excursion, especially camping, without lots of sunscreen!

At night, cleanse and use your **night treatment** cream. If you can take your eye cream, great. But if space is limited, use your night cream around your eyes. Again, this is less than ideal, but it is practical. When in doubt, improvise.

Don't forget **lip balm**. Carry it around wherever you go and use it often throughout the day and at night before you go to sleep. Lip balm will help save your lips from becoming dry and chapped. This is especially important if you are in high altitudes or in a desert climate. Try to find a non-petroleum lip balm and be sure to get one with SPF. Lips need protection from the sun's rays just as much as your skin does.

If space allows, I highly recommend taking your **toner in a travel-size spray bottle**. This step adds hydration (water) to your face as well as other soothing ingredients to help balance your skin. (Do I need to include that I am not talking about toners with SD or isopropyl alcohol in them?) Because toners are liquids, I recommend putting the bottle in a self-sealing plastic bag—just in case. You don't want any surprises when you open your pack.

If you are camping but have access to a bathroom, then you will be able to follow your regular at-home routine much more easily. You may not want to bring every skin care product you normally use at home, but you certainly can bring more than what I have mentioned. The previous recommendations are based on having very limited space and resources, yet allow you to keep your skin in pretty good shape during your time away from home.

Whatever your trip involves, have a great time, wear plenty of sunscreen, and do what you can to keep to some sort of routine, pared down as it might be. Happy trails!

Canker Sores

When clients come in who admit to eating sugar but have no outward signs of excess sugar consumption (like breakouts, for instance), I will not only ask if they get frequent headaches, which many times is a side effect of excess sugar, but also do they get canker sores inside their mouth or on their tongue? Your body simply cannot throw off sugar into thin air. The toxic residue from this white devil has to be eliminated somehow, some way, somewhere.

I believe these inner-mouth sores (sometimes called *ulcers* or technically *aphthous ulcers*) are actually similar to blemishes—like a zit inside your mouth. Why? Once again, from my own life experience, these sores arise in relation to the amount of sugar I have consumed. I am not saying that every canker sore's appearance is due to sugar. I am simply trying to give you my own personal experience with these problem spots and why I have discovered they occur. You may find other offenders and have a different experience than I have had.

Other causes may be vitamin deficiency, stress, or even a poorly functioning immune system. Since sugar depletes both vitamins in your body and immune function, sugar could very well be the culprit. Also, eating too much citrus can cause problems inside your mouth as well as little sores on the corners of your mouth. Some people think wheat or even dairy products could be to blame.

Be sure to notice why *you* think the sores are there. Sometimes I will get them but cannot find where I have had obvious sugar in my diet. Then, after really analyzing everything I've eaten, I usually can find a cause. It may be something as benign as a new brand of crackers or even a pasta dish I ate at a restaurant that probably had added sugar in.

Regardless of why they have appeared, canker sores are painful little beasts. There are several remedies I have found to be effective for relieving the pain of these irritated sores as well as helping them to go away faster. I don't have a lot of time or a lot of special ingredients in my home. I want to reach for something, apply it, and be done with it. So the following are simple and easy treatments to help the pain and suffering of canker sores.

Try rinsing your mouth with tepid **salt water**. Mix 2-3 teaspoons of table salt, or better yet, sea salt in a glass of warm water. Stir the salt until it dissolves, then swish in your mouth, paying attention to the location of the canker sore(s). Keep swishing for about 15-20 seconds, then spit and repeat. Salt water helps to reduce the swelling and irritation in these open sores. Do this several times a day for several days until the pain begins to subside, letting you know healing is starting to occur.

A less time-consuming treatment is to simply apply a drop of **peppermint essential oil** to the spots. Do this with a Q-tip. Otherwise, if you use a finger, you run the risk of accidentally putting that same finger with peppermint oil on it in or near your eyes later on. (I have done this in the past—*use a Q-tip!*) I recommend getting the oil on one end of the Q-tip first; then get a grip on your lip or mouth. Take the other, dry side of the Q-tip and place gently on the sore to dry it off. Next, put the peppermint on the area. Then, keep holding onto the skin to keep the area just treated from getting wet. Why? Because closing your mouth will cause the essential oil to mix with your saliva, rendering the treatment less effective. Keep the area open for 10-20 seconds so you can keep the treatment oil on the spot—alone—before it gets mixed into your mouth. **Clove oil** can also be an effective numbing agent for canker sores. Also used on toothaches, this essential oil has a strong analgesic (pain relieving) action.

Something else you could use to treat canker sores is **aloe vera juice**. Aloe vera has anti-inflammatory as well as antibacterial properties, which makes it a soothing yet effective treatment for canker sores. This juice can be found at most health food stores and is very inexpensive.

For canker sores, gargle (swish in your mouth) concentrating on getting the juice where your sores are. Try to keep swishing for 20 seconds or so, spit and repeat—two or three times, several times a day. If you work outside the home, take some aloe with you so you can swish and spit during the day.

Another remedy I used as a child and sometimes still reach for if a canker sore appears is **Campho-phenique**®. This is a "pain relieving antiseptic liquid" that can be found in any drug or grocery store. It contains 10.8% camphor and 4.7% phenol along with eucalyptus oil in a light mineral oil base. Although the package says it is for insect bites, scrapes, and minor burns, ever since I was a kid this is what I used on my canker sores. It tastes horrible (see ingredients), but it will numb the area as well as help the healing process. Use the same application technique that I recommend above for peppermint oil. Don't get this or any product in your eyes; read the directions and warnings on the label.

Whatever treatment you decide to use, don't forget to look to your diet and stress level to see if there are things you can do to help your body relax and defend against breakdown. Treating the symptom only does next to nothing to treat the system—your body.

A note of caution: If you have an oral lesion that you think is a canker sore but doesn't heal after 2 weeks time, it could be a sign of trouble. Even left untreated, an inner-mouth sore will usually heal completely within that 2-week time frame. So see your doctor if your supposed canker sore persists.

Capillaries

Capillaries comprise part of the blood network to the skin on the face. They are weak by nature and very susceptible to breaking or dysfunctioning. Unlike veins, arteries, and blood vessels that are very strong, capillaries are thin and fragile. Once damaged, the only way to reverse the damage is by getting them lasered. This does not truly reverse anything, but lasers can cauterize the capillary, rendering it invisible.

Capillaries are very susceptible to extremes in temperature. If you are exposed to cold weather or put cold water on your face, the capillaries will contract or constrict. If you are out in hot weather—especially direct sunlight, a hot tub, bath, or steam room, the vessels will dilate or expand. Exposure for long periods of time will weaken the capillaries, and especially going from one extreme to the other will really cause trouble for these weak-by-nature capillaries. Other extremes such as an excess of alcohol, smoking, or caffeine can damage the capillaries as well.

The moral of the story is be very moderate in the temperatures you expose your skin to. With hot or cold weather, there isn't a lot you can do, but you certainly can avoid putting either hot or cold water on your face. And if you smoke, drink alcohol, or are in the sun a lot, know that your capillaries are being adversely affected. Capillaries are very important to the overall health of your skin; be sure to take good care of them!

There have been many advancements in laser technology that have proved to be beneficial for removing damaged capillaries from both face and body. See **Intense Pulsed Light (IPL)** for more information on this type of laser procedure for broken capillaries.

Cellulite

I suppose I cannot write this book without including a discussion of the dreaded cellulite. My feeling about this "malady" is really no different than how I feel about wrinkles and the aging process in general. If you don't already have some cellulite, consider yourself lucky (or young). If you are a woman approaching your 40s who doesn't have cellulite, you soon will. If you are one in a million, you might not, but most of us ladies (and some men, too) will see the ugly monster present itself at some point in our lives. Cellulite isn't the end of the world; it is just your body going through the motions of aging and storing fat. It's doubtful you can get rid of cellulite completely, even with expensive procedures; in time the cellulite will most likely return. It is there, in women especially, for specific purposes, and fat is part of our body's composition. And although men do develop cellulite on certain parts of their bodies, I think it is predominately a woman's issue.

I doubt my point of view will make you feel any better, but it is an attitude that I have decided to adopt, knowing there isn't a lot I can do about cellulite. How I see it, since I can't see my own cellulite (the bulk of it is on the backs of my thighs), I just don't let it bother me. It's everybody else's problem to deal with, not mine. And I actually mean that!

Are you judging yourself based on how you judge others? Do you look at someone with cellulite and say "Ick," or "That is so ugly"? If so, then naturally when it comes to your own possession of this fatty substance, you are going to frame it the very same way. How about a paradigm shift? Stop judging others' cellulite and ease up on your own self-judgment too. If you try on this new attitude for a change, you may start feeling differently about cellulite.

If you have a lot of cellulite *and* you are out of shape, guess what? Maybe it's time to put things into perspective. You either need to get moving, get your muscles in shape, and burn some of your stored fat (aka cellulite), or you need to remember that the fat you see as cellulite is just your body showing you the fruits of your labor, or in this case, the possible fatty deposits of your non-exercising ways. Fat is stored (deposited) in the body to be used for energy at a later date. If you are not pushing your body to consume more energy, fat will accumulate. This is not to ignore those of us who have a genetic tendency to get cellulite, but in general keeping your body active and the calories burning can help keep fat from depositing.

Not everyone can be active and exercise to increase the mobility of his or her body. I realize some of you may have injuries you cannot overcome or are disabled in some way that decreases your ability to move. I am speaking to the majority of you who can exercise but don't. Or maybe you do exercise, but you also eat a diet laden with poor-quality foods. Finally, you may exercise rigorously, eat a low-fat, high-quality diet, and still be genetically predisposed to having cellulite. My condolences to all of us who fit under that category!

Rather than give a diatribe on exercising or diet, what I really want to say is that cellulite is here to stay, and there isn't a lot you can do about it. But be my guest: go and spend hundreds if not *thousands* of your hard-earned dollars trying to get rid of that dimpled fat. It's not unlike wrinkles: no matter how hard you try to get rid of them, they will find a way to make their presence known. You can fight and be defiant in your resistance, but somewhere along the way I hope you will ease up on your fight against cellulite (or aging) and turn your attention to helping your body become healthy and balanced from the inside out. The "out" may never be void of cottage cheesy-looking thighs, but if you are living a good life and enjoying it to the fullest, my hope is that those minor inconveniences will just pass in and out of your mind without stopping to be refueled. I'm hoping you will find a way to just let it go, to try and get over it and be happy!

As you are walking around, you cannot see your cellulite; it's other people who can. So let them bear the responsibility of liking it or not. Who cares what they think, anyway? If they are strangers, so what? And if they are your family or friends who love you, they love you, cellulite and all. Perhaps you have a friend or husband or mother who chides you about your cellulite. Create a good comeback for their insensitive comments and know you are doing the best you can to have a healthy body and a healthy outlook on life, cellulite and all.

Choose your battles. Is this one a worthy choice or could your time and energy be better spent pursuing more attainable goals? Maybe instead of seeking to eliminate the monster cellulite, could you settle for committing to a regular exercise program? Even if all it involves is walking—every day. Exercise is important and there are books, tapes, videos, and vast numbers of people who can help you put together a healthy routine to keep your body in good shape. For most of us cellulite is going to happen at some point—especially as we get older and especially if we gain weight and get overly fat. If you choose to spend your life trying to get rid of cellulite, I truly believe you are fighting a losing battle.

Chemotherapy & Skin

Chemotherapy is hard on the entire body, not just your skin. If you are currently undergoing chemo, you are undoubtedly experiencing severely dried-out, dehydrated skin among other things. Your face may look hard and dry, and the skin may be flaking. The two most important things to do for your skin while on chemotherapy are moisturizing and exfoliating.

Exfoliating will help to rid your skin of a lot of the dry, flaky cells while helping your moisturizer do its job. Because the chemicals being introduced into your body may make your skin very sensitive, finding an exfoliation process or product that works without irritating your skin may be a challenge. Usually abrasive scrubs will be too harsh and cause redness. You can try a scrub meant for very sensitive skin and see if your face will tolerate it. Gommage, listed in the **Resources** section, is a non-abrasive gel that does a great job of exfoliating. There are also enzyme peels that can rid dead cell buildup.

Along with exfoliation, you need to use a good moisturizer to ensure your skin stays well-hydrated all day long. During chemotherapy it is doubtful you will have many problems with breakout, so you may be able to use heavier moisturizers that might otherwise cause problems. Normally I don't recommend products with ingredients that are derived from petroleum. Why? Because they have a large molecular structure and sit on the surface of the skin, usually causing congestion along with possible breakout. In this case, while taking chemotherapy, some of these heavier moisturizers may be what you need to get your skin feeling hydrated. To most rules there are exceptions, and this is one of those exceptions. If your normal moisturizer just isn't doing the trick, opt for a cream that will get the job done—which may be a product containing petroleum.

While on chemotherapy you will probably go through periods of feeling tired with low energy. Why not get a facial? In the tranquil environment of the facial room, you can take care of yourself on two levels; you'll be helping your skin to feel smooth and healthy and helping yourself to relax on a deep level.

Chin Hairs

How can I prevent chin hairs? Why are they starting to grow, and how do I get rid of them?

Chin hair growth usually starts around perimenopause when a woman's hormone levels are starting to go through yet another change. During this time, estrogen levels start to wane, leaving more testosterone to run wild, creating such things as coarse, dark hair on a woman's chin. Who said getting older isn't all fun and games?

You can't magically prevent chin hairs any more than you can prevent hair on your body from growing. Electrolysis and laser hair removal are two procedures that can help keep hair from coming back once it is treated. Read the **Hair Removal** section to find out how to help get rid of these unwanted hairs. I don't recommend waxing the area; you will be removing too much innocent hair and may set yourself up for darker hair growth in the area. And tweezing usually winds up in disaster—especially if you are the type of person who doesn't know when to leave things alone once you've gotten started tweezing.

I have seen many clients over the years who are concerned about hair growth on their chin. When I inspect this area, may times I find they have been shaving the hair there. What this does is create a very obvious coarseness to the skin (a razor is too harsh for that delicate skin), and just like the stubble growing out of a man's face, stubble will result from shaving any area, including your chin. Usually the offending hair is dark, but I have occasionally seen white hair growth on the chin. Whichever color the hair is, it can be coarse and even causing some irritation, neither of which is desirable.

When I find a client who is shaving her chin for this or any reason, I implore her to stop shaving immediately! When you shave an area to get rid of a few (or many) stray hairs, you are indeed shaving off *all* hair in the area. And contrary to some people's belief, the hair then has the potential to grow back darker and thicker than it was before. Since it is usually only a few hairs that are growing in the area, you run the risk of stimulating even more hair growth if you shave. Some people are lucky and dark hair doesn't show up after shaving the chin, but it can affect the skin there as well as affecting all the hair in the area, not just one or two stray problem hairs.

My recommendation is to find a good electrolysis technician and to give this hair removal technique a good try. It would be more expensive than shaving, obviously, but the results could very possibly be long-lasting or permanent. (At the time of this writing, laser hair removal for light-colored hair is just becoming available, where in the past it was only effective on dark hair.) If you have experienced irritated skin where you have been shaving, this will improve if you stop shaving, and having electrolysis treatments can take care of the reason you were shaving in the first place.

When shaving (and waxing as well), you are getting rid of so many unoffensive hairs in the process of removing the few bad ones. I recommend looking into electrolysis or laser hair removal before using these other, less effective and potentially harmful procedures.

Chlorophyll

Chlorophyll is basically alfalfa juice concentrate. Chlorophyll loosens hardened fecal matter off the colon wall. Toxins abound in your intestines, and you want to keep as much old, hardened matter from hanging around. Even if constipation isn't a concern for you, I recommend taking a month's worth of chlorophyll as a preventative a few times during the year—every three or four months. As always, it is advisable to consult with your primary care health practitioner before adding or eliminating this or any supplement.

I read in your book to use chlorophyll; four tablespoons in water twice a day. So you recommend starting with eight tablespoons each day? Will I see results within the month? Also, do you have any ideas on making this more palatable or could I take the tablets? Are they as effective as the liquid?

I recommend taking four tablespoons twice a day for three to four weeks if you are experiencing a lot of breakout. This way you are getting a good deal of this clearing aid into your digestive system, and hopefully it will do just that—help to clear up your skin. (If nothing else, it should help your colon rid itself of toxic buildup.) Then, after that first month, you can take the dosage that is commonly recommended on the chlorophyll bottle, which is one tablespoon twice a day. This would be your maintenance dosage.

Your blemishes are not going to be "cured" by taking chlorophyll, and you may not see results that are earth-shattering. You ought to have a change in your daily eliminations, though. They should be more full and pronounced. This indicates that you are eliminating the waste your body has produced, which reduces the chance for those toxins to get into your blood and potentially cause problems with your skin.

As far as the tablets go, you have to take a bunch of them to equal the two to four tablespoons of liquid. The thing you have to understand about tablets (or capsules) is they are void of water. That's why they are in that hardened form: all of the water has been taken out. So it takes a lot of water to rehydrate them and bring them to the same hydration level that the liquid, for instance, would have. Personally, I think you are better off with the liquid. If you find it unpalatable, you can try taking the capsules or tablets, or perhaps try the mint-flavored version of liquid chlorophyll. You could even double the amount of water you are mixing the liquid with and see if that helps with the taste.

Is there any reason I should stop taking chlorophyll?

I don't know of any reason why you shouldn't take chlorophyll. My own personal routine is to take something for a period of time and then take a day, a week, or even a month off and let it clear out of my body. There may not be any reason—technically—to do this; it's just what feels right for me and for my body. You have to come to your own conclusion about taking supplements. What works for you may not work for someone else. Let your body be your guide. During the time you are taking chlorophyll, notice any differences there might be. Has your elimination changed for the better? Has your skin been clearer? Do you have more energy? If you answered yes to any of these questions, I would say keep taking it!

I used chlorophyll for about three months in an attempt to help my skin after taking Ortho Tri-Cyclen, which made my skin really break out. Although I didn't see as much of an improvement in my skin with the chlorophyll as I hoped I would, I did notice other benefits such as sweeter breath (even in the morning), and I was also very regular with the bathroom visits. I still keep chlorophyll in my fridge for occasional constipation, which isn't really an issue for me, but it's nice to know a healthy alternative is available.

This woman was experiencing cysts due to the birth control pill, which can be very difficult to clear up, and they would certainly not be cured by taking chlorophyll. The Pill, because it is delivering hormones to your body, can cause problems with some women's skin. Chlorophyll is not a match for serious hormone changes, but it did help her with other issues. Because chlorophyll helps to rid toxins and medications lingering in the body, it would be a good idea for her to continue using it. She may not see startling results, but internally her body will be better off.

A good question. One of my out of town facial clients, Judy, is in remission for breast cancer. She is diligent about her health care and is knowledgeable about what she is putting in her body, including supplements. She posed a very good question one day during her facial. Judy asked me, since reading in my book that chlorophyll "accelerates tissue cell activity and normal regrowth of cells," if she should take it based on her cancer history.

After asking different health professionals about Judy's question, I kept getting the same answer: there are few if any contraindications for the use of chlorophyll. For all intents and purposes, it should be good to take, especially if you are suffering from an illness. *However,* you must first and foremost consult with the people who are caring for you and who know the details of your condition. If you are pregnant or dealing with a health problem, like cancer or any number of concerns, you should always contact your doctor or health specialist and ask them about any supplements you are planning on taking—before you start taking them.

I am thrilled with the results I am experiencing by adding chlorophyll to my diet. I never felt that I had a problem with elimination, but with all the other positive attributes you listed for this product, I thought I might as well give it a try. For the past month, I have been mixing one tablespoon of chlorophyll and one tablespoon of flax oil in a cup of warm water for taking my morning vitamins, which also now include primrose oil! In the evening I mix another batch of this green drink but without the flax oil. Where I have really noticed a difference in my health since using the chlorophyll is my sinuses. I had been experiencing sinus problems for many years; taking a Sudafed® product had become a daily occurrence, which I hated, knowing that my liver and who knows what else was probably taking a beating as a result. Anyway, although I don't have any absolute proof, I think the chlorophyll has eliminated my sinus problems. The chlorophyll has really been the only change in my diet this past month. It has now been about two weeks since I have taken a Sudafed! This is BIG news for me, and I'll definitely keep you updated!

Clay Masks

What does a clay mask really do and why do I need one?

Clay, like earth, has an absorbing or drawing action that helps to clean superficial debris out of the pores. Even though you are cleaning your skin daily with facial cleansers, they are only removing surface oil and buildup from the day (or night). Clay masks help to pull out more material from the pores, leaving them clean and debris-free. Of course, given time the debris will once again collect in the pores.

Thus, you want to give yourself a clay mask at least once a week, more often (2-3 times per week) if you have problems with blackheads or breakout.

Clay also contains minerals and elements that are very soothing and healing for the skin. Most clay masks can be used on all skin types and are especially good for oily or problem/acne skin since these skin types tend to have a lot of congestion. You must keep the mask moist for proper results. (See the following question/answer for a more detailed explanation.) Try using a clay mask and see if you don't experience cleaner, brighter skin.

I have used clay masks before, but found them to be way too drying, especially now that it is cold and windy here in the northeast. I really feel the need for a more moisturizing mask, and I also want something to use at night that will help with a few little dry patches I have on either side of my chin that just won't go away.

The dryness you are experiencing with a clay mask is pretty common. That is why I recommend keeping the mask moist the entire time it is on your face. Clay does not need to dry on your skin in order to draw impurities to itself. If you keep the mask moist, this should solve your problem of dry skin after the mask.

Spraying clean, filtered water on your face is the cheapest and easiest way to keep your clay mask moist. Simply get a small plastic spray bottle at your local grocery or drug store and fill it with clean water. Once you have applied the mask, spray your face really well with the water, then have the bottle on hand to spray intermittently during the 15 minutes you have the mask on. Spray well enough to keep the mask wet, but not so much that water is dripping off your face. An alternative would be to spray your face with your toner, presuming you have it in a spray bottle.

Another tip is to lie in the bathtub with the mask on and the water bottle by your side. If you are a bath person, you know the relaxing benefits of a nice hot bath to soothe your muscles and indeed your soul. Having the clay on your face acts like a barrier and will protect your fragile capillaries from the heat of the steam.

Having dry patches doesn't necessarily mean you need a moisturizing mask. It really depends on how much oil you have in your pores and if your skin is dehydrated. Are you congested (clogged pores) at all or in any particular place on your face? If not, then using a moisturizing mask is fine. But if you do have clogged pores, the clay mask is what you need.

Although I am not a fan of using too many different things at one time, if you want to, you could use the clay on the places you need it and the moisturizing mask on the places you feel dry. Another recommendation would be to apply a layer of your moisturizer under the clay mask. This way you will be infusing the cream into your skin while the clay still has the ability to clean the pores and stimulate circulation. Also, don't forget to exfoliate (before masking). It will help with dryness and congestion. (See **The Extras**.)

Clay isn't the only kind of mask you can use; it just happens to be my favorite. It's effective and beneficial for most skin types.

HOT TIP: Apply a clay mask before hopping into the steam room. It's the perfect way to keep the mask moist while protecting your skin at the same time. Do not go into steam rooms bare-faced!

I have a lot of blackheads that are very stubborn around my nose and chin. I've used a scrub to help the problem, but I don't want to cause any damage to my skin yet I do want the blackheads to go away. Any suggestions?

The best product to super-clean your skin and the least likely to cause any damage would be a clay mask. If you have stubborn blackheads, I recommend using a mask more often at first and seeing how effective it is. With clay, and especially when using it frequently, you really need to heed my advice and keep the clay moist when it is on your face. Clay deep cleans and can definitely help to de-clog your pores. The more stubborn the problem, the more diligent you need to be about doing your routine.

I would be careful about using scrubs on stubborn blackheads. Why? Because when you have a lot of impacted material (dead skin and oil) held within the pores, you want to gently lift it out, not potentially drive it back into the pores. When using a scrub, the motion is to mash it into the skin—no matter how gently you are using it. If you do drive the debris back into the pores, you may cause infection, leading to all kinds of problems that are worse than stubborn blackheads. There is not a lifting action during the scrubbing process like there is with a clay mask.

I've heard toothpaste is good for clearing up zits.

Where this rumor got started I'll never know. Just like the myths about using common household cleansers for problem skin, the best thing to use on your skin is a product made for your skin. Clay mask and/or geranium (see section) is your best bet for clearing up blemishes. Try using toothpaste, but I am sure you will find it does nothing, except possibly irritate your skin. Toothpaste is for cleaning your teeth *not* for clearing your skin!

One of the tips I got from your book that I do religiously now and have benefited enormously from is the clay masking. I always have had dry skin and have avoided clay masks at all costs until I read your theory about keeping it moist. That has been a tremendous help to my skin. Once or twice a week I use a clay mask as well as geranium oil for overnight spot therapy on the occasional monthly blemish. Thank you for your helpful tips!

Cleansers & Cleansing

Is soap OK to use on my skin?

No, soap is not a good product to use on your skin—at least not your face. Why not? Because soaps, in general, are alkaline; alkalinity basically dries out the surface skin. It does this by stripping all the oil and water off your face. This not only makes your skin feel dry after washing, it also sets up a situation where your oil glands may produce more oil to compensate for the loss from soap use. What this can mean for you is congestion (clogged pores) as well as dry, flaky skin (dehydration).

What does a cleanser do and what should I look for?

Cleansers remove oil and debris from the surface of your skin and to some degree from inside the pores. Cleansers are not exfoliators and only do a surface cleansing. They are important in keeping your skin clean and free from built-up debris and oil. You should cleanse both morning and evening for proper skin care.

What you're looking for in a cleanser is a product that first and foremost gets your skin clean without causing any other effect, such as dryness or irritation. If you experience any negative side effect from your cleanser, I suggest shopping around for something else. Since you are using it at least two times a day—every day—you just can't afford to use something that isn't right for your skin.

I prefer milk cleansers to soaps. And no matter what you choose to use, you always want a pH balanced, non-alkaline cleanser. Also, you want to rinse the cleanser off with water, not simply towel off or use cotton. There are numerous products to choose from, and that is why I recommend purchasing Nitrazine or other pH papers so you can at least be guaranteed that the product you are using to clean your skin with is not stripping it, causing problems down the road. (See **pH**.)

My skin is so oily, I feel like I constantly need to wash my face during the day. Is this good or bad for my skin?

The answer to your question depends on what you are washing your face with and also why you feel the need to cleanse it throughout the day.

Washing your face in the morning gets the residue off your skin from the six to eight hours you were asleep. Even though all you were doing was essentially lying in bed all night, you were still eliminating sweat and toxins from the skin—albeit at a reduced rate compared to during the daytime. In order to start the day off right, you want to clean your face, just like you brush your teeth. At night, you have a whole day's worth of accumulated toxins—sweat, debris from the air, and possibly makeup. This has sunken into your pores throughout the day, and you definitely want to wash all of it off.

If in between your morning and evening cleansings you are washing again, you may indeed be washing too much. If you are washing with soap, more than likely it is alkaline, and it will actually strip your skin of all the oil and water, setting up the potential for more oil to be produced by your oil glands to compensate for the loss during cleansing. Can you see how this will immediately set up a vicious cycle? You wash (thinking it is a good thing) yet cause more oil to be produced; so you wash again to get rid of the oil, etc. One of the main things you want to be sure to use is a non-alkaline cleanser. Then hopefully you will not be experiencing the oiliness you are now.

If you have exercised during the day or for some other reason you have done something that has caused you to sweat, by all means wash your face. But if your skin just feels oily, consider changing your cleanser and continue reading to find out other things you can do to curb the oiliness.

Are you using too much moisturizer? Are you not using one at all? Either way, this can cause you to feel oily. If you use too much cream, obviously it is going to sit on your skin, then mix with your own oil from your face, which can cause you to feel greasy and look shiny or oily. If you didn't put a moisturizer on at all, again, your oil glands may be overcompensating for the lack of oil on the surface of your skin and pumping out more oil to balance things out. If you have true oily skin, you want to use a light moisturizer formulated specifically for your skin type. In some cases, moisturizers for oilier skin types can help inhibit oil production and even help to break down the oil sitting in your pores. This is especially true for products that contain essential oils. They are natural lipid (oil) solvents and help to balance the oil being secreted by your sebaceous or oil glands.

Finally, foundation can definitely make your skin look and feel oily by midday. If you do wear foundation, consider switching to powder—loose, *not* pressed powder. (See the **Powder** section to find out why you don't want to use this product.) Mineral makeup (see section) may be a good alternative to foundation as well.

To summarize, check the pH of your cleanser and make sure you are using something that is non-alkaline or acidic on the pH scale. Don't use soap; this will simply increase the oiliness of your skin. Be sure to cleanse morning and night, and in between if you have sweated. Don't use too much cream on your face, but do use some type of moisturizer to help keep your skin from becoming dehydrated. And consider not using foundation or switching to powder.

How much cleanser am I supposed to use? Enough so my face is white and then massage it in until I can't see it or just a small amount? Is it supposed to lather?

How much cleanser to use will depend on a few things. First, how big your face is and second, how much you prefer to use. Practically speaking, if you use too much, you're just wasting product. Conversely, if you don't use enough, you probably aren't getting a good cleanse.

So what's too much? Honestly, I think you will just know—it will probably feel like you are rubbing cleanser on cleanser rather than cleanser onto skin. If you use too much, it will just feel like you have too much product to work with.

If you don't use enough, you won't be able to spread the product across your face, leaving many places unwashed. Using too little may cause the cleanser to almost absorb into the skin like a moisturizer. This product is meant to remove surface debris from the skin, not to penetrate like a moisturizer. And you really don't want to massage it in until you can't see it. In fact, if you have massaged the product in too long or perhaps used too little, the cleanser may have gone into your skin. In this case, I would "bring it up" by adding a little water to it with your hands, then splash-rinse to remove.

I find that using about a half dollar-sized dollop of cleanser is enough, but you want to use an adequate amount in order to cover your entire face. The product I use has a pump, and I use about two to three pumps for each cleansing. If it doesn't feel like enough once I've gotten it on my face, I'll just add another pump or two. Sometimes just adding a little bit of water makes the cleanser go further. Just don't water it down so much that it can't clean your skin.

Experiment and see. The main thing is to use enough to enable you to spread the cleanser over your entire face and neck. To cleanse, simply apply the cleanser, massage for a few seconds, splash-rinse, and then towel dry.

Milk cleansers generally do not lather. Gel-type cleansers and most soaps will lather, depending on the sulfates in the ingredients. (Sulfates make soaps soapy.)

I read in a magazine that in order to save time in the morning, I can just splash my face with warm water. Is this true?

According to a skin care expert I saw quoted in a popular magazine, "...as long as you've cleansed thoroughly the night before, you can skip this [cleansing] step in the a.m. and simply splash your face with warm water for just 30 seconds." I want to ask this person if she just uses water on a toothbrush in the morning, skipping the toothpaste altogether. Why not skip washing your body in the shower while you're at it?

If you are going to spend 30 seconds splash-rinsing, why not put some cleanser on your face (8-10 seconds), massage it in for maybe 10 seconds, and then splash-rinse with tepid water, which would take another 10 seconds. Without doing the math, I think you can see my point. Why not cleanse? What is the purpose in skipping this important step? It doesn't really save you time according to this skin care expert's advise. I suppose if you just skipped doing anything to your face, that would save the 30 seconds it would actually take you to clean your skin. But is saving less than a minute in the morning that important? So much so that you may cause problems for your skin down the road?

Plain water, by the way, will not break down the oil that has accumulated on the surface of your skin during the night. Only by using a proper cleanser will you be assured of getting a good, clean start for your skin each day.

And finally, are you going to put makeup on unclean skin? *Wash your face*—both morning and evening.

I'm a fitness instructor and teach several classes each day, and it seems like I'm constantly washing my face. Is doing this really bad for my skin?

Due to your special circumstances as a fitness instructor, and because you are sweating throughout the day, you need to wash your face more often than the average person. What you are using on your skin becomes especially important since you are using it a lot. If you use the wrong type of cleanser (an alkaline soap or a harsh cleanser), you can be causing adverse reactions that don't need to occur. Wash with products that don't irritate or dry your skin, like a milky cleanser for instance, and take special care of your skin at home—namely exfoliating and using cleansing masks to get the pores super clean. Due to your job, you can't skip your added skin care routine. You should be fine if you just use products that are beneficial vs. harsh on your skin.

What about using cleansing towelettes for my daily cleanser?

The best use of these cleansing towelettes is after a workout, when you don't have somewhere to splash-rinse the sweat off your face. But as far as using these products as your regular, daily cleanser, I say no. This goes for the fitness instructor in the previous email, too. For an occasional emergency cleanse, I actually think these towelettes come in handy, but for everyday cleansing, use a regular facial cleanser. (Also see **Cleansing Cloths**.)

Some of these towelettes claim to cleanse, exfoliate, and moisturize in only a few fast swipes—without using any water. Some even have AHAs (alpha hydroxy acids), which claim to have "anti-aging" abilities. Beware of products that claim to do multiple tasks all in one. You may ask, "How can I tell if a product can do all it says it can?" Let's break it down and try to make sense of these claims.

A towelette or facial cloth by its very nature cannot hold much cleanser. It is prepackaged with a regulated amount of product on the cloth. No doubt it can exfoliate some dead cells—running *anything* over the skin will cause some exfoliation. So the cleansing and exfoliating can conceivably go hand in hand. AHAs do have exfoliating abilities, but how much can they really do as an ingredient in a cleansing product? Read my opinion about AHAs in cleansers coming up.

Many times these towelettes (and some cleansers too) claim to moisturize your skin. Now I'm all for moisturizing, but it really isn't the job of your cleanser to do this. Of course, you don't want your cleansing product to dry out your skin, but cleansers cleanse and moisturizers moisturize. And although a cleanser can have moisturizing abilities, it does not stand alone as a moisturizer.

Once again my question is how long does it take to cleanse, splash-rinse, spray toner and put moisturizer on? Thirty seconds maybe. Don't you have *30 seconds* for the health of your skin? Either you do or you'll use a cloth that may create problems later on—problems that may take considerable time to clear up.

AHAs in cleansers. Why do manufacturers put AHAs into cleansers? Cleansers are on your skin only briefly, 10-20 seconds tops. A moisturizing product is on your skin for almost 24 hours per day. If you are using alpha hydroxy acids for their intended purpose (exfoliation), doesn't it make more sense to use creams that contain AHAs rather than cleansers? If you are going to use a cleanser with AHAs (which isn't necessarily a bad thing, just superfluous), don't spend more money for these special ingredients.

Special additions. If you want to have extra help when you're cleansing (especially if you have breakout), **try adding clay mask to your cleanser.** After you have squirted or pumped your cleanser into the palm of your hand, take your clay mask and mix some into the cleanser. I would use two parts cleanser to one part clay. This will give you a little deeper cleanse, along with a slight exfoliating action. Due to clay's earth nature, it does have a semi-granular texture. So if you have a lot of infection to your breakout, don't use this or just be sure not to rub too hard. You never want to break open your blemishes, unless you are purposely extracting them.

Another recommendation is to **add equal parts of a facial scrub with your cleanser**. I typically use this mixture when I'm cleansing my face in the shower. I do this primarily for the circulatory benefits, but if you are sensitive to scrubs, try this suggestion. By adding some scrub of choice to your cleanser (only a liquid or milky kind), you can get a little bit of exfoliating without irritating your skin.

Cleansing Cloths

There are several companies that make daily facial cleansing cloths. These are meant to take the place of a liquid cleanser or even bar soap. My question is why? Do these cloths benefit the skin more than using a regular cleanser?

On one company's box of facial cloths, it suggests the cloth will "take the place of your normal cleansing routine, including bar soap, make-up remover, facewash, cleansing milk and toner." Although forgoing both cleansing and toning by using this product would never fly with me, I wanted to try these facial cloths to see if they could be used as a substitute for cleansing with a milk cleanser or wash.

Initially I liked this product. Before using one of the cloths, I tested it with my pH papers, and it turned out to be acidic, which was a positive. Then, as instructed, I wet the cloth, rubbed it to make it lather, then used it to cleanse my face. One side of the cloth is smooth while the other side has a slight texture, enabling it to exfoliate. I liked this feature because it was not abrasive, yet I could tell I was getting some exfoliation benefits. I removed the residue by splash-rinsing instead of just using the cloth as instructed. Splash-rinsing ensures getting all the product off; using only the cloth may still leave a residue. I used my spray-toner and moisturized.

While I was looking up the ingredients in my research books, I noticed my skin was beginning to feel taut and dry. I used my usual toner and moisturizer so I knew it was the cloth that was causing this result. The first two out of three ingredients are foaming agents, then a little further down on the list is a bad alcohol—benzyl alcohol, which is derived from pure alcohol (see **Alcohol in Products**). Just these ingredients alone could be what was causing my skin to feel dried out. Witch hazel is also listed and can be a drying ingredient.

By the time I had investigated all the ingredients, my skin felt dried out enough for me not to recommend these cloths for regular use. However, I think they can make a great addition to your workout bag or even something to take along with you camping. Because they come as dry cloths, you can stick them in your cosmetic bag (or even a sealed plastic bag) and take them with you rather than lug around your bottle of cleanser. I wouldn't use facial cloths as your daily cleanser, but for unusual circumstances when you may not have access to a regular cleanser, I think they will come in handy.

Comedone Extractors

I had a facial done back in early October. The lady who was working on me used some kind of tool to squeeze out blackheads and pimples. I asked her if [the red marks left from the extraction] would clear up right away because I had a singing competition in 2 weeks. She had said they would clear up fast.

My face did not clear up for my show, in fact there were still some rough areas at Christmas! Now, however, my skin has finally healed, but I have all these little dents in my face where she worked. They are purple in color and look like little pot holes that you see down dirt roads. I am somewhat depressed over this as my skin was always so nice and clear before, no scars from pimples like I've seen on other people's faces. Now unfortunately I have these places on my own face.

My question for you is: Is there any way at all to get rid of the pot holes?

I'm sorry you had this experience. The aesthetician probably used a comedone extractor. It is something I don't recommend using under any circumstances during a facial (or at home). These metal tools can cause a lot of damage. Mostly I see capillary damage, but depending on who is using it, scarring can also occur.

If what you are experiencing is truly scarring from the extractions done in your facial, there isn't a lot you can do. Definitely *do not* pick at those areas. If it has been months since your breakout, even though the skin may look purple, it is doubtful there is still infection after so much time. You want to be very careful not to get sun on your face. Those spots may pigment differently now that the skin has been altered, and that may cause dark spots from sun exposure. (See **Post-Inflammatory Hyperpigmentation**.)

If your pores are still clogged, you want to be sure to keep your skin clean—not just by daily cleansing but by exfoliating and using a clay mask as well. These two steps, if done on a regular basis, can really help to keep your skin in good shape.

There are currently lasers that may be able to help with the scarring. You would need to discuss this with a dermatologist to find out all the information on what is available. The doctor can evaluate your particular skin's condition and give you advice as to what to do for the scarring. Unfortunately laser procedures can cost a lot of money, and they aren't always 100% effective.

I wish I had a magic answer to your dilemma. Unfortunately scars are permanent, although their appearance may decrease over time and could look less noticeable. If you ever find yourself in a facial and see that a comedone extractor is going to be used, just tell the aesthetician that under no circumstances will you allow it to be used on your face.

Crow's Feet

How can I get rid of or prevent crow's feet?

In a word, you can't. Crow's feet are the lines and wrinkles that form around the eyes from years of expressing, including laughing, crying, squinting, and rubbing the area. Throughout our lives the eye area gets a good deal of sun exposure, too. This will increase both the speed of formation and the depth of the lines around your eyes.

You have no functioning oil glands directly under your eyes, so it stands to reason that this particular area remains dry throughout your life, coupled with the fact that the eyes are the most expressive part of the face. This gives just about everyone a recipe for premature lines and wrinkles.

Crow's feet are not preventable—unless of course you don't express and otherwise don't disrupt the tissue. Obviously, this is not going to happen. Even young people have the beginnings of crow's feet—they are a natural part of the evolution of our skin. You can't really get rid of them nor can you prevent them from occurring.

This is where Botox and other cosmetic procedures step in. And this is where I go my separate way. You get lines and wrinkles due to the natural aging process, like it or not. And my choice is to accept and move on. For others, moving on means reaching for cosmetic helpers that will help diminish or even eliminate the lines. I still contend the lines around your eyes cannot be completely eliminated, but Botox and laser procedures can significantly lessen their appearance. I don't subscribe to these procedures, but they are widely available.

I am not sure if 26 is the magic number, but I have started to notice the beginnings of the dreaded crow's feet (which is why I am stocking up on eye cream!). Is this normal? Am I aging prematurely? How can I make it stop?

The aging process starts when it does. It is different for every individual, but at 26 you are probably going to start seeing something. Because the eyes are so expressive, it is usually the first place you will see lines starting to form. You can't "make it stop," but using eye cream every day will help to keep the skin under your eyes soft and therefore discourage lines from forming due to dehydration. The lines will form there, and every year they will get deeper. Now in my 40s, I am of course seeing the aging process take hold. Gray hair, deeper lines, but I don't obsess or even pay too much attention to all that. I know intellectually those things are going to happen. So I choose to focus my attention on the things I can change like eating well, exercising, and in general continuing to learn how to relax through life.

At 26 this may all sound like a bunch of "who cares," but you can't change the inevitable. You can, of course, use good products on your skin and stay away from direct sunlight on your face. But nature will take its course. Try to enjoy the process! (I'm sure you are rolling your eyes right about now!)

It's doubtful you are aging prematurely, and yes, seeing some lines is normal. But how much sun you have had and continue to get will greatly influence how deep the lines get. For instance, do you ever sit outside to eat lunch? What about driving with your sunroof open? These are really no different than lying on the beach. Sun is sun, and it is the number one cause of aging, both premature and normal aging.

I would like to instill an air of confidence in younger readers. I encourage you to stop looking so hard in the mirror and live your life. You may see the wrinkles starting to form, but they aren't going anywhere! They will be with you for the rest of your life. Enjoy your youth; you have the rest of your life to worry about aging.

D

Dark Circles

What are dark circles? What causes them?

When you see dark circles under your eyes, you are essentially seeing the blood vessels—filled with blood—due to the exceptionally thin skin in that area. Stress and lack of sleep can cause changes in your blood circulation (it becomes slower), which can cause the tiny capillaries to expand. Thin skin or circulation that has slowed down can both cause dark circles to appear.

Then there are allergies. Airborne inhalants as well as food allergies can cause dark circles to form. So the short answer to that question is similar to what causes problem skin: diet, environment, and lifestyle habits. Genetics, as always, can also play a key role in whether or not you will have dark circles.

My story. Throughout my life, I have never really had a problem with dark circles under my eyes. Sure, once in a while if I was out too late or just didn't get enough sleep for some reason, they might appear temporarily. And, while I lived in Dallas, I had terrible springtime allergies, so during my annual two months of misery, the dark circles were generally always present. But by and large, I didn't consider dark circles a concern for me.

Then when I moved to Chicago, I noticed a marked difference in the dark circles under my eyes. In fact, I noticed that I constantly had them! At first I thought it was due to the stress I was under having recently moved my life to a new city. Then I thought it was the pollution here (although I think both cities have an equal problem when it comes to air quality). When I would go to Dallas on business I noticed the dark circles virtually went away, so I knew it was something to do with life in Chicago.

Now, months later, I think I have discovered the culprit. It was not so much the outside air pollution, it was no longer the stress of moving (I'd lived here long enough to smooth all that out), but what I think was causing the problem was the apartment I was living in at the time. It was extremely dusty there, and I'm not sure why. I could see the dust accumulate on everything—including my cats! I have never lived anywhere with so much dust! I put air filters in every room, including the bathroom, but still, the dust kept on coming. Dust is a very common allergen, and I believe it was dust that ultimately caused my dark circles back then. It was my body's allergic reaction showing itself.

Dark circles are there for a reason. But just like my dusty apartment story, it may take a sleuth to figure out why they are there. It's always going to be environmental—your *body's* environment. Our magnificent machines are always throwing off toxins, and when the toxic buildup is too much to take, the body starts giving signs of overload. So if you suffer with dark circles, look around and see if you can figure out what is causing them. I believe that common allergens, whether they be in your diet or your immediate environment, are causes for persistent or even temporarily dark circles.

I have very dark circles that are genetic and require concealer. I have had difficulties with eye creams that don't blend well with concealer or somehow increase the dryness or are too oily, making the concealer settle and crease in the wrinkles beneath my eyes. I was looking at an alpha hydroxy eye cream for wrinkle prevention. I also saw an eye cream that said it helped with the dark circles. But I am not sure whether either of these would work with concealer and makeup during the day. I was hoping perhaps you could help me.

I have very dark circles that are genetic and require concealer. Genetic is the operative word here. If you know your dark circles stem from a genetic predisposition, then please know that no product, miracle or not, is going to rid you of your genetic "gifts." How do you know if they're genetic? Look at your parents and even their parents. If you see dark circles wherever you turn, then you are just carrying on the family tradition.

I have had difficulties with eye creams that don't blend well with concealer or somehow increase the dryness or are too oily, making the concealer settle and crease in the wrinkles beneath my eyes. Eye cream shouldn't make the skin around your eyes feel dry. You may be having an allergic reaction or an intolerance to one or more of the ingredients. If the eye cream makes the skin too oily, you may be putting too much on (only use a small amount, but often), or it just may be too rich a cream for your skin. When you use concealer around the eyes, it will crease inside the wrinkles no matter if you use eye cream or not. Like foundation (both contain pigment), concealer will usually accentuate the lines and wrinkles.

I was looking at an alpha hydroxy eye cream for wrinkle prevention. I also saw an eye cream that said it helped with the dark circles. But I am not sure whether either of these would work with concealer and makeup during the day. Alpha hydroxy acids (AHAs) do help with lines and wrinkles because they decompose microscopic bits of skin, leaving the surface of your face smoother and the texture refined. They don't *prevent* wrinkles—nothing really does. Creams that say they help with dark circles might help, but only to a certain degree.

As far as AHAs or creams for dark circles working with your concealer, you will have to experiment and see. After applying your eye cream, try waiting at least 5-10 minutes before putting the concealer on. This might help with some of the creasing.

I am thinking of having surgery to remove my dark circles. Do you think there is something else I can do to get rid of them?

Surgery can only take adipose (fat) from that area; it will do nothing for the capillaries or blood vessels. I am not a proponent of surgery. Toxins in our bodies will contribute to the darkness around the eyes. The skin is very thin and shows vascular changes quite easily. So, if your internal health is optimal, usually the darkness will subside, unless of course you are genetically predisposed to dark circles.

I know from personal experience that on the morning after eating sugar, I have noticeable dark circles under my eyes. I believe this is due to an inflammatory response (similar to an allergic reaction) that sugar causes in my body. The same holds true for alcohol consumption. I see the same response (dark circles) after a night of even moderate drinking.

Eating sugar, drinking alcohol, smoking cigarettes, not getting enough sleep at night, and other environmental factors can all contribute to your problem. Change what you are putting in your body (really, give this serious consideration) and see what effects it has on your dark circles.

Products for dark circles. Although there are many products on the market that profess to remove dark circles, I would caution you against spending too much of your hard earned money on them. I'm not saying you won't find relief with one or more of these creams, but I have not found one product that stands out from any other. I believe if there was a product that really got rid of dark circles completely, we would all know about it. The manufacturers would be rich and no one would have to walk the earth with dark circles! But that isn't the case. If you want to try a product said to help reduce dark circles, don't hesitate! But don't be surprised if it doesn't do all you want it to do. If the product helps, great! If it doesn't, return it if you can. For less severe cases of dark circles, products truly may help. But if you are genetically predisposed and/or have a lifestyle that doesn't support your best health, you may not find the results you are looking for in a cream designed to help with dark circles. And do try looking at your diet to see if you may be contributing to the problem.

Dehydrated Skin

Dehydration is not dry skin or what I call *true-dry* skin. Dehydrated skin *feels* dry, but technically dry skin is lacking oil versus dehydrated skin that is lacking water. Dehydrated skin generally has a large buildup of dead skin cells. If there are too many dead cells on the surface, more water is needed to keep all the cells moist. By eliminating the buildup (achieved through exfoliation), your cells are better able to retain moisture and less likely to become dehydrated.

What's the difference between dry and dehydrated? I'm confused.

A definite misunderstanding surrounds these two separate conditions that are thought to be the same. No wonder you are confused! Many people think they have dry skin because it *feels* dry, when really they're simply dehydrated. Although true-dry skin and dehydrated skin *feel* the same, their causes are totally different, and the treatment of each separate condition is also very different.

Dehydration means there is an excessive dead cell buildup on the surface of your skin, and therefore you need to exfoliate (manually remove the dead skin). No amount of moisturizing will truly fix the problem, but through regular and thorough exfoliation, you can greatly reduce or eliminate dehydration.

True-dry skin is *oil* dry. It simply does not emit much or enough oil. Therefore this skin does not have blackheads, usually doesn't have whiteheads, and almost never has breakout. True-dry skin needs moisturizing to help add oil to its oil-deficient surface. Exfoliation can help, but what is really needed is proper moisturizing.

A common mistake people with dehydrated skin make is to over-moisturize. Because their skin feels dry, it seems logical to give the skin more moisture. But this is where the problems can really begin. You start off with dehydration and can end up with congestion or breakout on top of the dryness (dehydration). Making the distinction between dry and dehydrated skin is imperative. Without knowing which skin condition you have, you could really cause problems down the road.

A case in point is my client Bridget. She came in for a facial, complaining of congestion all around her nose and cheeks. She had experienced this for over a year and was unable to get any clear answers as to what might be going on with her skin. During the treatment, I asked her what had changed in her life a year or more ago—especially with her skin care routine. She did change skin care products right around then, but she didn't feel this was the problem. After looking at her skin, I agreed that it was indeed congested. I really felt it was product-induced rather than a problem with too much oil. Why? The pores were clogged in a way that just didn't seem consistent with an over-production of oil from within. Her skin had a spongy quality to it, like it was getting too much moisture. It looked puffy and felt oversaturated.

Bridget admitted to using too much product when she moisturized. Step one: stop using so much product! She was doing this because she felt "dry," which we now know (because she doesn't have true-dry skin) is really dehydration. Step two: start using products for combination-to-oily skin. (She had previously switched to dry skin products.) Step three: she needs to use a clay mask as often as possible.

Two to three times per week would be a good start, and then once a week after the congestion has diminished. Clay can greatly improve the condition of her pores, helping to clean out the superficial debris and keep her pores from enlarging.

Bridget did what many of you have probably done—treated your dehydrated skin like true-dry skin by overmoisturizing. Understanding the condition of your skin is crucial to treating it properly. Hopefully, you have a better understanding about the difference between dry and dehydrated skin. Now, after applying this knowledge, you can enjoy the benefits of proper skin care.

Bridget's skin, by the way, has dramatically improved. After switching to a more appropriate moisturizer and using less product, the spongy quality to her skin has all but disappeared. And the congestion she was experiencing has been cut in half at least.

I've been meaning to email you since we met in December because I've been so excited about my skin! I loved talking with you, and I have to tell you how my skin has improved!! After we figured out that the dry skin formula was probably the cause of my breakouts, I stopped using that specific moisturizer immediately. The breakouts soon stopped, and my skin started to clear up within a few days! (I was getting a new breakout almost every day.) Now I might get one small breakout a week, mainly because I started eating sugar again over the holidays. (I've got to wean myself off again!) I'm also so thankful I met with you before I was in my cousin's wedding this past weekend. My skin looked great for pictures, and I was even confident enough not to wear foundation for part of the day. Thanks again for everything!

Amanda came into my office and had a lot of "unexplained" congestion. After asking her a series of questions, it was pretty obvious what the problem was: she was using products for dry skin because her skin *felt* dry even though she didn't have true-dry skin. This is a big mistake. If you have anything other than true-dry skin (skin that emits little to no oil), you can really create a lot of problems using dry skin products—namely congestion and possibly breakouts. If your skin is producing enough or too much oil and you add oil on top of that, watch out! From your point of view, your skin feels dry. It may be flaky and just feels tight. It does make sense that perhaps you need products for dry skin if, that is, you don't understand the difference between true-dry skin and what you most likely have—dehydrated skin.

I have clients who come in regularly and say their skin is dry when the truth is it is simply dehydrated. And I have taken a number of clients off their dry skin products and helped them have healthier, less oily skin. Just like Amanda's comments illustrate, if you are using the wrong products for your skin type, it can have disastrous results.

If you are having problems with your skin, there is a reason. *Something* is causing the problems. And if you don't focus on the *cause* (in Amanda's and perhaps your case, using dry skin products when you don't have true-dry skin), the problems will no doubt persist.

I wanted to let you know that my skin has cleared up beautifully, and I have a question. My skin doesn't seem dry, but when I smile my cheeks (where the skin is very thin and scarred) have dry-looking lines. What should I use for this? Now that I have stopped breaking out, the scars are better but the skin is still thinner in that area. I certainly don't want to aggravate my skin with something that will make me break out—lines are better than blemishes for now!

If your skin doesn't *feel* dry, I don't recommend doing too much in terms of adding heavy moisturizers. You may just be noticing your skin there, whereas before you were looking at the breakouts. Perhaps it's not your skin that has changed, but your perception of it.

However, if your skin actually feels dry on your cheeks, you can try adding a glycerin-based hydration booster to your creams. I wouldn't recommend applying something directly to the area; there is too much of a risk the product might go on thicker than you realize, and breakout may result. I usually recommend a booster for people who have oily and/or problem skin that *feels* dry but is really dehydrated. Try it and see how this works for you. (See **Glycerin** for information on hydrating boosters.) Exfoliating, too, will help relieve the surface of any dead cells that may be hanging around and causing the dry feeling.

Dehydration needs to be attended to, but remember, you always want to treat the oil content of your skin first, whether there is an overabundance or lack of oil production. Dehydration is easily diminished by exfoliating. If you have severe or deep dehydration, you may need to use hydrating elixirs or a more effective exfoliator. If your skin can tolerate AHAs, then this type of ingredient may work to rid your skin of dehydration. I caution you, though, if you have sensitivities or are prone to redness, AHAs can be more detrimental than beneficial depending on your skin. Be sure to take care of dehydrated skin so it doesn't develop into a more severe condition. Exfoliate more regularly and see if this alone helps your problem. Understanding the simple difference between these two separate conditions (dehydration and true-dry skin) can keep you from experiencing a skin care catastrophe when purchasing your skin care products.

DermaNew™ Personal Microdermabrasion System

When a leading magazine asked a popular actress how she took care of her skin, one of her choices for exfoliation was using a "mild home microdermabrasion process" called DermaNew. I hadn't heard a thing about it before, but ordered this machine after reading the article. I figured that sooner or later someone would be asking me about this home microdermabrasion machine, so here is my assessment of DermaNew.

The literature says their machine is state of the art microdermabrasion resurfacing technology. I think the company is stretching things by calling this microdermabrasion system state of the art. What you get in the basic kit is a jar of DermaNew Creme and a resurfacing tool that has sponge applicator attachments. It says it is a safe and effective alternative to chemical and laser peels. This infers that the results could be similar, yet chemical and laser peels are completely different animals compared to DermaNew, which is simply exfoliation with the aid of sponge applicators powered by a battery-operated rotary tool. The advertising just doesn't match up to the reality of what this system can really do.

I tried the DermaNew system out several times over a few weeks. After each session, my skin felt irritated, which I know was from the cream. I had to use my milk cleanser to actually get the product completely off my face. I found just using water to get the cream off caused too much irritation. Why? Because in order to successfully remove the product, there is massaging involved as you splash-rinse. Even if you used just the cream on your face without the machine, it would still irritate some skin.

This system is exfoliating and therefore resurfacing your skin, but at what cost? Actually, it costs around $80, and I don't think it was worth the shipping charges. This machine offers exfoliation with the expectation it will be more due to the machinery involved. Some of you may have a different experience and get some true benefits from DermaNew, but my experience left my skin feeling irritated afterwards. This kind of product just makes me go back to the same speech I use in many different scenarios: Do your Basics 1-2-3 skin care routine morning and night and add The Extras for special maintenance. Don't veer off course and spend a lot of money in the process—unless, of course, you want to.

Dermatitis

Dermatitis is an umbrella term describing a general condition of inflammation (*itis*) of the skin (*derma*). If you think you have a form of dermatitis, go see your dermatologist. He or she will be able to prescribe medication (usually topical) that can help get rid of this often annoying skin condition. Let's look at the different types of dermatitis.

Allergic contact dermatitis. This dermatitis goes by the names contact dermatitis, allergic dermatitis, and allergic contact dermatitis. No matter which name you prefer, the symptoms are the same. Allergic contact dermatitis is an inflammation of the skin caused by contact with a particular allergen. It can cause a rash or even blisters, usually confined to a specific area that often has clearly defined borders. These allergens can be anything from ingredients in cosmetics, metals found in jewelry like nickel, and plants such as poison ivy, oak, and sumac. Even some chemicals used in clothing manufacturing or laundry detergent can cause skin inflammation.

Many of my clients have intolerances to nickel in jewelry, sometimes called earlobe dermatitis. This shows up as crusty, scaly skin on the earlobes. Nickel is usually a component of inexpensive jewelry, not solid gold, platinum, or silver. As long as cheap earrings are worn, the dermatitis will persist. Because this irritated skin can be unsightly, once you realize you have an intolerance to nickel, you will choose not to wear the cheaper type of jewelry—out of necessity.

Rubber is another common allergen causing allergic contact dermatitis. Latex, like rubber gloves, and spandex, usually found in elastic wastebands in pants, bra straps, and underwear can cause this type of skin allergy. Exposure to some rubber found in shoes can also cause parts of your feet and toes to have problems.

Ingredients in skin care products can cause allergic reactions in some people. Irritations and reactions are two different things. Allergic contact dermatitis will show up as a rash or a scaly, even crusty patch of skin, whereas an irritation from a product may simply cause an unpleasant sensation.

I have a client who came into my office with a strange red patch of skin near the right side of her mouth. It wasn't a blemish or anything that resembled problem skin, but it was persistent and bothering my client. After questioning her, I found out she talks on a cell phone—a lot. She said her phone got wet one day and ever since then she has noticed this skin irritation. Bingo! No doubt there was some type of reaction with the wet metal constantly pushing against her skin, and finally she developed allergic contact dermatitis. Even without water being a factor, just constantly pressing a phone against your skin is enough to cause a reaction—if you are susceptible.

Truly, there are numerous offenders that can cause allergic contact dermatitis. The best way to treat it is to keep the offending substance away from the skin. As long as the allergen is present, the skin will continue to react. If you think you are having an allergic reaction to jewelry, clothing, skin care products, or something else, make an appointment to see your dermatologist. Then you will know for sure what you can and cannot wear, use, or be exposed to.

Eczema. Sometimes called *atopic dermatitis*, eczema is yet another form of skin inflammation. Eczema comes in many shapes and sizes. Most commonly, I have seen it on the eyelids. Next (and this is where I tend to get eczema) is the cheeks and outer nose area.

It can show up as red, blistering skin, and oozing or weeping can even occur if it is left untreated. Eczema usually looks and feels scaly, can be red or brownish in color, and there tends to be a thickening of the skin where the dermatitis exists. When found around the eye area, the lines and wrinkles there seem to increase overnight. The skin is red and irritated and almost always the affected skin itches.

Technically, the origin of eczema is unknown. Many times skin conditions are thrown into the "unknown cause" category. But the truth is, something is causing the condition, although it may be too difficult to figure out what. The word *unknown* usually says to me that something other than an allopathic medical explanation is needed. I try to look from a wholistic viewpoint—looking at the body as a whole, not just the symptoms it is producing. This includes looking at lifestyle and the possible stress it may be causing in your body. Physical symptoms can be caused by many things, including something as intangible as mental stress. Therefore, I believe eczema is stress-induced. In other words, it happens due to stress—whether it be internal body stress or emotional stress from the outside world.

If the body is unable to produce gamma linolic acid (GLA), sometimes eczema is the result. Taking evening primrose oil, which is rich in GLA, can help to alleviate symptoms of this type of dermatitis. You may want to give this supplement a try and see if it helps you. Evening primrose oil is so good for your body in general, if it helps specifically with eczema, so much the better! You could even open one of the capsules and massage a drop or two onto the affected area for some relief.

Aloe vera gel is another treatment you can try. The soothing nature of the gel can ease your irritated skin as well as help to heal the area. However, what works for one person may be irritating to someone else. Using creams and salves on the eczema may bring relief, but be prepared that your experience may be different.

Commonly, topical cortisone creams and ointments are prescribed for eczema. You can also purchase cortisone over the counter (OTC), although the strength will be less than the prescription kind. If cortisone helps, the skin condition could have been eczema; if cortisone doesn't help, it probably is something other than a dermatitis.

I have eczema, and my skin is extremely sensitive. I was wondering if I should exfoliate.

By definition eczema is inflamed and irritated skin. You don't want to do anything active like exfoliating or masking, but do use either a prescription cream (if you have one) or an over the counter cortisone cream until the irritation has gone away.

Even water can irritate skin that has eczema. As wild as that sounds, it's true. This just exemplifies how sensitive skin with dermatitis is. So doing less while you have this malady is probably the best course of treatment. Don't neglect your skin care routine, but try to avoid any areas that are sensitive even to your normal products. Use your topical cortisone cream and wait for it to clear up.

The stress factor has to be taken into consideration when judging the time it should take for eczema to clear up. Eczema, like so many things, is a symptom of a bigger problem; the dry skin is just what you are able to see. The skin truly is a window into your internal health. So pay attention! And have patience.

I always tell my clients to use the cortisone cream for at least three days, even if after a day or two the condition improves or clears up. Kind of like a round of antibiotics (usually ten days), the doctor will tell you to keep taking the pills even if you start to feel better before the ten days are up. This way your body will get a full dose of the drug and get over the bug completely with a lesser chance of it lingering— if you take the full round. I say the same is true for topical cortisone on eczema. If you keep using it for a few days after your problems have cleared up you will better ensure a full recovery without a recurrence. So use the topical treatment for at least 72 hours and then a few more days after the eczema seems cleared up—just to be sure. If you are using a prescription product, follow your doctor's instructions.

I have eczema on my eyelids. What strength hydrocortisone cream should I be using? Should I be concerned about using it so close to my eyes?

Prescription steroid creams are always going to be stronger than OTC brands. That's why they are prescribed by a doctor. In the over the counter variety, you usually have the choice of .05% and 1.0% topical cortisone creams. Prescription are usually around 2.5%.

You definitely don't want to get this or any cream in your eyes. And unfortunately, eczema commonly manifests on the upper eyelids and under and around the eyes. So you must use extreme caution if you are going to use a medicated cream around your eyes. During the day you wouldn't want to put anything on your eyelids. Due to the fold in the eyelid skin, the chances of the cream migrating into your eye is pretty high. At night you could use the cream or ointment sparingly to help treat the upper eyelid area. If using prescription strength, consult with your doctor to get his or her professional advice. No matter where you purchased the cream, strictly follow the instructions on the cortisone product label.

Perioral dermatitis. A client wrote, "I get this red, scaly, bumpy stuff under and around my nostril area." This is a good description of perioral dermatitis. It is a red, sometimes bumpy rash around the nostrils and sometimes down around the mouth. *Peri* means around or about, and *oral* indicates the mouth. So *perioral* means surrounding the mouth, although this condition pertains to the redness around the nostril area as well.

Applying a topical cortisone cream or ointment to the affected area is going to give you the best results. This type of dermatitis can be very persistent and sometimes hard to completely clear up, and you may want to get a dermatologist's prescription for the stronger form of cortisone.

I was reading a medical book explaining some different treatments for perioral dermatitis. One of the recommendations, tetracycline (an oral antibiotic), was said to be a good treatment—one of the best. Unfortunately, dermatitis is stress-induced. Therefore, if you continue to be under stress and even if your perioral dermatitis cleared up after taking the antibiotics, more than likely it will return when your body's immune system is weakened by the stress. Antibiotics, by their very nature, distress and suppress the immune system, so taking tetracycline seems to me like it might keep you moving in a vicious circle.

In this same manual I was reading, perioral dermatitis was listed under Sebaceous Gland Disorders, leading me to believe that this type of dermatitis also includes unusual sebaceous activity along with the rashy dermatitis of the outer skin. This makes sense due to the usual location of perioral dermatitis—around the nostril area and sometimes going down to the outer edges of the mouth. The nose has so many active oil glands and the folds of the nostrils can become clogged with oil, so this is an easy place for problems to occur.

As I mentioned, tetracycline or even minocycline (another antibiotic) are prescribed to treat perioral dermatitis. And just like with acne (another condition these oral antibiotics are commonly prescribed for), taking medicine orally does next to nothing to help figure out the actual cause of the problem. And it is by finding the cause that you will find your greatest and most long-term relief.

Seborrheic dermatitis. This condition is an inflammation of the upper layers of the skin, causing a red, scaly, itchy rash in various locations on the body. The eyebrows, eyelids, scalp, sides of the nose, and even the skin behind the ears are the most common places to find this form of dermatitis. Other areas where the skin folds (under the arms, breasts, and buttocks) may also be affected. This condition may cause not only flakiness but greasy or oily-looking skin. Dandruff (flakiness on the scalp) is actually seborrheic dermatitis.

Weather seems to affect this condition. You may find seborrheic dermatitis worsens in the winter, and improves in the warmer months.

Seborrheic dermatitis is most common in people who have oily skin and oil-prone hair, although it is not limited to these oily types. Sometimes even infants can develop seborrheic dermatitis due to the hormone changes after birth. Babies can also develop what looks like diaper rash, but really may be a case of seborrheic dermatitis.

Treatment consists of hydrocortisone (as in most cases of dermatitis) as well as a medicated shampoo for cases of seborrheic dermatitis affecting the scalp. As with any and all cases of dermatitis, consulting with your dermatologist is the best course of treatment. He or she will be able to guide you to the best medications and can track the progress of your skin.

Dry Skin/True-Dry Skin

Dry skin, or what I call *true-dry* skin, is a condition where your sebaceous (oil) glands are not producing enough oil to lubricate your outer skin. The outer skin is kept moisturized by both water at the surface (and from the air) as well as sebum being excreted from your oil glands. Simply put, true-dry skin does not produce enough oil to keep the outer skin moist.

True-dry skin needs to be artificially lubricated with moisturizing creams, so you want to keep high-quality moisturizers on at all times. True-dry skin needs exfoliation as well since any dead cell buildup will make the skin feel even drier.

True-dry skin can be a frustrating condition, especially if you are not using products that are moisturizing enough. Once your skin stops producing enough oil to keep the surface of your face moisturized, tightness and perhaps even flakiness can be a part of your everyday life.

I'm not a soap lover, but someone with true-dry skin really should avoid soap at all costs. This alkaline product will just make your already dry skin feel drier. Many gel cleansers have a foaming action, and these can also be too drying if you have dry skin. The best cleansers to use are cream washes or milk cleansers. These generally will not strip your skin and shouldn't leave your face feeling dry after cleansing.

Always use a toner (without alcohol—of course!). I recommend finding one with moisturizing ingredients in it, like glycerin. And your moisturizers (day and night creams) should have quality vegetal oils in them that will ensure a good all-day or all-night hydration for your oil-deficient skin.

Note: If you don't have true-dry skin, none of the above recommendation are for you! Even if your skin *feels* dry. (See **Dehydrated Skin**.) Dry skin—*true-dry*—simply doesn't produce enough oil to lubricate the skin's surface and therefore needs special products to super-hydrate and moisturize.

I recently purchased some products for dry skin as well as an oil-based serum for hydration. I have been mixing a drop of the serum with the moisturizers and have even tried using the night cream during the day. I have also been exfoliating and using a glycerin-based toner for dry skin. My skin is still very dry and flaky. I have been using Ponds® cream during the day and Vaseline® at night. A dermatologist told me to use the Vaseline, and it worked pretty well, but my pores stayed clogged.

Instead of putting one drop of the serum into your creams, try putting five or so drops on your face *before* applying your creams. In other words, cleanse, tone, apply five or more drops of serum to your entire face, massage the oil in, and then apply your day or night cream over that. And if you feel like you need it, go ahead and add some of the oil to your moisturizers as well. If you are using a glycerin-based serum or even a vegetable oil-based product, these shouldn't cause you to become clogged (as long as you have true-dry skin).

Vaseline and anything else that has a high concentration of petroleum will usually clog the pores. These substances have a large molecular structure and aren't able to penetrate the skin. They remain on the surface as occlusive covers. This not only can clog the pores, but it also inhibits your skin's natural elimination and absorption action. See **Petroleum.** Also see **Dehydrated Skin** for more information on "dry" skin.

Enlarged Pores

Enlarged pores are a big concern for a lot of people. I have to say that when a client comes in complaining of enlarged pores, once I see their skin under the magnifying light, many times I don't consider the pores enlarged at all. This is a very subjective matter. But assuming you truly do have enlarged pores, there are some things you can do to keep their appearance less noticeable and other things not to do in order to avoid future enlargement.

What causes large pores?

It's pretty simple, really. Time and debris are what causes enlargement of the pores. Genetics do play a part, and some people are seemingly born with large pores. But generally pores enlarge over time and due to how oily your skin has been in your life. The more oil that is lodged inside the pores, the larger the pores can become. Not all oily skinned people have large pores, but generally if you have larger pores, at some point in your life you probably had oily skin.

> *I have purchased a few moisturizing creams that contain elastin and collagen. The creams are great for most of my face, but I have always had enlarged pores on my nose with lots of blackheads and an oily forehead. So far these products have not helped that problem at all. What can I do to decrease those pores and get rid of the blackheads?*

This client is definitely using creams that are too heavy for her skin. The symptoms of an oily forehead and lots of blackheads are the indicators. The enlargement she already has will probably not really change, but if she keeps her pores clean, they can appear smaller.

Usually creams with elastin and collagen are made for a drier skin type, sometimes what is termed *mature skin*. That term, to me, is relatively meaningless. It is the oil content that I am most concerned about when classifying someone's skin. Mature (older) people can still have oily skin.

If she has problems with blackheads on her nose and an oily forehead, she doesn't have true-dry skin. Her skin is producing enough and in some cases too much oil naturally. She doesn't need to use heavy creams—even on the rest of her skin. Just changing her moisturizer could mean an end to the problems she is experiencing.

To answer this client's questions, she should stop using those heavier creams and instead find something that is for combination or normal to oily skin. To decrease the pores and to help get rid of the blackheads, I suggest a clay-based mask, and regular exfoliation to keep the dead skin to a minimum.

Can skin care products help at all in making the pores less obvious, and if so, which products?

Keeping the skin clean and debris-free will make the biggest (and most realistic) difference in how big your pores look. If you have a lot of congestion (dead skin, oil, perhaps even makeup) sitting in your pores, not only will this be apparent visually, but this congestion will also further the very problem you are trying to fix: enlarged pores. Congestion or clogged pores is the biggest cause of enlargement in the first place.

Using a clay mask regularly is a good way to super clean your pores, along with achieving other benefits as well. (See **Clay Masks**.) Exfoliation (getting rid of the dead cells on the surface of the skin) will greatly decrease the amount of debris nestled in the pores. And just making sure to get your skin clean (especially makeup-free) every day, morning and night, is an important routine. If you are not getting your skin clean with your daily cleanser, you may be causing cumulative congestion that can cause enlargement down the road.

Men are more prone to enlargement than woman. At least this is what I have found to be true. Men tend to take minimal care of their skin; they are prone to oily skin, and their skin is thicker in most cases than a woman's skin. Thicker skin tends to produce enlarged pores more so than a thinner skin. Although men overall may have more enlarged pores, their apathy about what their skin looks like makes this a non-issue in most cases!

Some skin specialists recommend using oil-free products, but others even advise not using moisturizers on enlarged pores to avoid shininess. What are your thoughts on this?

Enlarged pores are one thing, clogged pores are another. The question you need to ask yourself is: are your pores just enlarged with no congestion, or are they filled with debris? Debris means anything that may be nestled in the pore, which could be oil and dead skin or environmental debris from the air. Congestion, therefore, is stuff (debris) clogging your pores.

There isn't much you can do about the enlargement that has already occurred. Once the pore is stretched, it can't shrink down to a smaller size. However, using appropriate moisturizers can help cut down on future enlargement. If you are using a moisturizer, oil-free or not, that is too much for your pores to handle, you could cause enlargement to occur.

If your pores are clogged, it will determine what type of moisturizer you will use, or rather what type of skin the moisturizer should be for (oily and possibly problem). But to forgo lotion altogether is a mistake. You want to use moisturizer, just be sure it is appropriate for your particular skin type.

If shininess is a problem due to oily skin, you want to avoid lotions that employ mineral oil or petroleum as ingredients. These will simply add to your already oily skin and could be the reason for your self-described shininess. In general, oil isn't bad as an ingredient, but petroleum-based oils are not desirable. Due to their occlusive (heavy) nature, they don't absorb into the skin and therefore just sit on top causing your skin to look shiny and even causing the potential for enlargement of your pores. Search for a moisturizer that has vegetal oil or nut oils. These will add moisture to your skin without creating an oil slick on your face.

Another tip for avoiding shininess is to watch how much moisturizer you are using and how you are applying your lotion. You want to use about the size of a dime. Place this amount in the palm of one hand, rub your hands together, and then spread the lotion over your entire face and neck. Avoid putting the bulk of the cream on the facial axis or t-zone. This area tends to produce more oil than the outer edges of the face.

Generally I don't tan outside or use tanning beds. I have, however, tried self-tanning creams. The only problem is my enlarged pores usually become more obvious after putting the cream on.

Self-tanners have ingredients that essentially dye your skin. If you are experiencing an increase in the appearance of your pores after using a self-tanning cream, you may not be able to use one on your face. There aren't any magic solutions. Perhaps you can experiment with different tanners and see if one of them doesn't cause this problem. Some self-tanners have less dye and more ingredients that help stimulate the melanin in your skin to produce a tan. Maybe one of these would work for you. I commend you for using self-tanning products versus going to a tanning salon. That is a great choice!

You might want to try exfoliating your skin before applying the self-tanner. This way you will clean out your pores and lessen the potential for debris held inside to be dyed from the product.

HOT TIP: After spraying your face with toner, then apply your moisturizer. This way you get good spreadability as well as an even application.

Essential Fatty Acids

Human beings can make nonessential fatty acids. This means we don't have to get these particular nutrients from our food. There are, however, a group of *essential* fatty acids (EFAs) that, as their name implies, are essential for our health and vitality although they are *not* produced by our bodies. Therefore, we must get EFAs from outside sources, either in our food or through supplementation. If you are not getting enough EFAs, deterioration, inflammation, and improper functioning of certain systems of the body can begin to occur. Day after day, year after year, this will lead to your body's downfall. Just like a car that has run out of oil, your body will eventually break down. Essential fatty acids are necessary in order to maintain not just physical health, but also mental and emotional wellness.

Two of the classifications for essential fatty acids are omega-3 and omega-6. Within these categories are both short and long chain acids. It is important to remember that you want to concentrate your efforts on getting the *long* chain omega-3 essential fatty acids more than any other. Short chain EFAs have to be converted in the body into long chain; therefore, depending on whom you ask or what book you read, taking anything but long chain omega-3 is a waste of time. However, there are many sources that recommend flax oil, for instance, as a good way to get omega-3s even though it is the short chain variety. Long or short, another important point is to get twice as much omega-3 as omega-6, or a ratio of 2:1.

The best source for long chain omega-3 fatty acids is cold-water fish like salmon, mackerel, sardines, and tuna. DHA (docosahexaenoic acid), an important component of the brain and also a long chain omega-3 fatty acid, is found in fish oil (from food or supplements). Dr. Barry Sears, in his book *The OmegaRX Zone*, likens trying to maintain proper brain function without enough DHA to trying to build a sturdy brick house without enough bricks—it just can't be done. So if you take anything away from this section, I hope you will research DHA and figure out how much you are currently getting in your diet. Not enough? Consider supplementation with fish oil capsules.

Cod liver oil is an excellent source for omega-3 fatty acids. I take a lemon flavored cod liver oil from Norway that contains the omega-3s DHA 500mg; EPA (eicosapentaenoic acid) 460mg; and ALA (alpha-linolenic acid) 45mg. It also has vitamins A, D, and E. Taking cod liver oil, to me, is the easiest way to supplement these all-important nutrients into your *daily* diet. The recommended dosage is one or two teaspoons daily. (I highly recommend taking a lemon flavored brand. Cod liver oil on its own tastes *very* fishy.)

Because you need to get twice as much omega-3 than omega-6, you want to limit the amount of foods you eat that contain omega-6 fatty acids—especially the "bad" kind. These foods include red meat, dairy products that are high in fat like butter, fatty cheeses and ice cream, along with margarine, and partially hydrogenated oils found in many snack foods. Corn, safflower, soy, or other hydrogenated oils are also high in omega-6 and should be limited or avoided when possible.

Sometimes I take flax oil; it is rich in omega-3 essential fatty acids. Even though they are short chain omega-3s, I still think it is beneficial to take this supplement. Flax oil is unique because it contain both omega-3 and -6, but in the correct 2:1 ratio. The flax oil I take is high in lignans. These are fiberlike substances that are also powerful antioxidants. Lignans help balance the metabolism of estrogen, so for women this can help with PMS; it may even help with hot flashes and other conditions associated with perimenopause.

For those of you who take evening primrose oil, although it is a source of omega-6 fatty acids, it is one of the "good" omega-6s, unlike the undesirable omega-6s from hydrogenated oils and fatty foods. Among its many other attributes, evening primrose oil is high in gamma linoleic acid (GLA), another fatty acid that is hard to come by in the average diet. GLA is vitally important for healthy cells (including skin) and cell function. Borage oil and grape seed oil are two more good sources for this essential nutrient. It is doubtful you are getting enough in your diet, so supplementation may be required.

Essential fatty acids is one of those subjects where the more you learn, the more complex the subject seems to become. I am just skimming the surface in hopes of giving you the most important points when it comes to EFAs, but I highly recommend reading up on this subject.

There can be no doubt that for most of us living in America (surely for anyone reading this book) there is no lack in the quantity of food available. It is the *quality* of food that is lacking. Genetically you may be blessed, but if your cells are not healthy, you are not going to be healthy. Good health is not an accident, so expand your awareness of the quality of your diet and if you need to, supplement—for your health.

EFAs at-a-glance:
- You want to get a 2:1 ratio of omega-3 to omega-6 fatty acids.
- Whenever possible, you want to get long chain omega-3s vs. short chain omega-3s.

- You want to avoid "bad" omega-6 fatty acids, like those found in snack foods and hydrogenated oils. *Start reading labels!*
- DHA is super-important to the brain. Unless you are eating cold-water fish every day, taking high-grade (pharmaceutical grade) fish oil is a good way to get enough DHA.

Evening Primrose Oil

If you have read the previous section, you learned how important it is to get essential fatty acids (EFAs) in your daily diet. Evening primrose oil is one way to get these essential nutrients. I recommend it for clients who have PMS, oily skin, breakouts, and dermatitis' like eczema. It even works as a hangover cure. There are many ways to get EFAs, but read on to learn more about evening primrose oil.

> *I started using evening primrose oil capsules and have noticed a great change not only in my skin, but a lessening of symptoms of PMS. I used to get cysts on my jaw and neck area, which I know is hormonal, and since the evening primrose I now only get one small pimple every 3 or 4 months around my period.*

Evening primrose oil is not for everyone, but I have seen it work really well for a lot of people. I include this email because it mirrors the experience of many of my clients.

Evening primrose oil can help with the balance of estrogen in the body during menstruation (when estrogen levels naturally lower). It can help to elevate estrogen levels and in some cases eliminate the pain and tension of a woman's period. I like to take it when I am ovulating, to help lessen the sometimes erratic emotional and physical changes during PMS. Then, by the time my period starts, I am feeling more in balance and experience less pain from cramping.

In your book you recommend evening primrose in capsules for oily or acne skin. I was wondering what milligrams are you talking about per capsule?

I personally use capsules I purchase at a large health food store that are 500mg each. They look like vitamin E capsules, or perhaps a bit bigger. Years ago, evening primrose was a little hard to find. Now there are many brands to choose from. I don't recommend one brand over another, but I do suggest talking with the people working in the herb department at your local health food store. Ask them which primrose oil would be the best for you.

I started taking evening primrose oil, but I'm not sure if it's really helping my skin. I've been taking it for 3 months now. Should I continue, or should I stop taking it?

The thing with evening primrose oil is you may or may not notice a big change. Some people do; they notice a lessening of the oil in general in their skin, or they may even notice their breakouts have diminished—if not in frequency, then in size and number. The essential fatty acids found in evening primrose oil are essential to healthy cells, yet they are hard to get through food. So for me this is reason enough to take evening primrose oil regardless of noticing big results.

When and how many evening primrose capsules do I take? Since it helps PMS, do I only take it during menstruation or should I take it daily?

I recommend experimenting to find out what works for you—especially if you are taking evening primrose oil to offset symptoms of PMS. For problem skin, try 2-4 capsules twice daily and increase if you don't see any noticeable results. For cramps due to PMS, try 1-2 capsules twice a day from the time you start ovulating, then increase by one or two capsules (3-4 twice daily) until you have finished your monthly cycle. I usually take more on the days I feel the emotional roller coaster that premenstruation can bring.

> *I have been using evening primrose oil to help with my acne and hormones, and it's been fabulous. I now want to become pregnant and wonder if I should continue or stop the primrose oil?*

I was advised by a doctor that evening primrose oil should be very good to take during pregnancy. He suggested the baby will like it and utilize its nutrients, and fish oils, too (if you take those), to build healthy cell walls. Evening primrose oil should be very good for a growing fetus. Conversely, evening primrose may not be advisable to take if you have or have had cancer because it may help those cells to grow. *Please* consult with your doctor before taking this or any other supplement.

Evening primrose oil may be contraindicated if you are taking Premarin® (a common medication taken for hormone replacement therapy after menopause). Because evening primrose oil can help promote the production of natural estrogen, coupling it with the estrogen in Premarin may result in an excess of this hormone. Whether or not you are taking hormones or any other medication, check with your health care practitioner to find out if you should or can take evening primrose oil.

Last night I was having a drink with some coworkers and the topic of evening primrose for hangovers came up. Anyone who has tried it now swears by it. Thanks again for that information!

Exfoliation

Exfoliation helps to remove surface dead cells, giving your skin smoother texture and a healthy, well-nourished glow. Getting rid of dead cells also helps keep your pores from clogging, and the act of exfoliation helps to increase circulation, which always services the skin. Improved circulation helps with cellular respiration, which is how your skin really breathes—through the oxygen carried in the blood. Toxins are dumped into the bloodstream, so stepping up circulation helps with this exchange as well. I tell my clients when they can't come in for a facial, exfoliate! Exfoliation is certainly not the be-all and end-all of healthy skin, but it can take away layers of stress from your face, revealing the natural beauty hidden beneath. If you aren't currently exfoliating, I recommend finding a suitable exfoliation system that works for your skin, your lifestyle, and your pocketbook.

You talk a lot about exfoliation and how important it is for the skin. Does using a Buf-Puf count as exfoliation or is it cleansing?

Buf-Puf™ is a type of facial sponge made from polyester fibers that is meant to exfoliate the skin's surface. I have two concerns about using this product. The first and most important one is Buf-Pufs can be irritating. Even the type for very sensitive skin feels rough to the touch; once you start rubbing this on your skin, it can irritate even the most non-sensitive skin. My second concern is about cleanliness. Buf-Pufs, like loofah sponges, harbor bacteria. No doubt some of the dead skin that is being exfoliated is also sticking around in the sponge itself. Without thoroughly rinsing the Buf-Puf after every use, you may run the risk of bacteria multiplying inside the material. Overall, I find that this product is simply too rough to use on the face.

Another way to exfoliate is to use a **gommage**-type product. In French, *gommage* means to remove or erase. In this case, removing dead skin and erasing dehydration. The secondary benefit of this type of product is it is a gel and is therefore hydrating to the outer skin. So not only do you get the exfoliation benefits, but you are actually helping to moisturize your skin as well. Since there are no abrasive particles in this gel peel to irritate red or inflamed skin (like acne), gommage is well suited for even the most sensitive skin.

A **scrub** is probably the best-known product used to exfoliate. Scrubs contain abrasive particles from either organic or inorganic sources that, when rubbed over the skin, help to dislodge pieces of dead skin, which helps to make the skin feel smooth. Sometimes scrubs, because they take oil and water off the skin's surface, can make your face feel dry although it is really dehydration (surface water loss) you are feeling. Scrubs don't offer the most effective type of exfoliation, but they surely are the easiest products to find.

Sometimes I like to **mix equal parts of my cleanser with a scrub**. This way, there aren't as many granules to irritate my skin, and I still get some circulatory benefits as well as some exfoliation. Try this if you have sensitive skin or don't have luck using a scrub by itself.

I don't recommend using washcloths as your exfoliator of choice. They can harbor bacteria, they are not gentle on your skin, and they can move around a lot of skin without you being aware of it. Once in a while, this wouldn't be a problem, but day after day, year after year, this can't be good for the elasticity of your skin. If you have to use a washcloth, be gentle and try not to rub your skin too hard. Also, use a fresh (clean) cloth every time; don't just let it dry out and reuse it time after time. Bacteria may accumulate in a used washcloth.

No matter what you choose to use, exfoliation is paramount to healthy and healthy-looking skin. So when in doubt, exfoliate!

HOT TIP: If you want your skin to look radiant before you go out, so beautiful that you probably wouldn't even want to cover it with foundation—exfoliate.

Extractions

Extraction is the procedure that eliminates impurities from your skin. Usually through applying pressure, a plug nestled inside a pore is encouraged to come up and out of the pore.

Extraction, if done incorrectly, can cause scarring. Don't take this statement lightly. If you insist on doing your own extractions but refuse to do them correctly, you are setting up the perfect environment for injury or scarring of your skin to occur.

I recommend having extractions done professionally within the context of a facial treatment. I have heard in certain states across America aestheticians are not allowed "by law" to perform extractions. This is ridiculous, and I can't believe there is policing of this procedure. Without being able to extract a client who needs this deep cleaning, the facial is only partially effective and thus incomplete. There are also aestheticians who refuse to extract as well as some technicians who spend too much time extracting—to the detriment of the client's skin.

Hopefully you have or can find a qualified professional to do the extractions necessary for your skin. If not, I am including instructions for doing it yourself. If you don't think you can follow these instructions to the letter, don't extract your skin! Get a professional to do it or treat the blemish or blackhead by reading their respective sections and getting some alternate ideas.

There are slight differences when extracting blackheads, white-heads, and pustules. Read through the description of what you are contemplating extracting to get the right idea of what to do and what to look for. But no matter what you have decided to extract, there are specific rules that must be observed. The overall comment I want to underline is **when in doubt, don't extract!**

The must do's. If you decide to forgo these recommendations, don't bother extracting your skin. You will discover that without following these rules, you will cause further damage to your blemishes, making them more noticeable rather than helping them to go away.

First, you want to do this procedure on **clean skin**. If you don't wash your face first, you are just asking for trouble.

Next and most important: **wrap your index fingers in tissue** to ensure you won't get any tears in the skin from your nails. I cut my nails down to the quick, but I still use this finger-wrapping technique when I do extractions on my own skin at home. If you have nails, know it is very difficult to perform extractions, and depending on your intent to extract, it could be damaging to your skin. If you have to, use your knuckles, still wrapped in tissue. The tissue also helps to keep bacteria on your fingers away from your skin. Now, *be gentle!* Need I say more?

Finally, you must always **treat the places you've just extracted**. The best thing to do is to immediately put a dot of geranium oil on the spot. Let it sit for a minute. Then, once it has absorbed into the skin, put a little clay mask over the blemish. Let that dry and once again put a drop of geranium over the clay. Just let all this sit on the skin—hopefully overnight. It will help to close the opening you just made (no matter how small) and keep bacteria away, which is very important.

Extracting blackheads. Blackheads are the easiest to extract—as long as they are ready. Sometimes even blackheads have some dead skin grown over them, making extraction next to impossible. But generally, all you need to do is wrap your fingers in tissue and locate the blackheads you want to extract. With your two index fingers on either side of the blackhead, gently push the debris out and onto the tissue. It may take a few tries, but generally the plug will come out. After extraction, I recommend liberally applying your toner to help soothe the skin. Then hopefully you have time to apply clay mask— either to your entire face, or at least the areas extracted.

Extracting whiteheads. Whiteheads can really be frustrating, even for me, a "professional." Why? Because although you can usually see them quite clearly and may think they will extract easily, this is not always the case. Different thicknesses of skin can really cause the whole extraction process to be an exercise in futility. And no matter how close to the surface the oil bead may be, sometimes whiteheads just don't want to come out. This is when the true test of willpower begins. If at first (or second) try you don't succeed, you must walk away.

When extracting whiteheads, just like pustules listed below, you must make an opening in the skin for the debris to exit the area. This can be done with the end of a thin, obviously sharp needle or a lancet, an implement used in facials. If you don't feel you have the restraint to use a sharp tool on your face properly, don't even attempt to extract your skin.

You should not dig with the needle point. You are going to angle the point parallel to your skin, to the whitehead. You are going to use the sharp point to create an opening for the debris to come out of. That's it. Gently make an opening with the needle, set it aside, and place your wrapped fingers on either side of the whitehead. Apply pressure and nudge the debris out of this tiny opening. Depending on the size of the place, it may take a few passes with the lancet to get a hole big enough to allow the debris to come out. Apply geranium oil and/or clay mask to treat afterwards.

Extracting pustules. Remember, pustules contain pus that you can see. Sometimes even when I'm in a facial with all the necessary elements to make extractions go smoothly, I still cannot get the debris out of the blemish.

I'm not a believer in warming the area before extraction. If the blemish is infected, this just aggravates the situation. But I realize this warming method is ingrained in many people, so if you have to use heat, keep it to an absolute minimum.

You want to angle the needle so you are simply poking a small hole on the weakest part of the raised skin, which is usually the peak of the blemish. Sometimes the debris will come out immediately; sometimes it will require a little nudging.

With your fingers wrapped in the tissue, gently press on either side of the blemish simultaneous with your fingers, and hopefully the bulk of the infected mass will come out. If the debris doesn't come out after one or two tries, give the needle another go; then press again with your fingers. If by this second try the blemish is not moving, it may be too deep within the follicle to actually be extracted manually. It may just need another day to come further up to the surface, ready to be extracted.

This is where restraint comes in. If the blemish is not ready to be extracted, and you decide to try anyway, you will lose the fight. What you will "win" is more infection inside the blemish. Trying to extract a place that isn't ready, or even just over-extracting (going at it too hard) can cause more damage within the follicle walls and thus cause more infection. The bacteria will proliferate, and you will end up with a bigger, more obvious red spot on your face than what you started out with.

Hopefully the pus will come out of the blemish and onto your tissue. Give another gentle push to make sure all the debris has come out, and then treat the blemish with geranium and/or clay. Without completing the process with this crucial last step, you will run the risk of creating more infection than you began with.

Do this extraction process if and only if you can see a clear and defined white or yellow pus-filled head on the blemish. If the spot is just red and raised, *leave it alone!* It isn't ready even if you are.

You mention that skin picking can cause damage. What kind of damage, and is it reversible?

Picking can but doesn't always cause scarring. Scar tissue doesn't just go away (it's usually irreversible damage). When you pick without care, you are basically causing a little tear or injury to the skin. It has to heal, and in that healing process, a little scar could form. Not always, but it's definitely possible. You must at least utilize the basic steps I have described earlier in this section, or you are asking for trouble. But even then, even if you do everything right, you still may cause scarring. It all depends on how careful you are when you extract your skin and also how skilled you are at doing it. Remember, part of the "skill" of extraction is knowing when to quit.

The Extras

As their name implies, The Extras are additions to your Basics 1-2-3 routine that can help to keep your skin clear and healthy. These two extra steps are exfoliation and using a facial mask, usually a clay mask. You can do The Extras together, as an at-home facial, or you can do them individually. However you decide to incorporate these steps into your skin care program, using them is important and will give you benefits whenever you do them.

> *I bought a clay mask because, just like you state in your book, I have seen an improvement in glow and cleanness from exfoliating and masking weekly.*

At-home facials can make a big difference in your skin. You may be wondering what exactly an at-home facial involves. The basics of this treatment consist of exfoliating and using a cleansing or hydrating mask. Although a professional facial involves a lot more than this, the point of an at-home facial is to get some of the results of a professional treatment in the comfort and convenience of your own home.

You can get elaborate if you want to, drawing a bubble bath and lighting scented candles, and even playing relaxing music. Clean your face, use your exfoliator of choice, and then apply the facial mask. If you have problem skin, a clay mask is a must. Even if you don't have problems, clay is beneficial for all skin types. If you use clay, you need to keep it moist (see **Clay Masks**), so take your spray toner or water in a spray bottle with you into the tub. Spray intermittently during the 15 or so minutes you have the mask on to keep it from drying on your skin.

Take as much time to relax as you can; after all, this is part of the at-home facial experience. Doing an at-home facial once a week would be great, but however often, whenever you can fit The Extras into your schedule, it will benefit your skin.

Whether you elaborate on my suggestions and create the at-home facial experience or just exfoliate and mask, doing these Extras once a week (or 2-3x a week if you have problem skin) will give you good results and help to maintain clear and healthy skin.

Eye Cream

Does eye cream make a difference? Should I use it?

Absolutely! Eye cream is an essential component to your Basics 1-2-3 skin care routine. After cleansing, toning, and applying face moisturizer, then apply your eye cream—every day at least twice a day. The difference eye cream will make is to keep the skin directly under your eyes soft and hydrated, something that doesn't happen naturally. You have no functioning oil glands there, so applying cream is the only way to keep that skin moisturized.

Can I put vitamin E around my eyes for eye cream?

I'm sure the reason you are asking this question is because you know the benefits of vitamin E. I reach for manufactured products when it comes to my skin. My eye cream might actually have vitamin E as one of the ingredients, which is a good thing, but it also contains numerous other ingredients that will help to soothe and moisturize this delicate skin. This is *my* preference. If using vitamin E as an eye cream works for you, then I don't think it is a bad thing. I just think it has limited capabilities vs. a cream that is produced specifically for the eyes. Perhaps for a happy medium, you could mix your eye cream with a drop of vitamin E oil. Mix these two in your palm and then apply to the eye area. This way you will get more than just straight oil on your skin, which could eventually get into your eyes and cause problems, or might even cause puffiness.

I am 34 and looking for something that will help combat these ever-increasing wrinkles under my eyes.

As I tell all my clients, the lines are only going to get worse! Seriously, it's true. The natural aging of our bodies includes lines and wrinkles where we are expressing the most. At 34 years old, you are probably just beginning to notice the lines around your eyes because they are probably just beginning to form. Using eye cream, if you are not already, is important. It will keep the skin soft and maybe even make the lines look less noticeable. Eye cream will *not* decrease the wrinkles—even over time.

> *I have so many lines around my eyes. I use eye cream every day, but still the skin around my eyes is so dried out. Is there a super rich cream I can use to keep this area from drying out?*

My recommendation is not to use a thick cream, but to use eye cream throughout the day, not just morning and night. The skin directly under the eyes has no functioning oil glands, so you need to keep a lipid substance there at all times to keep this skin soft and supple. In fact, you don't want to use a super rich eye cream. Usually these will make your eyes look puffy due to the heavy oils they contain. The thin skin around the eyes absorbs the oil, which can produce edema or puffiness. I recommend using eye cream vs. face creams around the eye area. These have been formulated specifically for this delicate and sensitive tissue and are going to be your best bet.

Something you can do which can be very effective is to add a drop of oil to your eye cream, mix and apply. Like the recommendation for the reader asking about vitamin E as an eye cream, mixing just one drop of this or another oil can really enrich your eye treatment and successfully help with dryness around your eyes. I find this recommendation particularly helpful in the winter months.

> *The skin around my mouth and eyes is very dry and kind of flaky. Once I put my moisturizer on, it's not as noticeable, but then*

when I wash again the dryness is back. It doesn't happen any-
where else on my face. It happens a lot; it even happens during
warm months and stays around for a few weeks, then sort of goes
away until the next time. Any suggestions?

You may be experiencing eczema, or it may just be a severe case of dehydration. Usually dehydration happens across a wide area, while other maladies such as eczema would be more localized. If you use a cortisone cream on the area for at least three or four days (consistent-ly) and the dryness goes away, it was more than likely a dermatitis. If the dryness is still there, try exfoliating the area and see if that helps.

Remember, if your body is deficient in certain vitamins and essen-tial nutrients (like essential fatty acids, for instance), your skin may be showing the signs of this. Don't just look to treat skin problems topi-cally. Also look at your diet and stress levels to get a clue as to what may be going on inside, which is showing up outside.

I never go without eye cream now. I cannot believe what a dif-
ference it has made. Thank you for your help!

Eye Makeup Removal

What's the best thing to remove eye makeup with?

Your facial cleanser will probably adequately remove your eye makeup. However if you are wearing waterproof mascara (and some non-waterproof brands), you will need to use an oil to remove this "glue" from your lashes. Baby oil is an inexpensive option. (Make sure not to get that or any oil in your eyes.) I don't recommend Vaseline, however.

It might take off a lot of the makeup, but because of its gooey nature, you might inadvertently pull the delicate under-eye tissue when using it to remove your eye makeup or when trying to remove the Vaseline from your skin.

Obviously you want to be careful not to use anything that will irritate your eyes. Also you want to be sure not to rub or pull the skin around your eyes when removing your makeup. Assuming you wear it every day, you can really do a lot of damage day in and day out with excess pulling and tugging at this tissue in order to remove makeup. So, be careful!

Removing mascara. In terms of saving the undereye skin from harm, the following is the best recommendation for removing your mascara.

First, wet a cotton pad and fold it in half. Then wet both ends of a Q-tip. Place the cotton under your bottom lashes, with the straight line of the fold directly up against your eyelashes. Take the Q-tip and with one eye closed (this is why it is difficult), gently rub the Q-tip on your upper lashes. The mascara will go directly to the cotton pad, and this will not disrupt the delicate skin around your eyes. Another possibility is to place either a cotton pad or a towelette folded under your lower lashes and use a towelette in the same way you'd use a Q-tip—gently going over the lashes to remove mascara. This might be easier considering you really don't have your eyes to guide you. Once you have done both eyes, simply do your regular evening Basics 1-2-3 routine, remembering to include eye cream.

This surely isn't the easiest way to remove makeup from your eyelashes, but if asked what is the least harmful way to do it, this is how I would suggest removing makeup. If you are constantly tugging your delicate undereye tissue, along with rubbing your eyes inadvertently during the day, squinting, and along with exposure to the sun, then this tissue may show signs of aging faster.

Something else to note: At the end of one of my skin care talks, one of the ladies in the audience brought up a great point that I wanted to pass along to you. Recently she realized that as she was putting on her mascara she was wrinkling her forehead due to the angle of looking in the mirror and using the mascara wand. She then took into account how many years she had been applying mascara and thought this may be one reason she had so many lines and wrinkles on her forehead.

Remember, all wrinkles are formed through expression, and raising your eyebrows to apply mascara causes expression lines that usually show up on the forehead. So use this as a reminder to try and find a way to apply your mascara or any makeup you may wear that does not reinforce or even create lines and wrinkles.

F

Facial Brushes

The sales clerk at my department store told me to start using a facial brush because it would reach into my pores to clean them better.

Facial brushes do have the ability to reach down into the pores. Therefore they can cause damage, like particles in scrubs. Presumably, the reason you are using the brush in the first place is for exfoliation benefits, yet you can exfoliate in other ways without causing harm to your skin. Of course it depends on the actual brush and what type of bristles it has. I'm sure there are some facial brushes that won't cause any harm to your skin, but why use them? They harbor bacteria, they can cause irritation, and then there is the potential to "reach into your pores" and do some real damage. Use brushes on your body if you want to—this skin is far less susceptible to irritation than on your face. But bottom line, I don't recommend using these brushes on your face.

A *good* use for a facial brush would be under a beard or even just a moustache. Due to the dense hair growth, the skin underneath doesn't get any action and certainly little if any exfoliation. This can cause itching and possibly bumps under the skin, although you may not be aware of their existence.

To exfoliate the area under a beard or moustache, take a facial brush and gently nudge it underneath the hair onto your skin. Use this brushing technique prior to washing your face. Gently massage with the brush until you can feel the stimulation on the surface of your skin. Go over the entire area under your facial hair. Afterwards, take some cleanser and wash your face as you normally do, paying extra attention to the areas you just brushed, and work the cleanser into your facial hair. Be sure to get a thorough rinse to finish. Use your spray toner, and moisturize your skin as usual. Do try to get some moisturizer under your beard, but don't glob it on there. Just massage a little bit into the hair to help moisturize the skin you brushed underneath. By using a facial brush under your beard, you are benefiting the skin by exfoliating that untouched area.

HOT TIP: Brush your teeth, not your face.

Flying & Skin

Have you ever wondered what the effects of air travel are on our bodies? Certainly humans were not designed to fly. Our digestive systems, for instance, work in conjunction with the earth's gravitational pull. So what really happens to the digestive process 30,000 feet up in the sky? Perhaps you've even experienced indigestion after taking a flight somewhere. Other than the possibility of bad airplane food and dehydration, isn't it possible poor digestion comes from the change in altitude?

Not only do our inner organs have to adapt to the altitude, but our outermost organ—our skin—seems to take the brunt of all things bad in an airplane as well. Although this environment isn't ideal for optimum health or healthy skin, there are several things you can do before, during, and after your flight that will do wonders for keeping your skin in tiptop shape and help to make your traveling experience more enjoyable. Follow some or all of the suggestions in this section and you may find your skin (and body) feeling better when you fly.

Curbing dehydration. Dehydration is the number one concern when you are flying. Ask any flight attendant and they will tell you, dry (dehydrated) skin is a chronic problem. **Misting your face with water** is the best and most immediate way to get moisture to your thirsty skin. You can purchase small Evian® water bottles that spray, or you can make your own. Get a travel-size plastic bottle at your grocery or drug store and fill it with clean, filtered water. I mention clean water because why spray chlorinated tap water on your face? You are trying to improve the conditions for your skin during your flight, not reinforce negative ones.

If you have already put your **toner in a spray bottle** (something I highly recommend), you can use this instead of plain water to mist your face with. Not only will you receive superficial hydrating benefits due to the toner's high water-content, you will also get the benefits of all the other soothing ingredients from your product. Obviously, if you are using an astringent-type toner that contains alcohol—something I do not recommend—this would not be appropriate to spray on your face. Even the word *astringent* brings to mind something that would be drying.

The next order of business is **exfoliation**. I will repeat that word over and over again since it is one of the most important things you can do to help your skin survive air travel. Getting rid of the dead cell buildup will go a long way to helping your skin retain water, which you lose a lot of when you fly. Lessening the dead skin also allows any hydrating products you've put on your face do a better job of moisturizing. The fewer dead cells a moisturizer has to penetrate, the better it will work, and the more hydrated your skin will feel. Finally, while exfoliating improves and refines the texture of your skin, it also increases the blood circulation to your face, bringing out the natural, healthy color of your skin. You should consider exfoliating the day of your flight, getting your skin ready for what's to come. Exfoliating ahead of time will diminish the amount of cell buildup on your face so anything you do to hydrate the skin will be more effective. Less dead cells equals better quality hydration.

You may not have thought of doing this, but if you are on a long flight (I consider long over five hours), you might try exfoliating en route. When I went to Australia several years ago, I was in the bathroom of the plane exfoliating (a couple of times) during the 15-plus hour flight. Although the quarters were cramped, exfoliating helped my skin combat the extreme dryness from the airplane. I even have a client who exfoliates right at her seat! She always flies first class and her attitude is, "If someone thinks it's weird, so be it. At least my skin will feel good!" She puts a towel on her lap and does a gommage right then and there on the plane. I choose to exfoliate in the bathroom, but however or wherever you feel most comfortable doing it, do exfoliate on long (or even short) flights. Your skin will reap the rewards. And if you do it at your seat, you might even strike up an interesting conversation with someone sitting next to you.

I also recommend exfoliating upon arrival at the hotel or wherever you are staying. Obviously you can wait until you are getting ready for bed, but do exfoliate before retiring on the day you reach your destination. Your skin will benefit from getting all the dirt, debris, and unclean air out of your pores along with lessening the dry, dead cells on the surface of your skin. *Don't hesitate—exfoliate!*

For some additional insurance to keep your skin hydrated during your flight, try using a **hydrating elixir or mask under your moisturizer**. An elixir might come in the form of a special oil or serum, which will not only add a lot of moisture to your skin but will also act as a humectant, drawing in moisture from the air. Elixirs (especially oils) are best used by those of you with normal to dry or true-dry skin. If you have an oilier complexion or problem skin, I would recommend using a gel-type hydrating mask or glycerin (see section) underneath your moisturizer. These will essentially do the same thing as an elixir without adding extra oil to your already oily skin. (Actually, *any* skin type can use the gel mask or glycerin approach, but oils should only be used only by those of you with drier skin types.)

Although using products topically will help keep your skin feeling good, I have some suggestions for things to do for yourself internally that can help with the stress your body might go through during travel time.

When you fly, not only does your skin become dehydrated, but you can suffer from internal dehydration as well. The best way to keep your insides hydrated is to **drink lots of water**. This may seem obvious, but whenever I fly it seems to me people are drinking sodas and coffee more than plain water. Some airlines offer prepacked lunch bags on your way to the airplane. (If you fly first class, you don't have to suffer though these prepackaged meals.) I rarely, if ever, eat what is offered in these bags, but they do usually have a little bottle of spring water, which is nice. Drinking water doesn't necessarily (and certainly doesn't immediately) hydrate your outer skin, although a lot of people think it does. But drinking water is good for you internally; all organs benefit from drinking plain old water. This includes your eliminating organs (namely the kidneys, liver, colon, and of course your skin), which definitely need this extra hydration to help combat the drying effects incurred on an airplane.

If you are going to have cocktails on your flight, please be sure to drink extra water with them. Alcohol is a diuretic, and the last thing you need to do while you're traveling is to leach water out of your body. The 2:1 rule definitely applies here. Try to drink two glasses of water for every one glass of alcohol. And try to only drink clean, bottled water.

Another way to get water into your system along with good nutrition is through eating **fruit**. Fruit is loaded with antioxidant vitamins and *water*. And fruit is self-contained. You can just throw an apple or orange into your bag and there's no preparation needed. Or you can spend a few minutes and cut up your favorite fruits, put the pieces in a small plastic container and you're set. They'll have napkins and utensils on the plane—all you need is the food.

Fruit—most fruit—is digested in the small intestine, so it doesn't take a lot of energy to process. This is important because, as I've said before, I believe flying at such high altitudes makes it hard for your body to process food. Add to the dehydration factor poor digestion, which can easily equal constipation, and this is enough to ruin your entire trip.

Supplemental help. As we all know, the air in an airplane is poor-quality at best. Add to that the potential of sitting next to someone who is sick with a cold or flu, and you have all the ingredients for coming down with something yourself. I recommend taking some type of immune system booster before and during your flight to help your body fight off foreign invaders.

There are many herbal supplements that can help boost your immune system. **Garlic** has well-documented antibiotic properties, and most brands have special coatings on the pills to inhibit giving you garlic breath. **Astragalus** is another immune system helper that can be taken in capsule or tincture form. (Tinctures are liquid concentrates that are usually taken mixed with a little bit of water.) **Echinacea and goldenseal** are both excellent immune stimulants, helping to fight off germs that may have infiltrated your body during the flight.

Antioxidants are another way to help your body fight off the bad air you are breathing in an airplane. **Vitamin C**, probably the most widely known antioxidant, comes in many forms and is easy to take with you on a trip. You can pop chewable vitamin C tablets throughout the flight, or Emergen-C powder can be mixed with a glass of water as a refreshing, thirst-quenching drink that also helps you internally.

Sleeping can be a concern when flying, and not getting restful sleep can adversely affect your skin. For a simple way to help your body relax, take a bottle of **essential oil of lavender** on the plane with you. Lavender is known for its sedative effects. By just sniffing the soothing aromatics of this amazing mood shifter, you can truly help your whole body relax. If you carry a pillow when you travel, dab a few drops of lavender on it, lie back and relax. You could also use a handkerchief if you prefer. Lay it on a pillow the airline provides, and you've just created an opportunity for some shuteye during your flight.

If you know you aren't able to fall asleep on an airplane, you might want to inquire at your health food store for supplements that might help. There are many homeopathic and natural products that help induce sleep without giving you a prescription sleeping pill hangover.

Creating a mood. Sound pollution (in this case the constant noise in an airplane) not only stops your body from relaxing, it can create tension for some people as well. The healing power of music is widely believed by many people. Consider using music to help create a mood of relaxation while flying. **Take soothing music** to listen to on the plane. You'll be able to cancel out the airplane's noises and soothe your mind at the same time. To be certain you will be able to listen to something you like, bring your own portable tape deck or CD player. They are relatively inexpensive and can be used for other activities besides flying. Music truly is the doctor, so don't forget to partake in some soothing tunes to help you relax and enjoy your flight.

If you won't or can't listen to music, try **writing in a journal**. Gratitude journals in particular help you to reflect on all the blessings in your life, which surely will help to calm you down. Even writing down three good things that happened to you that day or that you appreciate about your life can go a long way to helping you relax. It may sound silly, but it's true. Try it and see for yourself. I'll bet there are dozens of things you can think of right now that you are grateful for in your life. Maybe being grateful for a safe flight would be something you could jot down in your journal. No matter what you write about, using a journal to help remember the good things in life can in turn help you relax on any flight.

There are many things you can do to relax your body and to take care of your skin while traveling. Add to my list and do as much as possible to make your traveling experience more enjoyable.

A final note about your skin and flying: *Don't assess your skin in the plane's bathroom*! I always laugh when I see myself in the bathroom of an airplane. I look at least 10 years older! I see things there that on a normal day, in normal light, under normal circumstances I *don't* see. You are looking very close up, your skin is severely dehydrated, and you are looking at yourself under the worst kind of light possible: fluorescent light. Please do not use these reflections as real and valid. You are in unusual conditions, and these images of your skin are *un*real!

Folliculitis

Folliculitis is a persistent infection caused by either bacteria or possibly a fungus within the hair follicle. It occurs due to shaving, long-term irritation, or even restrictive or tight clothing. Folliculitis should not be confused with *pseudofolliculitis barbae*, otherwise known as ingrown hair. This happens due to hair curling back down into the follicle wall instead of coming up out onto the skin's surface, which is the reason pseudofolliculitis barbae tends to occur with African-American males or any men with curly hair.

Believe it or not, there is a condition called hot tub folliculitis or *pseudomonas folliculitis*. Like standard folliculitis, it is a bacterial infection within the hair follicle, but as the name implies, it is contracted by sitting in a hot tub! Usually the infection is located where the water meets the skin; around the neck, upper arms, and upper back areas.

I actually know several clients who have experienced this condition. It starts with a hot tub that is not well-ventilated, perhaps sitting inside a garage, and fungus multiplies in the water. Although poor ventilation seems to be a common factor, I have a client who was in an outdoor hot tub at a resort, and everyone who participated developed pseudomonas folliculitis, which looked like little red bumps all over their upper bodies and faces.

Regardless of how you got folliculitis, getting rid of it is what is important. Mild cases of folliculitis will respond to topical antibiotics that you can get either from your dermatologist or over the counter. Remember, the prescription treatment will be a stronger version than the store-bought kind. Don't wear tight or restrictive clothing over the affected skin, and I would steer clear of using harsh products on the area—even sunscreens. Due to the chemicals in sun products, this may further irritate the skin and cause a longer recovery period. However, if you are going to be exposed to the sun, you obviously need to use a sunscreen, but if at all possible avoid these types of products until the skin condition clears up.

For a man who has folliculitis on his face, shaving can delay the healing process. Every time you go over your face with a razor, you are probably causing further irritation. Be sure to prepare your beard and use a softening shaving cream or gel. It would be best to shave in the direction of hair growth. This won't give you the smoothest shave, but it will help to lessen the irritation caused by the razor. After shaving, apply a soothing aftershave product, and then apply your antibiotic cream to the affected area. If you don't use an antibacterial treatment, the bacteria inside the hair follicle will persist.

The timetable for recovering from folliculitis varies with the individual. Sometimes it can take months for this condition to clear up, so be patient and follow your doctor's recommendations.

Food & Skin

Let food be your medicine and medicine be your food.
—Hippocrates

This marvelous machine that we walk around in takes us wherever we want to go. We are not just a bunch of muscles and bones built for locomotion; we are so much more than that. *We are what we eat.* Food equals fuel. How are you fueling your machine? Cars need gas, oil, window wiper fluid, etc. They need certain types of products in order to perform optimally. If we are looking to burn fuel efficiently inside our own bodies, then why would we put junk and poison in our mouths? We've all done it, but when are we going to realize the connection between fuel and energy? Stop, take a look at what is going from your hand to your mouth and then how you feel. Do you see and/or feel a connection?

I like equating our bodies with cars because for some reason we take into consideration how a car works and take for granted our own machine, our bodies. You would never dream of getting into your car for a long drive with the gas gauge on empty. Every time you skip a meal, this is essentially what you are doing. Do you eat to live or live to eat? Either one is valid, but do you eat to fuel the machine, or does the way you eat have a detrimental impact on your body?

People are always asking me, "What are the best foods to eat for my skin?" I am not a nutritionist or a doctor, but I believe in following common sense and becoming aware of how certain foods are affecting our bodies. If we eat a healthy, balanced diet filled with all the "right" foods and very little of the "wrong" foods, our bodies will do well, and therefore our skin cells will also reap the benefits of this healthy diet.

Instead of focusing on what foods to eat for your skin specifically, I recommend using food to keep your entire body functioning at its best; this will in turn have positive effects on your skin.

Connect with your food. If you are wondering what to eat for your health and for healthy skin, ask yourself this question: Am I about to eat health-producing food or health-reducing food? Of course, there are many healthy foods that may not be healthy for *you,* but start at the beginning and acknowledge whether the majority of the food you are eating is providing an environment for your body to benefit from. Are foods that are alive, foods that contain a lot of vitamins and minerals, and foods that are health-producing foremost in your diet?

Packaged or manufactured foods (generally found in boxes or cans) are not going to contain the high volume of nutrients that live food does. One benefit of packaged foods is they are required to list ingredients, and many provide a helpful nutrient guide that includes calorie, fat, protein, and carbohydrate content. You can learn a lot about the foods you eat by reading these labels. In the **Sugar** section I explain how important it is to read labels. You will be amazed at how many poor-quality ingredients are used in the manufactured foods that you eat.

As with skin care, exercise, or in this discussion about food, keeping things simple is best. Keeping it simple with food means grilling rather than frying, eating fresh fruits and vegetables instead of canned, and steaming or stir-frying veggies rather than sautéing them in butter. Try drinking water instead of sodas and caffeine-laden teas and coffee drinks; and why not skip dessert once in a while, or skip it altogether. Use sweets as a separate treat to have every now and then.

I believe in moderation. One of my favorite sayings is "Everything in moderation—including moderation." Sometimes you have to break away and have some "bad" foods or drinks. But don't make these poor-quality choices a mainstay of your diet. Make them a treat.

Something that you look forward to—especially since you've been so good about what you've been eating. Remember, your body is a machine and food is its fuel. How are your fueling your machine?

Foundation

What foundation do you recommend to your clients? Which brand?

I am frequently asked that question. There are so many different products and colors of foundation and so many different colors and types of skin. Even if there was a brand I thought was good, it wouldn't work for everyone. That is one reason why I don't recommend any company's foundation. But it's mainly because I don't want to promote something I don't think is a good thing for the health of the skin in the first place. I understand some women want to or have to wear foundation, but I do not have one product to recommend.

If you have to wear foundation, try a water-based product vs. an oil-based foundation. The oil-based product will stick inside the pores more than a water-based type. Many times when I have a client who comes in for a facial with an oilier foundation on her face, it will take me more than the normal two cleansings to get it all off. Sometimes I see small bits of foundation sitting in the pores after cleansing and even exfoliating during the course of a facial, which indicates she is probably not getting her skin clean at home. I always let my client know if she isn't doing enough to get her skin clean—namely getting all the makeup off. Cleaning at least twice at night is in order if you wear makeup. The first cleanse is to get the makeup off; the second cleanse is to get your skin clean. Without doing at least two cleansings, you are increasing your chances of getting clogged pores—at the very least.

When a foundation has a label that says it doesn't clog pores, does that mean it doesn't clog even if you wear it all day long, or is there a time limit?

There is no time limit for how long a foundation can stay on your skin without clogging your pores. Just know that whether you are wearing an oil-free coverup product or not, if it is sitting on your face all day long, it is contributing to clogging on some level. Be sure to get it all off every day. Also try to do The Extras (exfoliating and using a clay mask) once to several times a week to ensure your pores are getting sufficiently and regularly cleaned out.

Can I use my spray toner over my foundation during the day?

It would be more beneficial to spray your toner on *before* applying foundation or powder. If you spray afterwards you may set the makeup further into your pores. Why? The moisture from the toner will bind with the makeup and then set or harden onto your skin. Spraying toner throughout the day if you aren't wearing foundation or powder would be a great thing. You'll get the benefits of the toner whenever you spray.

For an alternative to wearing foundation, see **Mineral Makeup**.

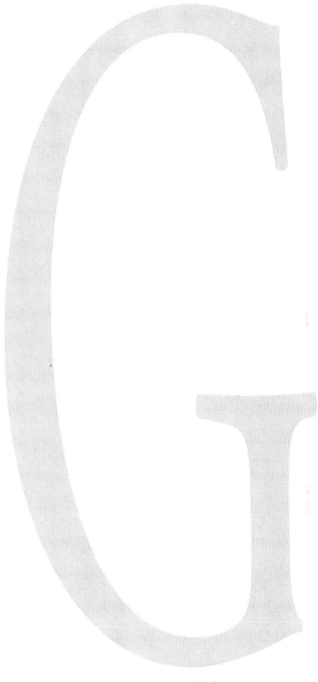

G

Geranium

I'm looking for a spot remover that will help with my occasional breakouts. I've used something in the past that stung a little when I put it on, but it was great for drying out the blemish. I can't find it now. Do you have any recommendations?

The best thing to use as a spot remover for problem skin is essential oil of geranium. The product you used may have had benzoyl peroxide as its main ingredient. Sometimes it can sting a little. If it worked for you, great. But drying out the skin isn't the best way to get rid of blemishes. I prefer the gentle yet highly effective effects of essential oils. They are generally antiseptic and antibacterial but do not dry the surface skin out. They are concentrated extracts from plants, herbs, or flowers, so they are quite aromatically intense. Give essential oils a try—they are better for your skin then benzoyl peroxide spot treatments.

Can you use geranium oil "neat" on the skin? I was under the impression only lavender and tea tree could be put directly on the skin?

I realize the box of geranium oil I sell says not to put it neat (straight or undiluted) on the skin. However, the way I tell my clients to apply the geranium is just to put a single drop on each blemish. If anyone was to put geranium all over his or her face, that would be too much. I only recommend putting it on the blemishes themselves, and there is no harm in doing this.

Any essential oils in the mint family (like peppermint, for example) should definitely not be used in very large amounts on the skin—neat. These oils are way too potent and can cause burning as well as redness.

But other than these, most essential oils, used in very limited amounts, are fine to use neat—providing caution is used around the eyes and sensitive tissue of the inner nose and mouth.

I suppose anything can be misused, and perhaps that is why the manufacturers label their products with that warning.

How often should I apply the geranium and where? Do I dab it on my blemishes or put it all over my face?

Do not mix geranium or any essential oil in with your creams, and *under no circumstances* should you rub it all over your face! In reference to the previous email, this is no doubt why manufacturers say not to use it neat—as a precautionary measure because someone may unwittingly put it all over their skin.

Geranium is best used on infected blemishes *only*. If the spot is red, which generally indicates infection, use the geranium. If not, don't. In other words, using this essential oil on blackheads won't do you any good. Just dab it on infected places for 2-3 days or until there is improvement in the spot(s). Apply it at night after your Basics 1-2-3 or right before bedtime.

Can I mix water and geranium oil together to make a spritzer toner?

I have read in several books on essential oils to do just that—to mix essential oils and water to make your own toner. The essential oils, however, will not truly mix with water and may cause burning. If you choose to make your own, be sure to have the toner in a glass or metal bottle and remember to shake it well before spraying each time. Hopefully this will help to mix the oils and water together. Personally, I prefer a manufactured toner with essential oils.

*If I put geranium on overnight, should I wait until the mask dries
then put on the geranium, or can I put both on at the same time?*

I recommend waiting until the mask dries. Otherwise, when you
apply the geranium to the wet mask, your finger will usually take the
mask off. So, wait a few minutes after applying the mask, then put a
drop of geranium on the clay.

*My husband says the fragrance of the geranium oil is "stout." I like
it because it helps clear my breakout and clears my sinuses too!*

Another client writes:

*The geranium oil seems to be helping with the healing of my
blemishes although my husband and I agree—it stinks!*

If you like the results of the geranium oil but just can't stand the smell,
try lavender essential oil. Truly, almost any essential oil will be good at
a base level for healing spots since essential oils all have antibacterial
abilities. Many people like tea tree oil, although this is not one of my
personal favorites. Not only do I not like the smell, but I also have better
results with geranium, juniper, or even lavender on skin problems.

Although using geranium on your spots is of great benefit, if you
have breakout anywhere near your mouth (lips), I would skip the
essential oils and just put clay mask there instead. Essential oils might
irritate the lip tissue, and worst of all, it will taste horrible!

As an experiment, I used geranium oil on a few tiny places right
near my mouth one evening. I knew the oil would seep into my
mouth, but I'm a scientist at heart, and I wanted to see what would
happen. The geranium did indeed get into my mouth and, as expected, it tasted awful! So I went into my bathroom and gently rubbed the
essential oil off my skin, knowing it wouldn't just magically come off.

Essential oils are very vaporous and easily absorbed into the skin, so there was very little to actually come off. Next, I reached for my mask and dotted the small places with the clay. Clay will stick wherever you put it and won't migrate like an essential oil will.

My advice is if you have blemishes (large or small) anywhere near your mouth, just apply clay mask. It won't cause a bad taste in your mouth, and the clay won't irritate the lip tissue like an essential oil can. Hopefully you don't need me to tell you to keep essential oils away from your eyes.

I do not recommend the following—remember I am experimenting for your benefit. I put peppermint oil in the same area near my mouth. I did this knowing the results, and I wanted to see how much it would burn. Less than a minute later, the entire side of my mouth and outer skin felt like it was on fire! Peppermint oil is great to use *inside* your mouth (see **Canker Sores**), but should never be used near your eyes or mouth or any other sensitive area.

I wanted to let you know I've been using your tip about putting the clay mask and geranium oil on places where I have breakout, and it clears everything up so quickly! I'm feeling so much better about my skin. Thank you!

HOT TIP: Geranium makes a great "spot remover!"

Glycerin

Glycerin is an important ingredient—especially for dry skin. It is a humectant, attracting moisture to itself; it has emollient properties, meaning it helps to make the skin feel smooth; it has a binding action, which helps to hold a cream together; and it is an excellent moisturizer.

My toner lists glycerin as one of the first ingredients. Is this a good thing for me to be using?

Glycerin is an excellent ingredient in a toner for dry (true-dry) skin—skin that doesn't produce enough oil on its own. I have found, however, that this ingredient in a toner for normal to oily skin can be too much for this skin type. And although this seems to hold true for toners, glycerin is not necessarily too much for oilier skins if it is in a moisturizer. It really depends on the product and where the glycerin is on the ingredient list. As you will read below, I recommend pure glycerin or glycerin-based products to help with hydrating skin, even oilier skin. But in general, glycerin makes a good ingredient for normal or normal to dry skin types.

Hydration boosters. I like to apply hydration boosters to help with the dehydration that inevitably occurs from the indoor heat and the cold wind of winter. I purchased a bottle of glycerin at my local grocery store—in fact, it was the store's own brand. Although I have more expensive glycerin products, I wanted to experiment and see if I could use this inexpensive brand with the same results.

In the winter, when my skin is feeling drier, I like to apply this hydration booster to my skin. I add enough to cover my entire face and neck, after cleansing. Then I spray my toner, and apply moisturizer. If you have true-dry skin, you can add more glycerin in with your moisturizer. If this mixture doesn't help your dry skin, you can try adding a few drops of true oil, but with glycerin you tend to not get the clogging effect that sometimes occurs with true oils.

H

Hair Removal

One of the leading health magazines called, asking me to contribute to an article for "painless at-home hair removal." The first words out of my mouth to the interviewer were, "There is no such thing!" Truly, there really are very few painless ways to get rid of unwanted hair. But there are several ways of removing hair that vary on the pain scale and are readily available to you. Some of these methods can be done in the privacy of your home, while others require going to either a salon or doctor's office.

You have hair covering your entire body—for several purposes. Not only does it help keep dirt and debris away from your skin, but hair also helps combat water loss and keeps you insulated, protecting you against extremes of hot and cold. The hair on your body plays a sensory role as well. The movement that occurs with the hair on top of your skin helps to detect the slightest change in temperature and touch.

If you think about it, hair protects you against all kinds of daily offenders you probably never consider. The hair on your head protects your scalp against the harsh burning rays of the sun. Hair, which is made from keratin (a durable protein that also makes up the outer skin and nails), has a high sulfur content, giving it heat-retaining properties. Did you know that up to 60% of heat loss comes from your head? So hair can keep you warmer on a cold winter's day. Eyebrows can help keep sweat from reaching your eyes, and eyelashes keep dirt, debris, and foreign objects away from the delicate eye tissue. Hair in your ears also keeps foreign offenders such as dirt and bugs away from the inner ear, due in part to the waxy substance this hair is coated with. Finally, nose hair filters out all kinds of debris from the air like dirt, pollen, and germs.

The bottom line is hair has an important function and should be looked at as an asset, rather than a liability. With that said, and although you may be able to live with some hair, there is still the problem of unsightly or objectionable hair that remains to be dealt with. The following are different tools and techniques available for removing unwelcome hair. One approach may be better suited to a certain part of the body than another, so read through this entire section to find the best removal process for you.

There are a few things I want to define before going further in order to bypass any confusion about the words being used. *Depilation* removes part of the hair from the surface of the skin. Depilation methods include shaving, trimming, and depilatory creams. Depilation has the shortest regrowth time; usually within a day or two you will start seeing hair reappearing on the surface of your skin. *Epilation* takes the entire hair or root from the hair follicle. Techniques for epilation include tweezing, waxing, sugaring, threading, and rotary epilators. Hair reappearance after epilation takes anywhere from several days to several weeks. Both depilation and epilation are considered to be temporary ways to remove unwanted hair. Permanent (or close to permanent) methods I will discuss are electrolysis and laser hair removal. The reoccurrence of hair growth with these more permanent procedures varies a great deal. It can take up to a year of treatments to keep the hair from returning, and even then there are no guarantees. More often than not, however, these techniques can permanently get rid of unwanted hair.

Finally, when I mention the upper lip or upper lip area, I am referring to the area where a man's moustache grows, the skin and hair above the upper lip. Using the term *upper lip* just requires fewer words, but I am not referring to the actual upper lip of the mouth. For instance, getting a lip wax is obviously not waxing of the actual lip, but the hair above it.

Bleach. Bleaching, of course, is not removing hair physically, but I include it here because it can remove hair visually. And sometimes this is all that is needed.

The most common reason (and my recommendation) for using a bleaching cream is for dark hair on the upper lip area. With bleach, all you are doing is lightening the hair, not removing it; so the hair doesn't change (get darker, thicker) due to this application. Other than a reaction to the bleaching cream itself, there aren't really any negative effects of using this method to remove dark colored hair. In short, bleaching is the least harmful way to take care of unwanted hair on the upper lip.

Jolen® is a brand of facial hair bleaching cream that has been around for years. There are other brands on the market as well. Full directions will be on the box or bottle of bleaching cream. Just be sure to read and follow those instructions to the letter. Also, since you are working with bleach, be careful not to get it on anything, especially clothes you care about.

Bleaching your upper lip is a painless and simple way to get rid of dark hair. I recommend doing a patch test first before using any bleaching cream. You never know if you will have a reaction, and you certainly don't want to find out after you've applied bleach to your entire upper lip area.

I recently had a facial, and the aesthetician told me not to wax or bleach my upper lip for a few days. What do you think— is that true?

I agree with your aesthetician. Waxing causes irritation for almost everyone. If the facial contained strong acid peels or a lot of active ingredients, your skin might be too sensitive to use chemicals like bleach. So, since the skin is susceptible to irritation in that area, although it may not cause a problem, play it safe and don't bleach either directly before or after a facial. And definitely don't get waxed there for a few days.

Depilatory creams. These are creams or lotions that contain a chemical that dissolves hair, basically causing it to break off. Like shaving, this method only takes the hair off at the skin's surface, so depending on how fast your hair grows back, the results won't last long (no more than a few days to a week), and repeated applications will be necessary for continued results. Most brands contain irritating ingredients such as calcium hydroxide and sodium hydroxide. *Potassium thioglycolate* (derived from thioglycolic acid compounds), one of the key ingredients in depilatory creams, causes hair breakage (depilation), but also has the consequence of severe allergic reactions in some people.

Depilatory creams have come a long way in recent years and many include soothing ingredients to help offset the rather harsh, caustic chemicals that remove the hair. Still, these products can cause even the most non-sensitive skin to feel irritated; they can possibly even cause a reactive chemical burn. As with any new products, especially those that contain harsh chemicals, you need to do a patch test on a small section of your leg. By doing so if you are allergic or intolerant to the cream, you will avoid having an allergic reaction on your entire leg.

The safest place to use a depilatory cream is the upper and lower legs. You can use it on other areas such as your bikini line, but you absolutely need to do a patch test first for this area. Depilatory creams tend to work most effectively on finer, lighter hair and since the hair in the bikini area is much courser and stronger, it may not respond as well as the hair on your legs. Add to this the natural sensitivity of the skin around your bikini line, and putting a chemical composition there may cause mild to severe irritation.

I rarely if ever use depilatory creams. As you will read, I employ other methods of hair removal. But if I have gotten out of my normal routine or don't want to shave for some reason, using a depilatory cream once in a while seems to work well for me. I am more apt to use this technique during the hotter summer months when I want to quickly get rid of the hair all over my legs, not just the lower half. By applying one of these creams, closely following the directions (or else irritation will surely follow), within a few minutes my legs are smooth without having to go through the possible nicks and cuts of using a razor.

Nair® is probably the most commonly known depilatory cream available. It's like Reynolds Wrap® is to tin foil; you think of the brand name as the product itself. There are several other companies that manufacture similar products so you will have a lot of variety to choose from. If one brand causes problems, you may want to try another company's product, and see if you can find one that works for you.

Using a washcloth in the shower is the best way to thoroughly remove the cream and hair from your legs. The slightly abrasive nature of the wash rag helps to complete the process of hair removal, and since you will be rinsing your body off in the shower, it makes for an easy cleanup. Just be sure you have a washcloth with you. Also, don't rub so aggressively as to cause irritation. Use just enough pressure with the washcloth to help the hair come off.

Your skin will probably be irritated after using a depilatory cream and anything, even a moisturizer, can cause further irritation on sensitive skin. So, you may want to skip applying moisturizer or at least wait a while. How long you should wait will be up to you to decide, but don't put lotion on immediately after removing the hair, or you may be sorry.

Also, I do not recommend using a depilatory and then immediately applying either sunscreen or a self-tanning product. And definitely don't be exposed to the sun directly after depilating. Given the many potential irritants involved in all of these products plus radiation from the sun, there is no telling how potentially problematic using all these chemicals at one time could be. If you're going out in the sun, do the hair removal the night before to ensure a safe outdoor experience.

I have hair above and below my lip and on my chin—yuck! I use
a cream remover from Sally Hansen® right now. What do you think?

Instead of using a depilatory cream on your sensitive upper lip area, try lightening it with a facial bleaching cream. If the hair bothers you and dying it is not an option, as long as this depilatory cream doesn't cause irritation on your upper lip (or chin), I guess that is the best option for you. Getting waxed is, of course, a very common practice, but I would use the depilatory cream before I would have those places waxed. If the hair is really something that bothers you and needs constant attention, you may want to research getting either electrolysis or laser hair removal to eliminate the hair altogether. These are sometimes painful and expensive procedures, but either one can alleviate the need to be concerned about removing the hair once it is permanently removed.

Remember this important point: If you use a depilatory cream or wax the area, you will be taking off all the hair in that area, not just the hair you are concerned with. Read **Shari's waxing story** later in the waxing section to get more information on why you may not want to take this route of hair removal.

Electrolysis. Electrolysis has been around for a long time and used to be the only permanent method of hair removal. It is now running neck and neck with laser techniques in popularity. Electrolysis works by sending an electrical current from a needle down into the hair shaft, affecting the root and effectively destroying it. Electrolysis is not foolproof, and the effectiveness rate varies from person to person. Some clients have an 80-100% success rate, while others have less than 50%. You have to go back for repeated visits for best results, and electrolysis can be expensive. When I was working for a spa back in my early years as an aesthetician, I had a client who was getting electrolysis on both of her legs. Imagine the time and expense of having this done! But I also picture this woman today, never having to shave or otherwise worry about unwanted hair on her legs. I'm sure she thinks it was worth every penny.

Electrolysis is not initially a permanent removal, but is a process of weakening the hair. With continued treatments, the hair essentially gives up and does not grow back, so you will need a series of electrolysis sessions lasting anywhere from a few months to a year or more depending on the location of the hair and how stubborn (thick) it is. This process varies with each individual, and you will have to discuss your specific needs with your technician. Don't think that going in for one electrolysis session will permanently eliminate your unwanted hair. The duration of your treatments will depend on your own personal hair growth cycles, how much damage you have done to the area (through tweezing and/or waxing), and how coarse the hair is, along with the depth of the hair within the follicle. Even medications you are taking can affect how the hair grows, which can in turn affect the success of your treatment process.

Generally, once you start getting electrolysis, the hair will grow back thinner and finer, setting the stage for permanent removal. Most electrolysis experts will tell you not to tweeze or wax the area— it makes electrolysis much more difficult. They need to work with "untampered with" hair. So if you decide to go through electrolysis, consult with your technician and obey their instructions, or the process will take longer and may potentially be more painful. Put your confidence in the professional you have chosen and leave your hair alone!

I highly recommend checking out more than one electrolysis facility. If you can, get some referrals from friends. If you don't know anyone who is getting or has gotten electrolysis, call a few reputable skin care salons in your area and ask them for referrals. If all else fails, get out the phone book and start calling around. Be careful when it comes to discounted electrolysis. Cheaper doesn't mean better. What you are looking for is a highly qualified technician who will help you get rid of unwanted hair. You don't want to waste your time and money on a person who may be charging you less than the rest, but is doing a less-than-effective job on your unwanted hair.

Epilation. This is a little known and highly painful way of removing hair from the root. I should know, I use this technique! It is basically a mechanical form of tweezing. A small, hand-held device made of a series of high velocity rotating spring-coiled discs operates like tweezers, trapping the hair and pulling it out entirely. This system can remove even the shortest and thickest hair by the root.

Epilady® is the brand name of the machine I use, but there are several companies that offer this device. If you choose to try this method, the first time you do it you might want to have a cocktail, anything to numb the pain you are about to feel! If you use epilation consistently, it becomes less and less painful, though the very first time is quite uncomfortable. This technique is a great way to remove hair from the root, giving you a smooth, hairless surface for a lot longer than shaving.

You may ask why I use the thing at all if it's so painful, and the reason is simple: I'm lazy. I don't like shaving my legs every day or even every other day, yet I want to have that just-shaved look and feel (this can be especially helpful during a vacation). The Epilady helps me achieve this; clean shaven legs without having to shave. I not only don't want to shave, but I don't like having my legs waxed either. It's just too painful—somehow more so to me than epilation. Maybe this is due in part because I can stop the machine at any time, which puts me at the controls vs. being waxed.

I try to use the Epilady at least once a week to catch any new hair growth that might be taking place. This way each time I use it, I don't have a whole leg full of hair to contend with. And this makes for much less pain; the more you use the machine, the less and less painful it becomes. I think you just get used to the sensation that occurs when the machine is turned on and turned loose on your leg hair.

There are machines on the market that allow you to epilate not only your legs but your bikini area and underarms as well. I haven't ventured that far in my quest for hairlessness, but I know there are machines available for these more delicate areas. I have a friend who has epilated in these areas and said it caused a lot of ingrown hair. I find this to be true, too, with epilating my legs. Still the benefits—for me—are worth a few stray hairs that have lost their way. (For more information, see **Ingrown Hair**.)

I have a few recommendations. First, whether you are a first-time user or just haven't used your epilator for a while, I recommend shaving your legs and letting the hair grow out slightly. Use your epilation machine when the hair is quite short—just long enough to be picked up by the coils; one quarter inch or a bit longer is ideal. If you try to epilate with a thick forest of long hair it is a much more painful process.

Second, use this machine after a bath or shower. However, do not use it in or near water—it is an electrical appliance so stay away from water! After bathing, the hair will be softer, which may make for easier elimination. As you will no doubt find out during your initial visit with the epilator, *easy* is not a term that comes to mind during this procedure.

And lastly—go slow! My first time using the Epilady I did a patch about 3" square, then gave up—until the next day. I just couldn't take it! But in my experience, over time you actually can get used to the sensation. Epilation is definitely not for everyone, but if you can get past the initial pain, the benefits are long-lasting and worth it!

Laser hair removal. This is yet another technique to get rid of unwanted hair. Laser technology is changing rapidly; what is available today will surely be improved as time goes by. For instance, until recently this laser technique wasn't effective on light-colored hair. Now, with advances in this technology, light hair can be removed.

During this procedure, a laser emits a pulse of light that is absorbed by melanin (the pigment in your skin) deep within the hair shaft, effectively destroying the follicle, making hair growth cease.

Because heat given off by the laser is coming in contact with your skin, there is a chance of scarring. Be sure you are going to a qualified laser hair removal technician (whether a doctor or a hair removal specialist), otherwise you may be left with undesirable side effects. And as I always recommend: ask questions! If you don't feel satisfied with the answers, I'd find someone else to do this procedure.

There are not universal results from laser hair removal. Some people have great results (see emails below), while others are left disappointed, expecting to have no hair left after as much as a year of hair removal sessions. Some people go through just a few sessions and are completely satisfied. No hair removal system is truly permanent, but surely you will have less hair than when you started, and hopefully even better results than that.

Laser hair removal is the best thing I've ever done! I have my chin, bikini, and armpits lasered. I recommend this to everyone I know. After just two appointments my skin is so much softer, and I hardly have to shave anything. (I purchased a package of six sessions per area.) I have to take some ibuprofen one hour before I go because the "zaps" [from the laser] can sting. However, there are no side effects (at least not for me).

I had the hair lasered from my legs and under my arms. I am thrilled with the results! I would definitely recommend getting it done. For me, it wasn't painful at all, and there were no side effects. Granted, 100% of the hair isn't gone, but what's left is hardly visible.

Shaving. We all know about shaving. Using a razor, the hair is basically chopped off on top of the skin, leaving a smooth, hairless surface in its wake—albeit for a very short time. Everyone's hair grows at different rates, but shaving offers the shortest amount of time between the removal and the regrowth of hair. Men generally only shave their faces, whereas women shave many different parts of their bodies. The most common areas for a woman to shave is her legs (some women only shave the lower legs, others shave the entire leg—upper and lower), the underarms, and sometimes even the bikini line. And then there are those of you ladies who shave your face. Shaving the face should be left for the men of the world—only. Let me reiterate that point: If you are a woman, ***do not shave your face!*** Read this entire piece to find alternative techniques to remove unwanted hair on your face. If you start (or continue) shaving, you are only going to be ensuring the need to do it forever.

Shaving is a relatively inexpensive way to quickly get rid of hair virtually anywhere on the body, and it is generally painless. If you aren't paying attention, shave too quickly, use an old or dull blade, or if you have problems with your skin, it can preclude a smooth shave.

Does hair really grow back darker if you shave?

It is my experience that once a particular area has been shaved (and I believe this holds true for waxing as well), the hair *does* grow back darker and possibly thicker than it was before. Some reports dispute this, but use your own experience as a measure of the validity of my observation. Perhaps for some people the hair grows back as it was prior to shaving. This has not been the case for me, however, nor most people I have spoken with. So in essence, once you shave an area, you will eventually become a slave to shaving it.

Usually women start shaving their legs as teenagers, many times as proof of maturation—a sort of rite of passage. I know this was true for me when I was a teen, around 13 or 14 years old. Like a young man shaving the peach fuzz off his face, I started shaving my legs long before I needed to. I was simply removing fine (and unnoticeable), light-colored hair from my lower legs. At this young age, noticeably dark hair had not become a problem. I don't remember specifically when I noticed the hair growing in darker and coarser, but it was. The hair also seemed to grow in quicker, probably due to the darker color being more noticeable. Now, of course, I can't go for more than a day or so without shaving, lest the dark hairs scare off my clients! The point is, don't remove peach fuzz from anywhere on your body unless you just want to speed up the process of being a slave to shaving.

Prepare or despair. Preparing your skin is of the utmost importance when it comes to shaving. For men, if you can shave in the shower, it will greatly increase your ability to get a clean shave, as well as make you less susceptible to irritation and razor cuts. The steam coming from the hot water does a great job of warming your skin and making it smooth, so the razor just glides right over your face. The same shower technique goes for women and shaving. Shave in the shower to ensure your skin is "warmed-up" for the process.

If the skin is dried out and flaky (dehydrated skin), shaving can cause irritation anywhere on your body. So in order to ensure a smooth shave, you'll want to incorporate these three components: Exfoliation, using a good shaving cream, and using a triple blade razor.

Exfoliating the area to be shaved is essential for good results. Exfoliation gets rid of dead cell buildup on the surface of your skin. This buildup is a factor if you are feeling dry. If you are a woman who has trouble shaving your legs, try exfoliating beforehand and see if this helps you get a smoother shave.

For men, you are actually exfoliating every time your shave, so it may not be practical to pre-exfoliate your face every time before you shave. Using an exfoliant (like a scrub or gommage) at least once or twice a week on your entire face will give your skin a smoother texture, setting up the optimum environment for shaving. Keeping your skin well-moisturized day and night will also help the cause.

Next I recommend using a soothing **shaving cream**. Aveeno is the brand I like best, and it is good for men and women alike. On the bottle it says, "Dermatologist recommended, therapeutic shave gel with natural colloidal oatmeal. For sensitive skin, irritated skin, razor bumps. No added fragrance." This is certainly not the only shaving product available, and perhaps you have already found one that works well for you, but if not, try Aveeno shaving cream and hopefully you will get better results.

I do not recommend using soap (especially bar soap) to shave with. Usually soap is alkaline, causing dryness on the surface of your skin. It also does not give you a thick, creamy-textured substance for the razor to glide across. Stick to shaving gels. You can even find some that heat up on your skin. In emergencies I have used cream rinse (hair conditioner) as a substitute shaving cream. I don't recommend this as a regular practice, but in a pinch it works better than soap, creating a smooth surface to work with without drying out the skin. Note: If you find your skin becomes irritated after using a shaving product, discontinue use and try something else. Irritation may be your skin telling you it is sensitive to something in a product, and irritation is not the goal. But before blaming a product, please make sure your razor has a sharp edge. A dull, overused razor spells disaster for even the best-prepared surface.

Finally a **triple blade razor** is a must in my opinion. Years ago, my friend, Jimmy (who shaves his head), came to town for a visit. I asked him what he used to get such a close shave without nicking his head. He said triple blades made all the difference in the world. A few days later one of my employees said about the same thing for shaving concerns for women. I immediately ran out and got a triple blade razor and have been singing its praises ever since. If you haven't ever used a triple blade, give one a try. Once you do, you won't go back to a double blade—I promise! Quadruple blades are also available now.

If you are shaving your bikini area, ladies, no doubt you have run into some problems—namely irritation and ingrown hairs. (Look up **Ingrown Hair** to find some ways to prevent this problem.) Shaving with a triple blade razor may bring some relief, but due to the delicate nature of that particular skin, shaving is not the optimum way to remove hair at the bikini line. It is, however, the cheapest way. So if money is a factor (and you don't experience the pain of irritation and ingrown hairs), shave on. But if you are a woman who does have problems when shaving this area, waxing or even electrolysis may be something to consider. These services will cost varying amounts of money, but will give you fewer problems than shaving that delicate area.

Aftershave. Whether you are male or female, using something on your skin after you shave (wherever you shave) will greatly increase your chances of having smooth and soothed skin.

As long as you are not allergic to it, **aloe vera gel** makes a great aftershave skin soother. Slather it over the area just shaved. Aloe vera has tremendous healing and soothing abilities; it is used for sunburns, so it will help with your after-shaving needs too.

Another alternative would be to use your **toner in a spray bottle** as an aftershave. As long as you use a toner without alcohol, this product will hydrate and soothe just-shaved skin.

Of course there are many **aftershave products** on the market, but be sure to use one without alcohol—the bad kind—in its ingredient list. Alcohol will be anything but soothing, although it does have antiseptic abilities. Alcohol will probably cause a burning sensation, which is the opposite effect you are looking for after your have run a razor over your skin.

Shaving tips for men. Remember, the softer the skin and hair, the easier the shave will be. Therefore, applying your shaving cream when you first get in the shower will give it a chance to moisturize your skin and soften the hair. If you can, leave the cream on for a few minutes and enjoy a smoother shave.

Use your shaving cream sparingly. If you use too much cream it can cause the potential for nasty nicks and cuts due to a dull (clogged) razor.

Next, shave the toughest areas on your face last. This will give the shaving cream time to soften the skin in these areas and hopefully make for a smoother and nick-free shaving experience.

If you have tried every technique and still have major razor bumps, you may want to try a few things. First is a product on the market called TendSkin (see section). It is also said to help with ingrown hair. I am not a fan of this particular product because it contains a high percentage of the bad type of alcohol, but I have heard from several people that it did actually help with their razor bumps. If you choose to use TendSkin, be careful and watch to see if your skin becomes dry and especially flaky. If so, discontinue use of this product and opt for something more soothing. If the places are red and infected, see **Geranium** and **Clay Mask** for more ideas on what to use on your razor bumps.

Secondly, alpha hydroxy acids have been found to successfully reduce razor bumps. Why? There is usually a lot of dead skin that interferes with the hair making its way to the surface of your face. AHAs help to decompose some of that dead skin, leaving room for the hair to make an appearance. There are moisturizers that contain alpha hydroxy acids, or even stronger AHA gels that can be used locally on the areas where razor bumps are a problem.

Tweezing. For women, tweezing is probably the most common method used to remove unwanted hair from the face, namely the eyebrows and chin. Using tweezers, the hair is grabbed and the entire shaft is pulled out. Because tweezing pulls out the whole hair shaft, it will take anywhere from two to four weeks for the hair to reappear.

Good tweezers are a *must* if you use this technique. Otherwise you will tear up your skin. Tweezerman®, available at most stores where makeup is sold, makes the best tweezers around and is the brand I use in my salons. Tweezerman tweezers get the hair easily, and they hold up well compared to other brands. Most professionals, including my employees, recommend buying tweezers that have a slant, not a flat or squared end.

Never buy tweezers with a sharp point. They can really cause serious damage to your skin and are unwise to use for a few reasons. First, because the ends are so sharp, they tend to break the hair off before you have a chance to pull it out. Then what will most likely happen is you will become frustrated and dig with these knife-like edges. Finally, you will have a wound where you were tweezing and probably a hair still within the follicle. So nothing gained and a lot lost.

Actually, even with quality tweezers, if you have the same inclination as a "picker" (a person who relentlessly picks at their blemishes), you could still cause damage. Because you refuse to be satisfied until you have gotten the stray hair, you will attempt, high-quality tweezers or not, to nab the hair, but you may just make a mess of your skin. Because tweezers can sometimes cut the hair off at the surface before you are able to fully pull it out, you may go in and try to get that darn hair. The result will most likely be a small tear in the skin, which leads to a tiny scab. This can make your skin look red and irritated for several days, at the very least. Restraint is a necessary factor for keeping the skin in the tweezed area looking healthy.

Please note that trying to tweeze the coarse, dark chin hairs you may have can be an exercise in futility. They are very strong and firmly planted inside the hair follicle, and if you have ever tried to use tweezers to pull these stubborn hairs out, I'm sure you have found it to be somewhat of a disaster. This is where I see most of my clients tearing up their skin. Not only are these chin hairs coarse, dark, and stubborn, they can sometimes cause irritation, which equals redness and sensitivity. My best suggestion is to look into electrolysis or laser hair removal to get rid of these unwanted chin hairs. These particular techniques can be permanent and are performed by professionals who won't leave the kind of marks you, the amateur, might leave on your skin from overzealous or ineffective tweezing.

Shaping brows is somewhat of an art form. Ask anyone who didn't have an "artist" shape their brows. If you aren't artistically inclined, you might want to find a professional to do this work for you, especially if you are shaping your brows for the first time. As with any profession, you want a qualified individual to perform this job. Remember, you will be wearing your newly shaped eyebrows for a long time. In other words, if you or someone else does a bad job of shaping your brows, it is still you who has to face the world afterwards.

A word of caution: Overtweezing is a common problem for the eyebrows. Although you may feel good about removing your unibrow, sometimes the hairs won't all grow back. As we age, the eyebrows may become less dense than they were in our youth. So be careful about overzealous tweezing—otherwise you may be faced with having to paint on your brows.

Another cautionary note: I have a client who said that plucking her chin hairs caused pigmentation spots. This was no doubt post-inflammatory hyperpigmentation (see section), which means that the injured area caused a pigmentation reaction when exposed to ultraviolet (sun) light. Be aware that this can happen and be careful when you tweeze!

In conclusion, tweezing is a quick and easy way to remove unwanted hair from your eyebrows, which is really the only place I would recommend using tweezers. For a stray chin hair here and there, no worries, but for anything more substantial, choose a different technique.

HOT TIP: The best time to tweeze and shape your eyebrows is right after a shower. Your skin will be softened by the steam heat, and your eyebrow hair will be easier to remove.

Waxing. Waxing is a popular hair removal technique. Your success rate with waxing will depend on the wax used (there are hot waxes, cold waxes, and some with special ingredients), the aesthetician providing the service (some people have more skill at waxing than others), and how your skin is attended to after the procedure (after waxing, a cream or salve that helps to soothe the skin should be applied). Hair regrowth is individual, but waxing should keep the hair away anywhere from three to six weeks.

Waxing is one of the least expensive ways to remove hair, but it is not a permanent removal, nor is it without side effects for some people. It is possible to have a reaction to certain ingredients in the wax itself, or the skin may become overly irritated due to the process. Welts can form, sometimes blisters, and although these are rare occurrences, they can happen.

Wax is applied to the area and a cheesecloth or cellophane strip is laid on top of the wax. Pressure is applied, and then in one quick movement, the cloth is ripped off the skin, taking with it a lot of hair pulled out from the root. As you may have guessed, or perhaps you have experienced this yourself, waxing is a painful procedure.

The hair needs to be long enough for the wax to grab hold of it. If you are waxing on an ongoing basis, this is not much of a concern; the hair grows in at different rates instead of all at once, making it less noticeable as you are growing it out. But if you're waxing for the first time, letting your hair grow out can be tedious.

I am not a fan of waxing. When I was an employee at a spa, I had to wax—or at least so my employer thought. I was so against waxing that I would try to talk a waxing client out of getting the procedure, especially facial waxing, and instead opt for an actual facial that had a host of benefits for their skin. Although facials and hair removal are mutually exclusive, I made the spa more money giving a more expensive service, so if I was ever found out, how could they complain? And I was providing the client with solid information about how to take care of his or her skin, which in my eyes was a much more beneficial thing to do.

I do offer waxing in my salons. Why? I know people (mostly women) are going to get waxing procedures done. At least I know in my salons I have done the best job I can to ensure every client will have a proper waxing experience. Call it quality control. I don't personally execute the service, but my employees do. They are, however, discouraged from waxing someone for the first time, especially a lip wax.

The reason I instruct my employees to not do a first-time lip wax is simply because they will be starting a never-ending process. They could be creating thicker, darker hair in an area that may actually be just fine as it is. And I don't want to contribute to that for any of my clients. What I have found throughout the years working on thousands of female clients is that they have a defective view of the hair that exists above their lips. Granted, some women do have a true moustache that contains thick, dark hair that may need to be removed. But for the most part, women just *think* they need to have a lip wax, when in actuality they have no real noticeable dark hair on their upper lip.

Because waxing can be lucrative for an aesthetician (employed or self-employed), this may lead her to encourage waxing even when it is clearly not needed. If you have been a victim of this practice and have only had one or two lip waxes, you are probably OK. But if you continue to wax, your hair may start to grow in darker and different than it was before. So please, take caution. Don't just go with the flow and agree to a service you are not sure about getting. And don't wax your lip simply because you think you should.

Shari's waxing story. Shari is a lovely 35-year-old mother of three. She has great genes for skin and has been coming to me for semiannual facials since 1996. Over the past few years, she has noticed one or two dark hairs on her chin—something that will probably get worse as she gets older.

Chin hair is one of those ugly secrets you don't read about in books. They usually start popping up around the magic age of 40, when so many other undesirable things start to occur. This phenomenon is due in part to waning estrogen levels in a woman's body as she is starting to phase out of her childbearing years. As the estrogen levels start to decline, the testosterone levels—although they may not increase—seem stronger due to the loss of estrogen.

Shari decided to get her chin waxed to get rid of the one or two stray hairs she had found. She later discovered that where she used to have peach fuzz on her chin, after waxing, the hair grew in darker and thicker than it was before. She was so disappointed she had begun this adventure (waxing) because now she had a worse problem than the one she began with: more dark hairs to contend with.

I recommended Shari stop waxing and look into either electrolysis or laser hair removal. Since she didn't have a lot of hair growth (the dark, coarse kind), it probably wouldn't be too expensive. *Expensive* is a relative term and completely getting rid of hair using lasers or electrolysis is not guaranteed. I also told Shari to try bleaching the area she originally got waxed if there was dark, fine hair there that bothered her.

Waxing can work for certain circumstances. But you have to understand you are taking off *all* the hair in the area, not just the problem spots. And sometimes that peach fuzz hair will grow in darker and coarser than before you waxed. It is something I see over and over again, and is one of the reasons I discourage facial waxing.

What do you think about waxing my entire face? I have a lot of hair and it's dark—especially on the side of my face to my hairline. I hate it and don't know what else to do but wax. Is that OK?

Please do not start waxing your entire face! Admittedly, there may be some women who can find no other relief for excessive, dark hair growth on their faces. But for most people, this is not why they wax the face. I have met many clients who are obsessed with every little hair they may see growing out of their skin. I know women who wax their lower arms to get rid of all the hair there—even light-colored hair. This is due to some belief that all hair, other than on the head, is bad. And I don't want you to get caught up in this and subscribe to the ultimate "solution," waxing.

Waxing your whole face can bring on a host of problems. Ingrown hair, irritation, small bumps that don't go away, stubble, obsession with your looks, and financial expenditures.

As with anything I may talk about, there are always exceptions. And with any of my recommendations or suggestions, they are only my opinions and may not fit into your lifestyle or needs. You will be the ultimate decision maker about what you do with your face, your skin, your looks. But waxing—especially your entire face—is something I strongly recommend *not* doing.

In conclusion, although there are many routes to hair removal, you must be careful to find the technique that is not only right for you, but for the area you are removing hair from. Not all techniques are right for all body parts. If you ever have a reaction from removing hair from your body and/or face, reassess your options and consider using a different procedure.

Hats

A client of mine was going to Arizona for a vacation one summer. I asked her if she had a good hat, and she said no. I knew this client didn't have a lot of money to spend on a hat, so I recommended she go to Target. They always seem to have good, inexpensive hats that I call Throw Aways.

I rarely spend more than $10 on a hat. It has to pack well (being able to fold and mash it is imperative!) and if I lose it, I am not out much money. Plus I know there are more where it came from. In fact, when I find a hat I truly love, I usually buy at least two of them. Having a spare for insurance means if I lose it or something happens to my beloved hat, there is always one waiting in the wings.

For me, this is very important. I don't want direct sunlight on my face—ever! Now that I am into my 40s, I am much more careful than I was 20 years ago—when I didn't really care unless I was at the beach. There, I always covered my face, but not while I was walking on the sand or the street or to and from my car. But now I always have something between my face and the sun. And I always have sunscreen on.

Keep your hats handy and try to have something for every occasion. Running, skating, walking, golfing, boating, snow skiing, biking, motorcycling, dressup, dressdown; you name it, you'll have a hat.

Of course, many of the above activities can share one hat. Sometimes a bandana is the only appropriate sun protection. If you water ski, for instance, you can wear a bandana tied around your head, at least covering your forehead. A hat would never stay on during this activity. Be creative and be well-protected. You'll thank yourself as you watch the years go by. Sun is the number one cause of premature aging.

Hydrating Masks

Hydrating masks are generally concentrated moisturizers. Some are creams, and some come in gel form. If your skin is dehydrated, using a hydrating mask can help to relieve the dryness you may be feeling.

Generally, hydrating masks are applied in a thick layer to clean skin and left on for 15-20 minutes. Sometimes, for overnight hydration, I apply my gel hydrating mask in a thin layer, after cleansing and toning. I massage this into my skin, then apply my nighttime moisturizer, apply eye cream, and then go to bed. In the morning, my skin feels much smoother and better hydrated. Using a hydrating mask this way really can help to add moisture to your skin. If you have an oilier skin type, I would avoid using a cream mask overnight and opt for a gel-type hydrating mask.

If all else fails and you're without a moisturizing mask and need one, put a thick layer of your day or night cream on your face, just as you would a mask. Leave this on for 15-20 minutes, then remove. Be sure to exfoliate beforehand if possible. This will ensure the cream does the best possible job of hydrating your outer skin.

Hydroquinone

Hydroquinone is an ingredient that is used in bleaching creams to help lighten discolored skin. It is available over the counter in lower strengths, usually 2%, or at your dermatologist's office in higher 4%-6% strengths.

Some doctors are reluctant to prescribe hydroquinone. Although it can help to even out pigmentation, some feel there is a risk in terms of the chemical composition of this ingredient. There are studies being conducted to see if hydroquinone has a carcinogenic (cancer-causing) effect. There are no conclusive results from these studies, but no doubt more information will be available in the future.

Hydroquinone can be a skin irritant, so if you are going to use it to help lighten your hyperpigmentation, do monitor your skin and be sure it isn't developing any redness or irritation.

Hyperpigmentation

Hyperpigmentation is a concern for many people. I have included several emails regarding this often misunderstood skin condition. I hope you find these questions and answers helpful in your quest for even skin tone, free from pigmentation spots.

About 3 years ago I began to develop melasma from birth control pills, which I discontinued. I have discoloration above the lip (like a dark mustache), on my forehead near the hairline, directly above my eyebrows, and various other patches. I went to a dermatologist, stayed out of the sun, and used two different prescribed bleaching creams and was scrupulous with sunscreen.

Both worked well superficially, but during the sunnier months the darkness came back as if it had never gone away. Then to top it off, one of the products gave me whiteheads, which I still have to this day. I no longer use the products. I still have hope that this condition may reverse itself. Can you make some product recommendations? Right now I use drugstore products. Have you ever had a client experience a total reversal of melasma? Do I have hope or am I doomed to wear this shadowy mustache for the rest of my life?

This email says a lot. She developed hyperpigmentation (also called melasma or chloasma) from taking the Pill; she tried, unsuccessfully, to use prescription bleaching treatments; she is frustrated and is looking for a miracle (reversal of this condition). The questions and their answers are important to understand if you are ever going to take hold of your hyperpigmentation and have more evenly pigmented skin. The answers, however, may not be what you want to hear. Let's break this email down into smaller pieces.

About 3 years ago I began to develop melasma from birth control pills. When you are pregnant, on the Pill (when your body thinks you're pregnant), going through perimenopause, or just having fluctuations in your hormones (perhaps showing up as irregular periods), the result may be the same: hyperpigmentation or brown spots. Hormones can and do cause photosensitivity. Translation: hormones make your skin sun-sensitive. And although men are subject to hyperpigmentation (men have hormones too!), it is the hormone fluctuations females experience that can really cause pigmentation irregularities.

I went to a dermatologist, stayed out of the sun, and used two different prescribed bleaching creams and was scrupulous with sunscreen. It is common for people to seek the advice of a dermatologist for help in lightening their pigmentation spots. She had the right idea as far as staying out of the sun and always using sunscreen. It is direct sunlight that is going to darken the spots; no matter how long you are in the sun—minutes or even seconds—it all adds up.

Both worked well superficially, but during the sunnier months the darkness came back as if it had never gone away. The prescription creams or even over the counter types are only going to work to change what is on the surface of your skin. They are not meant to go deeper. But, and this is important, trying to treat the pigmentation problems in the warmer months is almost always going to be a lesson in futility. During the sunnier months, the sun is literally closer to the earth, and therefore the UV rays are going to be stronger. It's just a fact. So the best time to try bleaching or lightening hyperpigmentation is during the cooler months of the winter. You are inside more, unless you live in Florida or another year-round sunny climate, and you just aren't exposed to the degree you are in the summer months. I tell my clients if they are going to try to get rid of the spots, wait until the fall or winter when their efforts will possibly give them some results. Unfortunately, trying to treat the brown spots in the summer—especially if you are outside a good deal—for the most part is going to be all for naught. Summer is for prevention, preventing an increase in the darkness and preventing new pigmentation; winter is for lightening, due mostly to less UV radiation and any lightening creams you may be using.

Then to top it off, one of the products gave me whiteheads, which I still have to this day. I no longer use the products. I'm not sure why whiteheads were forming, but perhaps there was an ingredient in these prescription creams that this reader's skin couldn't tolerate—something too thick and occlusive. Discontinuing use of a product that appears to be doing something negative to your skin is always a good thing. In this particular case, I would recommend that you get in touch with your dermatologist, explain your complaint (whiteheads from the pigmentation creams), and see what he or she says. Perhaps there is another prescription treatment you can try that would work just as well on the spots without causing other conditions, like whiteheads.

I still have hope that this condition may reverse itself. The reversal is only possible if sunlight is no longer a factor. Obviously I am not advocating not going outside, but you have to get used to the idea of covering your face physically. This is done with hats or even putting your purse up to block the sun on your face while you are walking to and from your car. You will have to become diligent and conscientious of any and all sun hitting your face if you truly want to reduce the color of these spots. I don't view hyperpigmentation as curable, but it can be managed by making awareness of the sun a habit—for life.

Can you make some product recommendations? Right now I use drug-store products. Again, my answer is not the one you are looking for. The "product" to watch out for is the sun. Try any and all of the products available for reducing the darkness of chloasma, but in my experience they don't give the 100% results most people are looking for. There are laser procedures constantly being invented, and lasers for hyperpigmentation are no exception. Check with your dermatologist to see if there is a laser that can help with pigmentation irregularities. But be aware: sometimes these procedures can cause more harm than good. Do your research and proceed with caution.

Have you ever had a client experience a total reversal of melasma? I will speak for myself here. I haven't seen a "total reversal" of my melasma, but because I am so hyperaware of sun on my skin, I have decreased the look of hyperpigmentation on my face a thousandfold. Most people can't see the pigmentation spots because they are so faint. I can because it's my face, but the spots are so light even I don't notice them anymore. In the summer, especially if I'm roller blading or playing a lot of golf, watch out! Even the most diligent person (me!) cannot keep all darkness away. But I choose to trade some discoloration on my face for the pleasure that being outside provides for me in my life. But please know, when I am out enjoying various activities, my face is covered in a waterproof sunscreen, and I always have a hat on. I don't want to tempt fate, and I know I am prone to chloasma. So hats are simply a necessary part of my life.

Do I have hope or am I doomed to wear this shadowy mustache for the rest of my life? If you are constantly controlling the amount of sun your face gets, your moustache can and probably will go away or at least lighten considerably. We tend to sweat more on the upper lip area than other places on our faces, so keeping sunscreen there will be a bit of a challenge. The drill is sunscreen is great, but it is direct sunlight you want to avoid.

I am concerned because I spent a lot of time in the sun when I was younger playing tennis, swimming, running, etc. Now as a result, I have brown spots. So what do I do now?

My question to this person would be are you still an active, outdoorsy-type person? If the answer is yes, you can spend a lot of money erasing the spots you have accumulated from the past, but as long as you are still in the sun to a large (or even a small) degree, the brown spots are going to keep occurring. If you have them now, you are prone to getting them. If you are susceptible now, you probably will be for the rest of your life.

Rather than viewing this as a life sentence of irregular pigmentation, accept it as simply a fact and a reality in your life. If you read this entire section on hyperpigmentation, you will know that avoiding direct sunlight is going to be your biggest help in stopping the brown spots from occurring in the first place as well as helping lighten the darkness you already have incurred. Several of the newer laser technologies have had good results with existing pigmentation irregularities. But please know that you truly control this situation by controlling the amount of direct sunlight that reaches your face. You probably were not aware of this in the past, but by using this knowledge, you can help the dark spots to fade over time.

I have a funny brown spot on my lower neck. Why?

This question could also be about a white or pigmentless spot on one or both sides of the neck. The number one reason for this, from all the clients I have seen, is fragrance application and sun exposure.

Where do you put your perfume? On your lower neck or the sides of your neck? Up near your ears? If this is the case and you receive sun exposure, you are begging for hyperpigmentation or possibly hypopigmentation, which is loss of pigment resulting in white spots. Perfume is highly chemical and can cause a chemical reaction when exposed to UV radiation. So there is your problem.

However, if this "funny spot" is an irregular mole—especially one that has changed recently or is new—and not hyperpigmentation, I recommend having it checked out by a dermatologist now.

I break out and also have dark spots on my skin that I would love to try to lighten. Is there a product I could use for that?

There are several products out on the market that say they lighten pigmentation. Some are actually bleaching creams, and others inhibit melanin production. Many of the creams to reduce pigmentation also contain glycolic acid or even retinol. To any of you who have redness in your skin like couperose and especially rosacea, I caution you against using these types of creams. I see redness worsen when using AHAs (glycolic is an AHA) or retoinoids. Don't take care of one thing, like hyperpigmentation, and cause another, like redness or couperose.

Even if you successfully use one of these bleaching or melanin-inhibiting creams, you still have to be ultra-sensitive to how much sun exposure you are getting. No matter how light your spots get, if you are prone to hyperpigmentation, then you are prone to hyperpigmentation. Lightening the dark spots does not change this tendency.

It's a drag I know because I have hyperpigmentation. When I was about 32 my fluctuating hormones created for the first time in my life dark spots (chloasma, melasma, or hyperpigmentation). Whatever you want to call it, I had dark patches all over my face—mostly on my cheeks and forehead. Now in my 40s, things have not changed; I am still susceptible to darkness unless I am ultra-careful not to get direct sunlight on my face. I wear a water-resistant sunscreen every day, rain or shine, and still if I am not careful, I will get the dark spots.

If the pigmentation spots this emailer is inquiring about are due to her breakouts, this could be a condition called post-inflammatory hyperpigmentation. See that section for more detailed information.

I have a problem with a pigmentation spot on my face that will not go away. I've had it since childhood and have tried everything to get rid of it—hydroquinone, Retin-A, AHAs, everything, but with no success. I assume the spot is caused by sun exposure. It looks very much like the age spots older people get. I have extremely fair skin, so sun damage really shows up on my skin. What would you recommend?

Your dermatologist may be able to remove the spot with a laser; you'll have to go have a consultation and see what your options are. But keep in mind, any amount of sun you receive will increase the pigmentation— the darkness of spots. So the best preventative measure would be to always have your spot covered, even if it is simply by your hand as you are walking to and from the car. And definitely wear hats and use sunscreen when you are outside for any length of time.

Is the spot located in a place where sun easily gets to it when you are driving a car or even sitting in the passenger seat a lot? This is a common occurrence and means every time you drive or sit in the car, the spot is going to receive a lot of UV sun exposure. This is true even if your car windows are tinted. Granted, this darkened glass may inhibit some radiation, but not enough to stop hyperpigmentation.

Consult with a dermatologist if you are truly looking to remove this spot; perhaps he or she will be able to assist you. Also, if you are prone to hyperpigmentation, even if you were able to remove a particular pigmentation spot, there is no guarantee that same place or another place on your face won't turn dark in the future.

I have noticed I am getting brown freckles on my forehead.

This is simply pigmentation. When we are exposed to the sun, and especially as we get older, pigmentation irregularities are bound to happen. With sun exposure comes sun damage, sometimes in the form of simple freckles.

Hyperpigmentation is not a fun thing to have; but luckily it's not life-threatening, just a nuisance. So make covering your face a daily habit. Be aggressive about keeping direct sunlight off your face and wherever else you have developed hyperpigmentation. To read more about pigmentation irregularities and procedures that may help, read **Post-Inflammatory Hyperpigmentation** as well as **Intense Pulsed Light (IPL).**

I

Ice & Skin

I heard that rubbing ice on my face would help kill bacteria. I have problem skin and don't know what to do. Is ice good for my face?

I was reading in your book that I should always be washing my face with tepid water, never cold. On a talk show I heard a celebrity say his secret to looking young was to put his face down in a sink full of ice every morning.

Warning: *Do not try this at home!* The extreme cold of ice will cause the fragile capillaries of your face to constrict—forcefully so—and over time this will damage or "break" the vessels and cause permanent redness. If that story about the celebrity is true, I bet if you were up close to his face, you'd see that his skin is red, *red, RED!*

I have a client whose daughter was going to an aesthetician who had been using ice on her face to kill the bacteria. This may seem good in the short term, but in the long run it will no doubt cause considerable capillary damage. Maybe a teenager's capillaries would be stronger than an older person's, but nevertheless, this is a bad practice that I highly discourage. *Don't use ice on your skin!* (See **Capillaries**.)

Ingrown Hair

Ingrown hairs are basically hairs that have lost their way. Instead of moving directly up the hair follicle, which is cylindrical like a tunnel, the hair curls around and remains either close to the surface of the skin or actually makes its way back down to the base of the follicle. This inability to reach the skin's surface and eventual exit above it causes an ingrown hair.

Ingrown hairs are a problem for many people, but men tend to have the most trouble with ingrown hairs on their faces, which look like irritated bumps on the skin. This is especially true for African-American men because dark-skinned people generally have curly and coarse hair. Curlier hair has a more difficult time finding the surface of the skin. These ingrown hairs may cause inflammation to occur, which is a condition called *pseudofolliculitis barbae*.

Ingrown hairs generally form after the hair in a particular area has been cut, waxed, or in some other way removed. Some say that pulling the hair out against the natural grain (most waxing procedures follow this rule) can cause the hair to break just below the surface. Then when the dead cells set in, the hair can't find an exit, causing an ingrown hair.

Exfoliation is really important if you're prone to ingrown hairs—no matter where you get them. If they occur on your face, using a scrub or other exfoliator on a regular basis should help to alleviate the problem. This is where alpha hydroxy acids (AHAs) may come in handy. Several of my male clients have seen good results with their ingrown hair problems by using products that contain this ingredient. AHAs help to dissolve the intercellular glue that holds cells together, which can be helpful in the case of ingrown hairs. AHAs may work well for women who find ingrown hairs are a problem in the bikini line area.

Women who get ingrown hairs on their legs can try using AHAs, but because of the large surface area of the legs this could get quite expensive. Using exfoliation gloves may be your best bet. The gloves give you the ability to regulate pressure and therefore not irritate the skin. Do be careful not to rub too hard with these gloves. They are abrasive and too much of a good thing can turn bad.

Exfoliation gloves can be found at most stores where cosmetics are sold. They're easy to use and are machine washable. Unlike a loofah, you can get them clean and bacteria free between uses. They aren't very expensive so you could get several pairs and just throw them in the wash after each use. They make great gifts too. Put them in a basket with bath and body products and maybe a scented candle, and you will make someone very happy.

If you have irritation bumps with the ingrown hairs, be careful when you shave over this area. You can easily break open the skin and cause further irritation and possibly spread infection.

A product called TendSkin (see section) has been helpful for some people with ingrown hairs. Be careful to follow the directions and do not use on a large area of the face. Men's skin tends to be less sensitive than women's, but even so, if you are a man and have ingrown hair in your beard area, be careful to apply this product appropriately. If you experience irritation with TendSkin, discontinue use immediately and refer back to some other products and techniques for helping with ingrown hairs. You don't ever want to use a product that is causing more harm than good.

In the end, no matter where the ingrown hairs are forming, exfoliation is the best course of treatment.

Intense Pulsed Light (IPL)

In your book you say there isn't anything that can be done about broken capillaries, but I had successful laser sessions a year ago that erased most of them from my face.

This email came from a client of mine. Indeed, she had severe couperose (broken capillaries), predominately in her cheek and nose area. She did achieve remarkable results from having her capillaries lasered. It took several sessions, but over 70% of the damage was eliminated.

Intense Pulsed Light (IPL) can be an effective treatment for mild or severe couperose, rosacea, or just getting rid of those pesky capillaries that have been hanging around on your face for so long. I have many clients who have had success with this procedure and are now enjoying less redness in their skin. One of the benefits of this treatment versus some of the older laser versions is it can treat tiny broken capillaries as well as redness deep within the skin where abnormal vessels are found, which is especially good for rosacea sufferers. Because IPL helps to alleviate the flushing associated with rosacea, treatments can really have a long-term effect.

IPL is also effective for getting rid of hyperpigmentation, making your skin tone even and free from pigmentation spots. Because sun exposure is what caused this condition in the first place, you will be instructed to be very aggressive with your sun protection program; it will not be just temporary care, but diligent sun protection for the rest of your life.

Although I don't believe in before and after pictures in most circumstances, in several books discussing IPL for redness, the before and after pictures speak volumes for this procedure's efficacy. The photos give a clear view of the patient's skin prior to IPL, which looks like skin with medium to severe capillary damage. Afterward, there is at least a 60% reduction in redness—the capillaries have disappeared. I have also seen these results in several of my clients.

Usually you will first go through a consultation with your dermatologist or a physician's assistant in the office. They will go over your needs and wants as well as procedural information. Then you will find out about cost. IPL is not cheap. On average, each treatment is around $500, and you have at least five treatments in a series. However, if you are suffering from severe hyperpigmentation, rosacea, or just capillary damage, and you are willing to truly commit to aggressively protecting your skin (especially your face) from sun exposure, then IPL may be the miracle you have been searching for.

Your skin may be red for a day or two, but (if you have rosacea) it was red already, so it may not look very different after the treatment. Once the redness subsides, what you should be left with is less redness and an overall improved condition.

Depending on your pain tolerance and the normal procedure at the doctor's office, you may have a topical anesthetic applied to the skin being treated. This is not a painless procedure, but the effects can last a long time, making it worth the small amount of discomfort you may experience.

> *I had a wonderful treatment called PhotoFacial™ that really helped to eliminate acne scars I've had for years, as well as hyperpigmentation from when I was pregnant. It's a bit uncomfortable, like a rubberband snap, but tolerable—and worth it! I had a series of 5 treatments, each one was about 2-3 weeks apart.*

PhotoFacial (developed by Dr. Patrick Bitter, Sr.) is yet another name for IPL therapy; FotoFacial™ and EpiLight™ are a few more. No matter the name, if hyperpigmentation, rosacea, broken capillaries, or perhaps even acne scars are a concern, investigate IPL and see if it works for you. Laser techniques are analogous to computers; the technology is advancing and expanding so rapidly that the lasers used today may be obsolete tomorrow. As with all procedures, please get more than one opinion, and *do your homework.* When it comes to your face, you want someone who has a lot of experience and a great reputation working with IPL.

Juicing   **262**

Juicing

Juicing is not to be confused with drinking juice. The two couldn't be more different. Juicing involves taking whole fruits and vegetables (skin, rinds, and all) and putting them through a machine called a juicer. What comes out is the liquid version of whatever you put through the machine. Drinking juice, orange or apple or grape, for instance, usually involves ingesting a manufactured product that has other ingredients in it, not just the fruit juice. Juicing is a way of getting pure vitamins and minerals into your body very quickly and without any preservatives or other chemicals.

I was given a juicer about four years ago as a birthday present from a dear friend. In all of those years, I used it once. In fact, I wasn't sure if I should pack it up and bring it to Chicago when I moved. Why should I? I had only used it once! At the time I didn't have a good book on juicing, and I wasn't very clear on the hows and whys of juicing. So, like many things in life, I just forgot about it.

Then a friend of mine who was a big proponent of juicing helped get me started on the juicing path. It came at a time when I was in the throes of writing this book and had been neglecting my dietary needs; if I wasn't skipping meals altogether, I was eating foods I don't often eat—things that were not contributing to a healthy body. My friend's enthusiasm about juicing spurred me on to develop my own enthusiastic pursuit of juicing for my health.

Most mornings I try to have a glass of cantaloupe juice, usually one quarter of a large melon. As with most fruits and vegetables, the entire rind of the cantaloupe is used as well as the fruit inside. At first this may sound strange, but almost all of the vitamin and mineral content is held in the rinds of fruits. So by drinking the entire cantaloupe, I am getting tremendous benefits, outweighing just eating the inside fruit alone. Cantaloupes are high in vitamin C and provitamin A (beta carotene) and contain high quantities of digestive enzymes. Cantaloupes are actually one of the most nutritious fruits available. Drinking this juice first thing in the morning is giving my body a good start each day. Because it's a seasonal fruit, I usually juice cantaloupes in the warmer months.

On a personal note: I adhere to several of the rules of food combining. One rule is never mix melons with any other food, including other fruits. So, although when I juice I usually combine several fruits and vegetables together to make one drink, I juice cantaloupe by itself.

There are many juicing machines available. I have a small, inexpensive one (under $100) that has a good motor. You can spend hundreds of dollars on a juicer, but you don't have to. It depends on how much you are *really* going to use the juicer. If you haven't done this before, you might want to go with a less expensive machine until you are sure juicing is something you are going to do regularly. Even if you can only juice once a week, it would be great for your health!

I highly recommend preparing what you are going to juice right after you get home from the grocery store. It doesn't take that much time, and it will save you the trouble of doing it when you want to juice. First I use a vegetable wash that helps to remove dirt, wax, and any pesticides from the produce. Even if you buy "organic," I recommend getting everything you can off the rinds and skins of the food so you won't be ingesting it. Next I clean the fruits and vegetables with a vegetable brush. Then I cut up all the produce I will be eventually juicing so I don't have to do this work later on. I put everything in well-sealed containers then into the refrigerator.

The cleanup after juicing is my least favorite part—or course! But you must do this soon after juicing to keep any residue from collecting in your juicer. Usually I rinse everything really well and only use soap on the plastic parts. For the metal disc the produce goes through, I have a brush (different than my vegetable brush) that I use to get all the pulp and debris out. You don't want bacteria forming because you didn't do a thorough job of cleaning your machine.

Because I want to get the juice into my body when it's freshest, I drink the juice I've just made, slowly but steadily, then I clean my juicer. This way the juice isn't standing around losing precious nutrients while I am cleaning up. I adhere to the adage, "Chew your liquids and drink your solids." So be sure not to guzzle the juice; let your saliva help to predigest this concentrated health elixir and let it go down slowly. (And enjoy!)

There are several books on the market describing what juicing is and how to juice different fruits and vegetables. I have read several of these books, but found one to stand out above the rest. You may have seen Jay Kordich, aka The Juiceman®, on TV infomercials. It is his book, *The Juiceman's Power of Juicing*, that is the one I use on a daily basis. I found the instructions about how to juice, what tools I would need, and even information on juicers to be the most straightforward and easy to understand.

Whether you choose to read his book or another book on the subject, I hope you will add juicing to your diet. It is a wonderful way to get powerful nutrients easily and readily into your body—for your health!

I couldn't end this section without telling you one more thing! As you will read in the **Sugar** section, I am sensitive to sugar and believe that sugar causes breakouts—not just in my skin, but in anyone skin-sensitive to sugar. With that said, when you start juicing be careful how much carrot juice you drink. I have found through trial and error that I am highly sensitive to the sugar in carrots and drinking carrot juice will (always) make my skin break out. It tends to give me canker sores (see section) as well. So, in your quest to bring the power of juicing into your life, do watch how your skin may be reacting to high-sugar produce like carrots. You may not breakout, but if you are sensitive to sugar, you may.

K

Keratosis Pilaris

What causes these small bumps on the outsides of my upper arms? I also find bumps on my rear and my upper thighs, again on the outsides.

This is probably a condition called *keratosis pilaris*, which is an inflammatory disorder characterized by an accumulation of cells surrounding the hair follicles, as well as a rough texture to the skin. It usually occurs on the outsides of the upper arms, thighs, and even the buttocks.

If you are experiencing these bumps on your arms (or legs), this is a case where I wouldn't hesitate to recommend a retinoid product or alpha hydroxy acid (AHA) cream or lotion to help this problem. Why? Because I wouldn't be concerned that the acids would be irritating the delicate capillaries that are found on your face. The desquamation (exfoliation) ability of these types of products might work very well on the bumps. One caveat: I would use an inexpensive brand because you don't need to use an expensive cream on the backs of your arms, thighs, and buttocks. Save your money for your face. Use one of these products consistently, and see if it helps the bumps go away.

I have evidently inherited keratosis pilaris (little red bumps on the back of my arms and on the front of my thighs) from my parents and grandparents. When I try to moisturize (because most of the literature mentions that it is a dry skin-related issue) it just causes more bumps. I am tired of my skin looking this way. The dermatologists either give me Tazorac® gel* and a greasy lotion, or they just tell me to live with it! Meanwhile I am embarrassed to wear a sleeveless shirt, and now I am nervous about wearing shorts. All of my reading seems to suggest that I must use some form of

Retin-A, which is extremely hard on my skin. I would appreciate any insight you can provide. It seems like there must be something out there that can help!

*Tazorac is the brand name for tazarotene, a retinoid product.

As with many skin conditions, keratosis pilaris is not one, in my opinion, that can be helped completely from the outside in. From my own experience with this skin problem, I believe it is related more to diet than being just a "dry skin-related issue." I believe your body can get rid of this condition once you understand what may be causing it. I don't usually live by the "get over it" theory of skin care. I have faith and hope for you! My first question would be how is your diet? Tell me what is *bad* in your diet—especially if you eat or drink it consistently. The response to my question was:

I was afraid you were going to ask me about my diet! I am certainly not as healthy as I should be. My two downfalls are anything with cheese, and sodas. Although I try to drink water, I am afraid I don't come close to what I should be drinking on a daily basis.

My personal experience is that when I eat certain things in excess, the bumps will appear. After I stop eating these foods, eventually the bumps will disappear. I find milk and dairy products cause keratosis pilaris, as well as sugary foods. Dairy products can not only cause bumps like keratosis pilaris, but I have also seen an excess of dairy consumption to lead to milia (whiteheads) on the face.

So, right off the bat I think this client's problem is too much dairy, along with too much sugar or sugar substitutes in her sodas. If these are both her downfalls, she has a somewhat long road ahead of her if she indeed wants to get rid of the bumps on her arms and legs. One way to find out if dairy is the offending substance is to eliminate it from your diet—completely—and see what happens. Understand that even though you may take something out of your diet, it may take time for your body to rid itself of the culprit. If the condition clears up during this sabbatical, you may have found the cause of your problems. However, to be sure, I recommend reintroducing dairy, for instance, and see if the bumps recur. You may be able to get away with eating some of the offending substance, but not to the degree you did in the past. If you monitor the situation, you can control it.

Without trying the elimination experiment, you won't ever know if something you are ingesting is literally feeding the problem. Simply applying topical medications does little at the source to stop the problem from occurring. Using retinoid or AHA creams may help the immediate problem, however, so do try these (as long as they don't irritate your skin). But to avoid future problems, look to your diet and do the elimination experiment. This will give you the long-term information you are looking for.

Last summer I purchased some AHAs from you for the bumps on the backs of my arms. The AHAs definitely helped, but nothing seemed to totally eliminate the bumps. I never had this problem until we moved to Chicago. Recently my husband and I moved to L.A., and the bumps were much better but not completely gone. Since the water here has a lot of chlorine in it, I bought a chlorine filter for my shower head. Within a couple of weeks, the bumps had almost disappeared! I thought if you have clients who struggle with this problem you could pass this information along to them. I just purchased a cheap filter attachment at the hardware store, unscrewed the shower head and attached it myself in about two minutes.

My belief is that keratosis pilaris shows up due to dietary excesses more than for any other reason. However, as this client found out, it can also be caused by other factors. I'm a big believer in doing what works—whatever that may be. So give the water filter suggestion a try. Chlorine is so bad for skin *and* hair, having a filter on your shower head is a good idea whether you have keratosis pilaris or not.

Kinerase®

Kinerase is the name for a nonprescription cream that is only available (currently) from a doctor's office. It is said to help retard the aging process. It utilizes the natural growth hormone in plants called *N6-furfuryladenine*. It is this plant hormone that helps the leaves stay healthy, moist, and alive. Kinerase is available in both a cream and a lotion; each contain 0.1% of the plant hormone ingredient. The lotion is lighter, for normal to oily skin types; the cream is for true-dry (oil-dry) skin. Kinerase can be used in conjunction with your regular skin care products, as well as with makeup or even sunscreens.

Unlike Retin-A or Renova® or other anti-aging counterparts, this treatment does not (according to most information available) cause redness, irritation, or flaking of the outer skin. In fact, it is often used after peels (whether strong or gentle) to help ease skin irritation or redness that might have occurred.

For the most part, Kinerase is best used on skin that has been damaged by the sun. In clinical studies some improvement has occurred in both wrinkles and pigmentation, although only modestly. It can be used by women who are pregnant or nursing, something some other topical anti-aging products prohibit.

Although I haven't used this product, the word from my clients who have is that they saw little or no improvement (or detrimental effects) with their skin. They didn't see any significant changes in their lines and wrinkles, or with the small amount of hyperpigmentation a few of them have on their faces.

I chalk this product up to the ravenous appetite of some consumers and the cosmetic industry as a whole for products that will stop, impede, or otherwise change the most natural act we will go through in life: aging. Out of 24 ingredients listed on the jar, the anti-aging component N6-furfuryladenine was the very last ingredient. Maybe that is enough to affect a change in the skin, but it seems like this is an expensive moisturizer with a little bit of the anti-aging plant hormone in it.

You may want to try this product as directed and see if it helps with either pigmentation or lines and wrinkles. Your experience may be different than the experiences I have heard about.

L

Lavender

Lavender is probably the most popular and widely recognized of all the essential oils. Lavender has numerous healing abilities. Probably the best-known is the effect of this essential oil on burns. Lavender is even used in burn units in some hospitals in France. I know if I had a severe burn, I would want essential oil of lavender as at least one of the healing tools used.

My friend Elizabeth called and said she had splashed hot oil on her face while cooking the night before. Although the spots were fairly small where the oil had met her skin, they were starting to blister and were red. She had Neosporin® (an antibiotic cream) in her medicine cabinet and used that until we talked the next day. I recommended she go to her health food store and purchase a bottle of pure essential oil of lavender. Lavender oil has excellent properties that help to alleviate the pain of a burn, and it also has a tremendous ability to help start the healing process for the damaged cells. And as with almost all essential oils, lavender also has antibiotic properties. I instructed Elizabeth to simply apply the lavender oil to the affected areas as often as she could, and no doubt it would help her skin to heal as well as soothe the pain, which it did. Elizabeth called a few days later and said all signs of the oil burns on her skin were gone. She agreed that everyone should have lavender oil in their first-aid kit.

I always travel with a bottle of lavender in my skin care kit. Lavender oil has natural antibiotic as well as antiseptic abilities. It is a mood enhancer, helping to calm you down during times of stress. It can even help you sleep if you put a few drops on a cloth or a pillowcase. As mentioned above, it is excellent to put on burns. Lavender is truly an important product to have in your medicine cabinet or travel kit.

HOT TIP: *After a smoke-filled night (in a bar or restaurant, for instance), you can take a shower or bath to wash the smell off your skin, but what about your hair? It's late and you don't want to go to bed with wet hair, so what can you do? Essential oils to the rescue! Take an essential oil you love (I think lavender, ylang ylang, or a citrus oil would be best) and put several drops (4-8) in the palm of your hand; rub your hands together and then go over your hair. Be sure to get the underside as well as the top of your hair. Just mix the oils in really well and you won't have to go to bed smelling like cigarette smoke.*

Lips, Chapped

Why do lips get chapped in the first place?

The tissue that comprises your lips doesn't have any oil or sweat glands like the rest of your body does, so the lips can quite easily become chapped. Did you know that simply habitually licking your lips can cause chapping? We may think that the moisture from our saliva will help hydrate our lips, but in actuality it dehydrates them due to moisture evaporation. Licking your lips just makes things worse.

Also if you are on medication you may experience chapped lips. Medications alter the body's natural functions and may induce dry skin on the body as well as the lips. As you may have read in the **Accutane** section, dry, chapped lips are a common occurrence while taking this drug. Also, if you are on chemotherapy, you probably have discovered that your lips are continually chapped due to the harsh chemicals that are infiltrating your body.

In addition, dry air (like in the desert) or the cold air of winter can cause chapping. You may find yourself wetting your lips with your tongue to overcome the dry feeling, and as I've already said, licking your lips actually *creates* dry, chapped lips.

Last of all, lipsticks in general have a lot of drying ingredients in them and if you wear lipstick, no doubt you have had chapped lips at one time or another.

What can I do about severely chapped lips? Are there any good lip products?

Although it is a common problem, chapped lips can become a thing of the past. What does it take? Diligence and consistent use of proper lip products. And in the case of severely chapped lips, a vacation from lipstick—a product that probably caused much of the chapping in the first place.

One reason I don't have chapped lips: I don't wear lipstick. I haven't for over 10 years, and when I did wear it, my lips were invariably chapped—if not always, then often. I am not advocating giving up lipstick altogether, but I am recommending becoming aware that lipstick could very well be a main culprit in your chapped lips conundrum. If you don't want chapped lips, you must be prepared to treat your lips—especially if you are a lipstick wearer.

Using a lip balm is going to be your best and safest bet to stave off chapped lips. I prefer non-petroleum lip balms, which can usually be found at health food stores. Buy several, and then put them *everywhere!* Typically they are about $2 apiece. So I buy five or six, and spread them out in my home, office, in my jeans, and regularly used jackets, so I don't have to worry about being without. They last for an eternity since I have so many in use at one time, and my lips are never chapped because I am consistently attending to them.

One last recommendation: don't bite your lips! Trying to bite off the chapped skin that is sometimes hanging off your lips just causes more problems. It creates tiny tears in the lip tissue, which can bleed and take a long time to heal. Instead of tearing that delicate skin, just slather your lips with a non-petroleum lip balm and stay away from lipstick for at least a few days and let your lips heal. I know it's hard to leave the lipstick off, but treat your lips as though they are injured, and give them loving care—and lip balm!

Although non-petroleum lip balms are the products that I recommend most for chapped lips, the downside is they don't add color to your lips; tinted lip balms do, but they don't have the coverage like a true lipstick. However there are some products on the market that can give you moisturizing abilities in a regular lipstick.

I have a client who has always had very dry, cracked lips. Aside from lipstick use, there doesn't seem to be a clear and definite reason for this severe condition. Because of her lip concerns, she has tried every lipstick and lip product known to womankind. I have seen an improvement in her lips since she started consistently using one of the newer **moisturizing lipsticks**. Try one of these moisturizing lip products and see if it helps with your dry, cracked lips. I recommend finding a moisturizing lipstick with SPF 15 (at least). You want to protect your lips from the sun—not just your skin. And to treat your cracked lips at night, do use a non-petroleum lip balm.

Cracking and dryness at the *corners* of the mouth is a different problem. The following was written by one of my clients in Dallas, Debbie:

In the past week, I have developed cracks in the corners of my mouth. I looked these symptoms up and have found that this can be a riboflavin deficiency. I take a lot of vitamins every day, so this seems odd to me. The only other cause that I can think of is stress.

Up until last week I was under a lot of stress. What do you think the cause is, and how should I treat this?

Symptoms of stress can be anything from looking and feeling tired to more severe problems like the kind Debbie has described. Many times stress will have a delayed response in the body, so even though the stress may be over (the wedding, the divorce, the new job, the event) the symptoms of a depleted body may keep on coming. It's as though your body takes the brunt of the stress for a certain period of time, then it crosses over the threshold of tolerance. That is when the symptoms really begin to show.

Cracking at the corners of the mouth is thought to be a riboflavin (vitamin B2) deficiency. The B vitamins are known as the "stress vitamins." When we are stressed out, vitamin B is easily depleted from our system. Because these vitamins are water-soluble, they are easily destroyed by alcohol, pollution, smoking, and stress, to name just a few causes.

Although Debbie was on the right track for figuring out why she was experiencing cracking at the corners of her mouth, it wasn't until another six months went by that she discovered the real culprit. After trial and error with vitamins and products put directly on her lips, Debbie returned to her dermatologist who said it could be *toothpaste* that was causing her troubles. Honestly, when Debbie first told me this I was skeptical, although I had recently read about toothpaste causing reactions like perioral dermatitis, a condition that I didn't link to Debbie's.

Debbie called me and said that she didn't want to jinx the results, but after switching toothpaste, her cracking problems cleared up within three days! Debbie's problems began in October and it was now April. I asked her if she switched brands anywhere near the time she was getting cracked lips. Due to an important event (the one she was so stressed about in the email), she wanted to have bright, white teeth and started using a special toothpaste made for this right around the time she started having the problems.

You really have to become your own private detective when it comes to figuring out why you have "all of a sudden" developed a skin condition—or a change in anything having to do with your body. I talk a lot about this in regard to sugar and breakouts. Without finding what the offending substance is, whether a food or in Debbie's case, a product, your problems may persist. If Debbie's doctor hadn't suggested this seemingly unrelated product (toothpaste) as being the cause, she would have continued to use it and continued to have skin problems. Or at some point, Debbie might have gone off the toothpaste, and her lip problems would have cleared up, but she might not have connected the two events.

Awareness is the key, along with being able to dissect your life in such a way as to figure out even the most mundane of activities or products used and how they may be affecting your health. I am happy to report Debbie's cracking problems have completely gone away, and needless to say, she won't be using teeth whitening toothpaste ever again!

You talked about a light-colored lip balm this morning on a TV news program. Could you please give me information about this product? Where can I get it, and what was the brand name? I don't wear any makeup at all, but there are times I would like a little color on my lips. The product you mentioned sounds perfect for me. I have been looking for something like that for a long time.

The items I was showing on TV were tinted non-petroleum lip balms. They are wonderful problem-solvers because they are treating your lips while at the same time giving them some color. The pigments in these colored balms are not as dense as in a real lipstick, so they don't give you deep color, but they do give you some color. The actual products I had on the show are made by a company called Un-Petroleum®, although they are not the only company with tinted lip balms on the market. They can be found at most health food stores, and I've even seen some at regular grocery stores.

Chapped lips no longer need to be a problem. Sometimes you can't avoid the causes, but you can always contribute to the healing of chapped, dry lips—primarily by using lip balms as often as possible. No matter what you use on your lips, do use something, and you can kiss chapped lips good-bye.

Lipstick

I've always wondered what happens to lipstick when it wears off—does it just evaporate?

In an article I read about lipsticks, it said that on average, women who regularly wear lipstick will consume (that means eat!) over 750 tubes of lipsticks during their lifetime! Where do you think your lipstick has gone when you look in the mirror and have to reapply? You may have just had a glass of wine and a good conversation, but you probably also ate your lipstick. And by unconsciously licking your lips throughout the day, you are furthering the ingestion of this product.

The article went on to say that according to the gastroenterologist quoted you swallow so little at a time there really isn't any harm to your body. He stated that the waxes and polymers in lipsticks are nontoxic and are broken down by stomach acids. Well, if the research for this article is correct, and a woman can conceivably consume as many as 750 full tubes of lipstick during her lifetime, I cannot see anything good about ingesting these substances. Lipstick contains a lot of questionable ingredients that you may want to think twice about before eating day after day. No doubt large amounts of lipstick go through your body to be digested, so if you can find alternative products that perhaps don't have as many bad ingredients in them, then I recommend giving these a try.

I've been looking for a moisturizing lipstick with sunscreen for years, but lipstick dries out my lips and makes them peel.

I recommend having your favorite lipsticks on hand to wear at night if you are going out and a tinted lip balm with SPF for daytime. This way you won't have to forgo lipstick altogether, yet you can have protecting products on your lips throughout the day. Tinted lip balms may be the best option for you. As I've said, they won't give you the coverage of an actual lipstick, but you won't have to contend with all the chapping you have now. Less color, but less chapping—hopefully this will be a happy compromise for you.

Ethylhexl methoxycinnamate, by the way, is a sunscreen ingredient commonly used in lip products with SPF. Avobenzone is also used in many products (see this section for more information).

Do treatment lipsticks containing anti-aging ingredients such as Kinetin* and vitamin C really work?

*Kinetin is a plant-based "miracle" ingredient that is supposed to help reduce wrinkles.

Are you confusing your actual facial skin with the tissue of your lips? These two different types of tissue don't age the same way. You cannot use an anti-aging lipstick on your lips and hope to help the wrinkles you may be concerned about *above* your lips. Using vitamin C on your lips would come under this same umbrella.

My recommendation is to stop looking for one product to solve many problems. Wear lipstick to color your lips. If it contains special ingredients and you find these helpful, great. But I wouldn't recommend searching for lipsticks that have "all the rage" ingredients in them and paying the high price for these types of products. If you want to keep your lips from drying and flaking, you may find a lipstick that helps with that specific concern. But I highly recommend wearing a non-petroleum lip balm whenever you aren't wearing lipstick, especially at night before bed.

HOT TIP: *Lipstick is one of the top offenders in making your lips chapped or keeping them chapped. Try switching to non-petroleum lip balms whenever possible.*

M

Magnifying Mirrors

At the end of Chapter One of *Timeless Skin* I wrote:

I strongly recommend not using a magnifying mirror when it comes to looking at your face. Unless you require one to apply makeup, there is no need to make yourself crazy with this unrealistic view of your skin. No one looking at your skin can see what shows up through magnification. Not even you!

Recently a new client, Diane, called me about her problem skin, wondering if I could help her. We spoke for a few minutes, and she booked a facial. She came in without makeup, and I noticed her skin looked to be in pretty good shape although she reiterated her concern for "all the breakouts" she was experiencing. At first glance I thought perhaps she had gotten a little too much sun over her lifetime, but all in all, she didn't have a lot of problems that I could see. Later I would look at her skin under magnification. That would tell me the real story.

I filled out a questionnaire and proceeded with the facial. I asked what her top concerns were regarding her skin and she replied, "I want to stop all the breakouts and stop my skin from aging." I stepped up onto my soapbox about the aging process, basically explaining to her my philosophy that "you will age!" And yes, certain things can be done to keep the process from speeding up, but certainly nothing can ultimately be done to literally stop the aging process from happening.

As I examined her skin, I wasn't finding the breakout she complained about. I could see some residual spots clearing from previous infections, but her skin looked good to me with just a few areas that needed clearing. She simply had normal skin with a few spots here and there, but nothing major. The first red flag presented itself.

I questioned her about her diet and found out she didn't eat well. Normally she ate lots of fast foods and was a consumer of large amounts of sugar. (She did have a few places on her nose that looked to me like sugar spots—tiny infections with sebum in the middle, but she was lucky her skin wasn't a mess due to her diet.) I thought to myself, "Something is wrong here; we are not seeing eye to eye." This is not to say that a client's view of his or her skin is always the same as my own opinion. But with Diane, she really had a very critical view of her skin, and I wasn't able to concur.

When I look at a client's skin, I am comparing what I see to thousands of clients who have come before. And in Diane's case, I not only wouldn't classify her skin as the worst I've seen, but she wouldn't even make the list of clients with problem skin. I was beginning to realize her problem was something other than with her skin.

Later in the facial she started asking me what she could do about "all the hair on her face." What hair? She meant the normal, everyday, run-of-the-mill peach fuzz we all have on our faces. "You need to leave it alone," I said.

Then it hit me: She has a magnifying mirror. I asked her if she used one and sure enough, I was right. She had been looking at her skin from the point of view of almost seven times its normal size. *Everything* looked huge—her pores, the hair on her face, any small blemish that might be present—everything! No wonder she had a skewed view of her skin. Nothing looks normal in those mirrors!

She said she needed to use the mirror to tweeze her brows. I asked Diane if she could restrain herself and only use the magnifying mirror to shape her brows and not look at her skin. She said she would try. It would take discipline, but I have faith that where there's a will, there's a way.

I wanted to tell Diane's story to illustrate how you can drive yourself crazy by looking at yourself enlarged. What would it be like if we magnified our voices seven times the normal volume or magnified pain seven times? Don't magnify your perfectly good skin seven times larger by looking at it through a magnifying mirror! Otherwise you are simply and completely setting yourself up for failure, disappointment, and ultimately for taking steps to solve a problem you probably don't even have. Trust me, don't use magnifying mirrors for anything other than applying makeup (if you can't see very well), shaping your eyebrows*, or for some other positive reason. And if you do have problems with your skin, looking through a magnifying mirror certainly isn't going to help clear it up. Looking at your lifestyle habits and making better choices will be a surer way to bring about long-term, permanent change.

*Using a magnifying mirror to shape your eyebrows can be equally disastrous for your skin if you don't use restraint. Once again, no one can see the stray hair of your brows unless he or she is standing extremely close to your face. What usually happens is you will see hair that no one else can see, perhaps hair that isn't even ready to be tweezed. You go after it, can't get it, and then have to get it. Due to your diligence you break the skin, causing a tear, which will cause a scab to form. You may have gotten that stray hair, but now you have a very obvious scab or scabs on your brows. You have just given attention to something you were trying to conceal.

Melanoma

Skin cancer is a real and lethal threat. Many people seem to have a lackadaisical approach to their skin and having moles checked. Even when it has been recommended to have a growth checked out, many times people don't heed the call. (See **Basal Cell Carcinoma** for examples of this.) The bottom line is, skin cancer—melanoma specifically—can kill you. And the good news is, if detected early, melanoma is usually totally curable. In fact, it is one of the only curable forms of cancer. It is also preventable to a large degree. Prevention involves being hyperaware of sun exposure and wearing hats, protective clothing, and sunscreen whenever (and however long) you are in the sun. Don't risk your life: go to your dermatologist. If you don't have one, get one, and have a full-body check done on your moles. Why wait? The following are some stories from clients and friends about their melanoma experiences. They are good examples of the importance of getting regular mole checkups. (See **Resources** to find a dermatologist in your area.)

Roxanne's story. I always recommend clients get a full body check when they go to their dermatologists, no matter what the reason is for the visit. During a normal office visit, the doctor might not check all of your moles, so be sure to ask for that service. Don't pass up any opportunity to get your moles looked at. Luckily my client, Roxanne, followed this advice.

I sent her in for a funny-looking mole on her forehead. The good news is the mole wasn't anything to worry about. The other news is rather shocking. As the doctor did a check of all of her moles, she noticed something on Roxanne's left forearm, on the underside. After the biopsy, this small mole turned out to be malignant melanoma—the deadliest type of skin cancer.

Poor Roxanne. She had just given birth to her second child and the news of skin cancer was understandably quite upsetting. Melanoma can kill you if gone undetected. It enters the blood stream, and unlike the slow growing basal cell carcinoma, it spreads rapidly and eventually affects the entire body if given a chance.

Roxanne is now sporting a rather large (compared to the size of the mole) scar on her arm. It's a small price for living a life fulfilled. Without the keen eye of a skin doctor, this mole might have gone unnoticed for years, eventually causing Roxanne more problems than just a long scar. Don't delay, get your moles checked today!

Sally's story. Sally went to her dermatologist for an annual mole check. During the examination, the doctor noted a small freckle on her back that she wasn't even aware of and had it removed to biopsy. Sally wasn't really worried about the removal of this spot—until the results from the tests came back: melanoma in situ, which is an early stage of skin cancer. She went in to get the area surrounding the original spot removed until no cancerous cells were found.

Sally is one of the lucky ones. Luck didn't have anything to do with the fact that she schedules regular visits with her dermatologist. That is simply smart on her part. Her story goes to show you that these regular exams are crucial in keeping skin cancer from having too long to proliferate. Without this exam, Sally might not have ever noticed this spot on her back, and that could have been fatal in time.

If you are in the sun on a regular basis, you really should have a regular mole check at your dermatologist. If you are not in the sun a lot, but are over 35 or 40 years old, I recommend getting a baseline check (the initial data recorded about your moles and skin irregularities), and then going in annually to be sure nothing has changed with any spots or moles.

Sally will now be visiting her dermatologist more often than once a year to be sure there aren't any more problem places and to keep an eye on the spot where the cancer was removed. This is a small inconvenience for keeping skin cancer away. Found early, skin cancer is treatable.

Ronald's story. My friend Ronald was in town on business, and we met for dinner one night. He asked me about how I was coming on the book and I told him I was currently writing the section on melanoma. He proceeded to tell me his father's skin cancer story.

His dad had a biopsy done on some unusual moles, and for whatever reason, never got the lab results back. The doctor never called him, and he just figured no news was good news. Unfortunately, he did have malignancies, and over time they took over his body, and he eventually died of malignant melanoma. This is one of those rare cases of an oversight, but it can and does happen.

I tell this story so you will be sure to get the lab analysis of any skin biopsies that are taken, even if the tests show the growths are benign (non-cancerous). This may seem obvious, but every once in a while a mistake takes place due to human error, as this story so tragically illustrates.

Men's Skin

What skin care advice do you have for a man?

This question comes from many different men I have spoken with about skin care. My short answer (and this is specifically directed to men) is: *use products!* Classically, men are not huge consumers of skin care products. That of course is changing, but by and large, men are not as educated in matters of the skin as many women are. The Basics (cleansing, toning, and moisturizing) would be about all I would ask a man to do for his skin. If he is truly looking to do more—great! The Extras (exfoliating and using a clay mask) would be excellent additions to anyone's skin care program, male or female. Most men just don't use any or many products on their skin, so I like to start them off slowly and see how it goes. Usually once they see a positive difference in their skin, they are more willing to do a few extras to further help the health of their skin. (See **The Basics** and **The Extras**.)

I would like some recommendations for men. My brother has some problem areas, and I would like to pass along some information to help him. What exactly should a man with problem skin do?

The recommendations for a man with problem skin are really no different than for a woman. The main difference in this equation is men are generally not accustomed to doing much with their skin. So for a man to treat his problem skin may mean using products when in the past he didn't use any. I think you have to take this into consideration when making suggestions. To recommend a lot of products to someone—especially a man—who isn't using anything is probably a mistake. It's just too much, and the routine is doomed to failure.

The Basics would be beneficial for any skin, especially if there are problems with breakout. You want non-alkaline skin care products, which includes your cleanser. Aveeno bar soap or Cetaphil liquid cleanser are both easy to find and are pH balanced.

A spray-on toner that has essential oils in it would be good to use following shaving and dabbing pure essential oils neat (straight) on the blemishes would make an excellent spot treatment for breakouts. Remember, breakout needs antibacterial products to help quell the growth and proliferation of bacteria. Without treating the blemishes, they will just take their own sweet time going away. I don't recommend oxy-type products, as they are usually too harsh and drying; essential oils are my personal products of choice. (See **Geranium**.)

Shaving may open up blemishes that are trying to go away, prolonging the healing process. If you are trying to clear up broken out skin, if possible try not to shave for a few days. Obviously this may not be something you can do, but by not shaving and treating the spots with essential oils, you are giving your skin the time it needs to heal. When you do shave, be very careful to avoid opening the blemishes up. I understand this is not an easy task. Try shaving *with* the hair growth in order to avoid too close of a shave and possibly nicking the blemishes.

Finally, using some sort of treatment cream (moisturizer) would be good. Many men are not accustomed to using creams on their faces. And some men might not like the way a moisturizer feels on their skin. However, if you want optimum resources for treating your problem skin, find a good lightweight cream specifically meant for problem skin. Use this day and night along with cleansing and toning. Hopefully this all will help you to have clear, problem-free skin.

I love the spray bottle idea for my toner (my husband likes it too!). My husband's skin is doing better than ever. I've got him into a daily and nightly skin regimen, and he hardly breaks out anymore. He used to have frequent breakouts, which runs in his family.

Attention men: If you just give your skin The Basics, it can and will make a difference! The total time spent on those three steps is less than two minutes. Surely you have a few short minutes in the morning and before you go to bed to take care of your skin.

Microdermabrasion

This procedure should be termed *micro*epiderm*abrasion*. *Micro* means very small or involving minute quantities or variations; *derma* refers to the dermis or inner layers of the skin, but in the case of microdermabrasion it is hopefully only affecting the epidermis or outer skin; *abrasion* means to wear away by friction, through abrading.

I would like to know how you feel about microdermabrasion. I am 35 years old and fine lines are starting to show, especially around my mouth (smile lines) and forehead. Do you think products would work just as well? The procedure is quite costly, $900 *for 6 treatments. I'm trying to decide if it's worth it or not. Any information would be greatly appreciated.*

Microdermabrasion *is* expensive. It is a superficial exfoliation of the outer skin. Anything more than that would not be allowed to be performed by a mere aesthetician. It can help to reduce the *appearance* of the fine lines, but not the actual lines themselves. Keeping your skin regularly exfoliated at home can help you achieve similar benefits as microdermabrasion at a fraction of the cost.

I asked this reader if she exfoliated at home, and her answer was no. She had tried Retin-A, but it burned her skin and made it peel, so she stopped using it. She wasn't actively exfoliating (vs. passive exfoliation like AHAs or Retin-A) on a regular basis—or at all. She wanted to stop wearing foundation but was having a hard time getting used to not wearing it.

I would recommend exfoliating at home first before you invest in microdermabrasion. This way you can find out the benefits of regular dead skin removal, which reveals soft, supple skin underneath.

I know many people enjoy the benefits of microdermabrasion, but I also have firsthand experience from some of my clients about negative experiences with this procedure.

I came into the facial room to see my client who hails from India. Gowri has beautiful light brown skin, and like many darker skinned people, she has some trouble with hyperpigmentation. She went to investigate what all the fuss was about microdermabrasion and had an unfortunate experience.

Apparently the aesthetician working on Gowri's skin was a little overzealous in wanting to get rid of her dead skin. There was a pimple in the middle of Gowri's forehead, a spot that had been there for a while, and it resisted leaving (clearing).

Perhaps in an attempt to "get rid of" the blemish, the aesthetician must have kept the microdermabrasion machine on that spot for a long time because what she actually did was create a hole in my client's skin! I couldn't believe it! Not only was there a visible hole, but since Gowri is from India, she is prone to post-inflammatory hyperpigmentation (see section). This shows up as dark brown spots at the site of inflammation or infection. In Gowri's case, she had a medium-sized dark spot at the site of this hole left by the microdermabrasion treatment.

Over time the skin healed, and because Gowri was diligent about sunscreen and covering her face in the sun, the dark spot went away as well. Both of these processes took some time, but I am happy to report her skin looks great. Needless to say, Gowri won't be getting any more microdermabrasion.

Another client of mine who likes to experiment with new and different procedures tried microdermabrasion. She said it actually hurt, and now she has red patches on her cheeks from the treatment. I have been giving her facials for over 10 years, and her skin is very delicate and sensitive. She is not a good candidate for any kind of abrasive procedures or products; no wonder she didn't enjoy microdermabrasion.

Microdermabrasion isn't for everyone. I encourage all my clients to experiment and see what works best for them. Microdermabrasion isn't—or shouldn't be—any more than superficial exfoliation, so it should be a safe procedure. However, any treatment given by someone who is unqualified could turn out to be disastrous, so be sure if you do get microdermabrasion you are going to someone who knows about skin and all the possible effects of this procedure—not just the benefits. I still think microdermabrasion is too expensive for what you get. Doing your at-home exfoliation, especially utilizing the gommage, can in my opinion give you similar results without compromising the health of your skin or your wallet.

Mineral Makeup

Over the years, I have had numerous women ask me, "If foundation is bad for my skin, what can I use for coverage?" Loose powder is one alternative to liquid foundation. And now there is something called mineral makeup that I also recommend.

Mineral makeup contains micronized minerals, which are concentrated pigment. This gives the skin very good coverage without causing the congestion you get with liquid foundation (or pressed powder). People with rosacea are particularly happy with the coverage mineral makeup is able to give their skin.

Unlike loose powder, mineral makeup does not generally contain fillers like talc. This helps with the efficacy of the pigments contained in this powder makeup.

Most brands contain both titanium dioxide and zinc oxide (see sections). These provide full or broad spectrum sun protection. Not all mineral makeup products have an SPF rating. Keep in mind, any sun protection must be included on the label.

There are several companies who manufacture mineral makeup. Some of the most popular are Jane Iredale, YoungBlood, and Bare Essentials.

My goal is to help you get your skin looking healthy so you won't want to cover it up with foundation, powder, or mineral makeup. However, if you feel you need coverage and don't want the negatives liquid foundations and pressed powders offer, give mineral makeup a try. Hopefully you will find it works well for you—and your skin.

Nails & Skin Care

Nails & Skin Care

What is a hangnail?

It is simply dead skin that has pulled away from the fingernail area. I am sure you have found that if you pull the dead skin off, it leaves a little tear in the skin. Due to a lot of nerves located at the ends of your fingers, these tiny little pieces of skin really can hurt when they are tearing off from the finger. So don't pull the skin off, but do cut it with nail clippers, and get as close to the surface as possible without cutting your finger. And if it still hurts, and to ensure infection doesn't set it, put a tiny drop of an essential oil (like lavender) on the area, then put a Band-Aid® on it until it heals. On the other hand, the cuticle around the base of the nail should never be trimmed off. It could lead to infection and overgrowth of the cuticle.

How can I best take care of the skin around my fingernails? I get lots of hangnails, and they hurt! Please tell me what I can do (or not do) to stop them from happening.

Frequently washing your hands throughout the day can create an environment for problems with the skin around your nails as well as the nails themselves. The absorption and subsequent drying of water on your hands (through washing dishes, baths, and even simply washing your hands in soap and water) can cause brittle nails and skin that tends to create hangnails. Wearing rubber gloves whenever possible is always a good idea. It may seem like a nuisance at first, but once you are used to wearing gloves, your hands will reflect this new type of care.

Putting a healing oil on your cuticles can help to keep hangnails away. Because hangnails are dead skin gone bad, keeping that skin soft and flexible will help to keep those painful tears from happening. After bathing or taking a shower is a good time to push the skin of the cuticle back, which helps to keep that tissue from tearing. Nighttime is the best time for this application. The oil will stay put longer, and that's when everything regenerates anyway!

Finally, getting regular manicures, even if you don't have long nails, is another good way to keep hangnails away and just keep up with overall maintenance of your hands. I don't have any nails since I have to keep them short for my work, but I love to get manicures. It keeps my nailbeds in good shape, and I love the massaging that comes with a professional manicure.

The following are two of the most frequently asked questions and their answers from my favorite nail professional, Sharon Bayles.

Why do my nails peel?

Many factors could be to blame for this annoying problem. It's usually environment or chemical stresses. Your nails are porous, so excessive washing can make them brittle, as mentioned before.

Never use polish removers with acetone (very drying) or polish with sensitizing ingredients like toluene, nitrocellulose or formaldehyde. If your nails have always peeled, you have your parents to thank for that gene! Buffing is an excellent option because it helps to hold the peeling ends together, and it shines like a polish would without the chemicals. Buy a good buffing cream and a chamois buffer and shine away! Note that buffing is great for most nails to diminish ridges and peeling ends, but should be avoided if skin or nail disorders like psoriasis or dermatitis are present.

How can I get my nails to grow?

Having regular manicures by either yourself or a licensed professional is the fastest way to healthy nails. Always incorporate a good massage to your hands and pull on the fingers to tips to get the blood circulating. You will see results with this consistent care. Second, don't think you have to have talons to have great nails. Be realistic and honest. Most of us know our nail length "limit." Keeping nails trimmed at or below this limit will eliminate a lot of breakage.

When looking for a manicurist, be sure to find a qualified professional. Ask her how many natural nail manicures she does. This is important because you could get roped into wearing fake nails before you know it. Believe me, this "quick fix" could take your nails years to recover from all the damage. Some damage could even be permanent.

And my last tip is to always wear sunscreen on your hands. In the years to come you'll thank yourself as you hear your friends complaining about their "spots."

O

Oil-Absorbing Sheets

Clean & Clear Sheets: Instant Oil-Absorbing Sheets by Johnson & Johnson

True to the advertising, these absorbing sheets will indeed temporarily remove excess oil from your skin. What I found when I used them is they also create a feeling of dryness—obviously due to the removal of the natural oils in your skin.

If you have excessively oily skin, it would be most helpful to figure out why you are so oily in the first place. This information is not the quick fix of these oil-absorbing sheets, but it can give you long-term relief from oiliness. However, these sheets will immediately take away the shine you may experience. I would say it is OK to use them on a temporary basis, but don't get addicted to them. My skin, after using them every day for just one week, went through a dry, flaky period until I stopped using them. I don't have severely oily skin; I do have normal skin with some excess oil in my nose area.

As with any new product you are using, monitor your skin. If you are beginning to see changes for the worse, stop using the new product and opt for something more beneficial. Sometimes products like these oil-absorbing sheets are convenient and seem like a good thing, but in the end, your skin will tell you if you can use them long-term or not.

Oils in Products

There is a misconception that oil in products (moisturizers) is a bad thing. I disagree. Oil-free products have to add fillers and emollients in order to make their product smooth and spreadable. If a product isn't using oil(s), it is probably using synthetic, nonnutritive ingredients to replace natural oils.

High-quality, vegetal (vegetable) oils are not detrimental to an oilier skin type; petroleum derived oils, like mineral oil, probably are. Please do not shy away from using "oil" in your moisturizers if you have oily or normal to oily/combination skin. If the product is made for your skin type, you should be fine—as long as it is a quality product. As I will talk about in the **Product Recommendations** section, cheaper products with cheap ingredients (like mineral oil) are probably not going to work well if you have problem skin.

Here is a short list of oils that can be found in moisturizers. These oils (vegetable and other) are preferable to mineral oil or petroleum derived ingredients. This list is not every oil that is available, but it gives you something to compare with the products you are using. Just because you are using a moisturizer with one or more of these oils in it doesn't mean it will turn out to be a great product for you. But if you find your creams have mineral oil or petroleum listed as the main ingredient, I would opt for a moisturizer that contained more organic, "natural" ingredients and vegetable oils such as these:

Almond Oil, Sweet Almond Oil
Castor Oil
Coconut Oil, Hydrogenated Coconut Oil
Corn Oil
Olive Oil

Palm Kernel Oil, Hydrogenated Palm Kernel Oil
Pumpkin Seed Oil
Shea Butter
Soybean Oil
Sunflower Seed Oil
Wheat Germ Oil

Please note: If you have internal allergies (food allergies) to any of the above, more than likely they will *not* make good ingredients in a topical skin care product—for *you*.

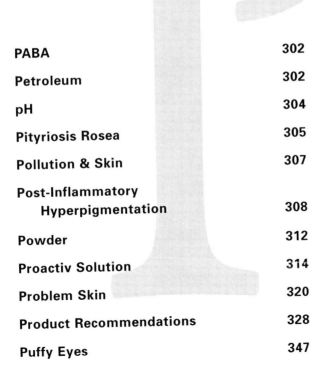

P

PABA

PABA (para-aminobenzoic acid) acts as a chemical sunscreen, helping to keep UVB rays from harming the skin. It was one of the original sunscreen ingredients. However, this once common ingredient in sunscreens has proved in the past to be a skin irritant. Not everyone has a reaction to PABA, but so many do that most manufacturers have taken it out of their ingredient lists.

If you have sensitive skin and tend to react to sunscreens in general, before you purchase your next sun product, check the ingredient list. If PABA or para-aminobenzoic acid is listed, I would look for something else. Avobenzone and both zinc oxide and titanium dioxide make good sunscreen ingredients and can all be looked up in their respective sections in this book.

Petroleum

Is there any good, "healthy" use for petroleum*?

*Note that when the word petroleum is used, it is referring to petroleum jelly.

Petroleum jelly, sometimes listed as *petrolatum* on ingredient lists, is a thick gel-like substance that has absolutely no nutritive content. It is void of anything actively healing. In other words, it is inert. Although, due to its gel consistency, it can feel soothing and even hydrating.

Petroleum has a large molecular structure (especially the lower grade types) and is not a good ingredient in skin care products for the face. This large molecule prohibits absorption into the skin. Therefore, if you use a moisturizer with petroleum in it, it will just sit on the surface of your skin, potentially clog your pores, and perhaps even make your skin look shiny.

If you ski, for instance, this might not be a bad thing. Under harsh environmental conditions, having an occlusive covering over your skin may be just what you need. But day to day, under normal circumstances, you won't want to have petroleum on your face.

If you go to the grocery store and look at the ingredient lists on products like Lubriderm and Vaseline Intensive Care, you will see that some of the first ingredients are petroleum and mineral oil. (Mineral oil is just another form of petroleum.) Both of these can really clog the pores on your face. But both of these make great ingredients in body products. Petroleum helps to lock in moisture, and it stays on the surface and helps to make skin feel smooth. This may sound like a favorable thing for your face, but because of the potential for congestion, I stand by my recommendation to avoid petroleum in your facial moisturizers. See **Oils in Products** to get an idea of some good alternatives to petroleum.

I've been taking mascara off for years with Vaseline and have used it on my lips also. Is it harmful, and if so, what should I use instead?

Vaseline or any other petroleum product in and of itself isn't harmful to the skin necessarily; these ingredients can clog the pores if contained in a moisturizing cream or foundation.

Whenever you are removing mascara, you have to be sure not to pull your undereye skin as you are wiping off the mascara. This tissue is delicate and should not be pulled or tugged daily. This is the number one reason using Vaseline isn't such a good idea. Due to its gooey consistency, it will naturally stick to the skin. Therefore, the potential for having to pull the skin near your eyes increases. Vaseline tends to stick around wherever it has been applied, so if you choose to use this as a makeup remover, you also add the potential for it getting (and staying) in your eyes. See **Eye Makeup Removal/Removing mascara** to find out the best way to remove your eye makeup.

pH

pH means the *power of hydrogen* and refers to the acidity or alkalinity of any given substance. The pH scale ranges anywhere from 1 to 14.

Your skin is naturally acidic. In order to maintain this pH balance, you only want to use acidic skin care products. The reasons for this are twofold. First, bacteria cannot thrive in an acid environment. Therefore, if you use acidic products, you help to fortify this natural acidic state, keeping bacteria away. Secondly, using alkaline products almost always strips the skin of its natural oils and surface water, causing the skin to become dehydrated. This can look and feel like dry, flaky skin.

Because it is so important to know the pH of all of your products, I highly recommend purchasing pH papers. This will enable you to test any product, whether for your face or body, and know if it's the proper pH for your skin.

One of the first things I did after reading Timeless Skin *was order Nitrazine papers. It's been a long time since chemistry class, and I don't remember if 4 is on the acidic side or the alkaline side. Exactly what numbers do I want my products to be on the pH scale?*

I just picked up pH papers from the local science store with a range from 1-14. So far all of my products have been a 4, 5, or 6. One Clinique® toner was an 8. Please refresh my memory: the products I check should be at what pH level?

If you are using pH papers, whether Nitrazine or otherwise, they will provide the pH values. When you put some product on the paper, it will turn a color that corresponds to one of these values listed on the packaging. You will know immediately if the products you are testing are what you want to use or not. Neutral is 7 on the pH scale. Acid is considered anything less than 7, and anything above 7 would be considered alkaline. In answer to these specific emails, anything in the 4 to 6 range is acidic and the proper pH for a skin care product. The toner at a pH of 8 would be too alkaline, and I wouldn't recommend using it.

Remember: it is alkalinity you want to avoid. I can think of no good reason to use an alkaline skin care product on your face. This is precisely why it is so helpful to have these papers to test the pH level of any and all of your products.

I used the pHydrion strips that I found in the chemistry department, and they worked the same as the Nitrazine papers you recommend.

You can buy a single roll dispenser of pHydrion much cheaper than Nitrazine papers. They do the same thing, but they do it for one third the cost. If you cannot locate these papers at your local pharmacy, ask them to order some for you. No matter which brand you are able to find, do make a point to locate pH test papers.

Pityriosis Rosea

Although pityriosis rosea (PR) isn't the type of skin problem I am focusing on in this book, it is a skin condition I have had myself, so I thought I'd write down my own experiences in case it might be helpful to some of you. It is described as an acute inflammatory skin disease, marked by reddish ring-shaped eruptions, predominantly on the trunk.

Just for the record, PR has no "known" cause. But I can tell you in one word why I developed this condition: stress. The year I was producing my first book was one of the most stressful periods of my entire life. I cannot begin to explain the inner stress my body and soul was going through. The outer or physical manifestation of this inner turmoil was, in my opinion, pityriosis rosea.

It started with the classic herald patch; mine was located just above my right hip bone on my backside. I noticed it immediately because it was big—about the size of a half dollar. It had an unusual and distinct border but that was the only spot I could see. That initial single spot changed within a few short days, and I started to get what looked like chicken pox-type red spots all over the entire trunk of my body. The number of spots increased by the dozens on a daily basis, yet I had no idea what was going on.

I happened to be on vacation with friends in Seattle during the time the increase of the spots was occurring. One of my friends, Julia, is a Physician's Assistant, and immediately classified it as *pityriosis rosea*. I had never heard of it, so Julia explained what she could: namely that there was nothing I could do for it but just ride it out. I put soothing creams with allantoin and aloe vera all over my body, but I can honestly say I don't think anything I did really helped the spots go away. Like Julia said, I just had to let nature run its course.

I was lucky—although the spots were somewhat unsightly, they did not itch. In some cases of PR, itching does occur. Due to the numerous red dots spotting my body, I can't imagine how awful it would have been if they did indeed itch.

If you are diagnosed with PR, be patient and know that the spots, whether they itch or not, will go away in time. Although I had what seemed like hundreds of spots, there were no scars left and looking at my skin today you would never know I had PR.

It is not a fun skin condition, but it is fairly harmless. If you are under a lot of stress, your body will do what it needs to compensate. For me during this particular period of time, I developed pityriosis rosea. It's not the end of the world, and the look of your skin is the worst part of this unusual skin problem.

Pollution & Skin

I live in [a large metropolitan city]. What does air pollution do to my skin?

If you live in a highly polluted environment, most likely a large city, you may suffer from the effects of air pollution—mainly congestion and debris in your pores. You may also experience dark circles and puffiness, which are common allergic responses due to inflammation. Pollution, obviously, affects the lungs as well.

If you live in a high-pollution city, you need to make sure you are getting your skin clean every day. You probably want to do more clay masking than the average person since clay will super-clean your pores and detoxify the skin. Two to three times per week is not too often as long as the mask you are using doesn't irritate your skin and you keep the mask moist (see **Clay Masks**). Exfoliating will also help to deep clean the pores, keeping them free from the daily buildup of dirt and debris.

Although pollution has an obvious effect on how dirty your skin may get during the course of a day, the effect it has on your insides is a bit more profound and perhaps not as obvious. We live in a world with a lot of airborne pollutants that can age us faster and compromise the health of all of our body's cells. Unless you change your physical environment, you will suffer the effects of pollution, whether you feel them or see them or not. Taking supplements, namely antioxidants, can help to keep cell damage from air pollution to a minimum. See **Antioxidants** for more information on these all-important health producers.

My best advice to you is keep your skin clean and debris-free and take your antioxidants!

Post-Inflammatory Hyperpigmentation

You are no doubt wondering, what is post-inflammatory hyperpigmentation? Yet I bet many of you suffer from this common condition. Another way to say post-inflammatory hyperpigmentation is after-infection dark spots. Some people think these are scars, but actually they are spots of pigmentation that occurred due to blemishes that received sun exposure.

Without UV sunlight, the infection from blemishes would come and go and the pigmentation of your skin wouldn't change at all. It is solely due to sun exposure that this hyperpigmentation condition occurs.

People who have darker skin, whether African-Americans, certain Europeans, and even Caucasians who have a lot of melanin in their skin, are all susceptible to this condition. Let's see what some people are asking about post-inflammatory hyperpigmentation.

I am a 30-year-old Asian-Indian woman and have occasional breakouts that always leave very dark pigmentation after healing. It will take 3 to 4 months for the mark to lighten and disappear.

I use concealer and do not enjoy being anywhere without having makeup on in order to camouflage the pigmentation. I want to be free of my makeup to enjoy a more athletic and outdoor life. Any recommendations?

You have a very common complaint, not that you should feel better by hearing that! The condition you are asking about is called *post-inflammatory hyperpigmentation*. The blessing is you no doubt have beautiful skin tone due to your heritage. The curse is you are susceptible to pigmentation irregularities.

Anytime you have blemishes, they are like wounds in the skin. The deeper the infection the more tissue that is damaged, and the longer these places will take to heal. Since you have so much pigmentation naturally in your skin, you will be prone to this condition more so than someone who has very white skin (especially redheads and those who burn but never tan).

I'm sure it is disheartening that these pigmentation spots take so long to clear. Three or four months is a distinct possibility, especially in the warmer months and especially if you are outside in the sun a lot. Whether or not you can be free from makeup may be out of your control if you continue to get these pigmentation places and want to cover them up. But being able to enjoy a more athletic and outdoor life is your choice. I don't think you have to curtail being out in the fresh air of nature; you just have to take precautions against sun exposure.

Being extremely careful about sun on your face is a lifestyle habit you will absolutely need to adopt. Any sun on your face will stimulate melanin and therefore darken all pigmentation, whether on healthy skin or skin that is damaged and healing from a blemish.

The truth is sunscreen is not enough to protect your skin. It is a manmade product with the ability to screen out only some of the harmful UV rays. Don't feel falsely armed if you wear sunscreen; you will also need to physically block the sun from reaching your face. You do this by wearing hats and sitting in complete shade if you are outside.

Be careful about products that claim to lighten skin. There are some prescription products available through your dermatologist that might help, but the reviews are mixed on how well these products actually work to lighten the skin. Some products bleach, and others inhibit melanin production; melanin is what is causing the darkness. In the winter or colder months, your skin will naturally lighten, or the spots will, due to a decrease in sun exposure.

My top recommendation would be to become hyperaware of how much sun you are receiving. I guarantee it is more exposure than you think you are getting. Always wear sunscreen. And keep hats with you or in your car so you won't be caught out in the sun unprotected.

Can you suggest something regarding scars (dark spots) that have been left by past pimples? I was thinking about either microdermabrasion or using products containing kojic acid* that promises to lighten scars. Any thoughts on these?

*Kojic acid is a skin lightening ingredient. It can inhibit the formation of melanin.

You could try microdermabrasion. It is expensive, but it may work for you. You could try kojic acid products and see for yourself if their promises are well-founded. As I have said, no product or procedure is for everyone. And many things out on the market may work for you. My belief, however, is that many will not.

True scarring from blemishes is a tissue-related problem. I think the scarring this reader is talking about is really post-inflammatory hyperpigmentation. Because the dark spots never seem to go away, it probably seems like a scar, but in reality it is an overaccumulation of melanin at the site of the blemish. This caused the dark spot and sunlight is helping it to remain there. What I know is that if you become diligent and hyperaware about sun exposure, your "scars" will lighten and go away—as long as you keep sun off your face.

I am in need of a spot lightener. Basically I suffered from acne when I was pregnant, and the blemishes caused dark spots on my face. I need something to make the spots lighten up. Do you have a product that will reduce the darkness? PS: Why did these dark spots appear in the first place?

As you've learned, when you have breakout, especially deep cysts or pustules loaded with infection, the spots are like tiny wounds, and this wounded tissue is subject to variations in pigmentation. For example: One summer I tripped on my office patio as I was leaving work. My right foot caught the fall, but I ended up deeply scraping the top of it. Once a scab had formed, I stopped wearing Band-Aids; when the scab came off, scar tissue was left in its wake. Since it was summer, the area received all kinds of sun exposure due to wearing flip flops and sandals, leaving the injured tissue full-on exposed to sunlight. When I thought about it, I would put sunscreen there, but for the most part I was a "bad client" and just forgot about protecting it from UV light.

Due to the amount of sun that area received, and the extent of the injury with its resulting scar tissue, a large dark spot existed where the scrape occurred. Some people even thought it was a tattoo! But in actuality it was hyperpigmentation around the outside edge of the injury along with pigmentless scar tissue inside. Had it been winter, the area would have received little or no exposure to the sun, and no doubt it would be less discolored. Now the scar is barely noticeable, but when summer rolls around the darkness will probably reappear and then fade again in the winter. This example is of a foot; imagine how much sun your face is getting in the summer (or winter), subjecting your "injuries" to the potential for hyperpigmentation.

One way to avoid some of the darkness of post-inflammatory hyperpigmentation is to *stop picking at your skin!* It's a bad habit and can cause damage to the area. With that said, a picker is going to pick. I can't change your predilection for doing this; you believe you are helping your skin by picking. Perhaps when you can install a different belief, you can change your behavior. Try the belief: "When I pick at my skin, I am causing further damage. And it will take my skin *longer* to heal. Picking does not help." Adopt this, and you are on the road to recovery.

I am not saying that extracting the infected mass from a spot isn't advantageous. It is. However, in my experience, most people have little or no restraint when it comes to self-extraction. And sometimes tools are needed to properly get to a plug; the use of which is best left to an aesthetician in the course of a facial treatment. If you can't get a facial, at least put healing products on the blemishes (geranium, for instance) and know this will go a long way to getting rid of the spots faster. Picking will only prolong the healing process and create the potential for post-inflammatory hyperpigmentation.

In conclusion, as long as you are experiencing breakout and receiving sun exposure (even limited amounts), you have the potential for causing dark spots where the blemishes are located. So, don't pick at your skin, always wear sunscreen when you are out, and find ways to heal the blemishes without causing further damage. Many tools for having healthy skin are listed throughout this book.

Powder

I know you say women shouldn't wear foundation, but what about powder? Is it also bad for the skin? I feel like I want to have something covering my skin!

Powder is preferable to wearing foundation. Loose powder is basically talc, which is the main ingredient found in baby powder. Talc is essentially (French) chalk, or a "finely powdered native magnesium silicate, a mineral," as defined in Ruth Winter's *A Consumer's Dictionary of Cosmetic Ingredients*. Powder can actually help absorb excess oil from the surface of the skin while giving you a finished look. So if it comes down to a decision of whether to use powder or foundation, I would recommend powder. I do understand your desire to have something covering your face, but I bet if I saw you, I would not see the imperfections you see in your skin. We are all too critical when it comes to looking at ourselves in the mirror.

I was at a convention where you spoke. I remember you saying something about pressed powder being bad for your face. I was wondering if all powder is bad for your skin or just pressed and why? Do you think powder is the reason why my pores are clogged?

Pressed powder is just like foundation when it come to how it functions on top of your skin. Look at the ingredients; there will be certain ingredients in pressed powder that are not in loose powder. Ingredients that help make it "stick" to your skin. It is simply liquid foundation in solid form. The following scenario happens over and over with clients who come in wearing pressed powder. I'll ask the client if she's wearing foundation, and the response is, "No, I just have a little bit of powder on." It then takes me multiple cleansings in order to get that "little bit of powder" off her skin and out of the pores. Pressed powder contains a lot of emollients and thickeners that are then *pressed* into the skin and can cause congestion in the pores. Yes, you get great coverage with pressed powder—because it is more like foundation than true powder. If you have to wear something to cover your skin, I would suggest a light-textured water-based foundation instead of pressed powder.

Many times women who wear pressed powder have some enlargement of the pores, especially on the middle forehead, around the nose and cheek area, and near the corners of their mouths, similar to foundation wearers. If this is true for you and you are wearing pressed powder, try using loose powder for a while. Also try using a clay mask to unclog the pores and get your skin in better shape. See if the combination of these two things helps with the quality of your skin. I really find pressed powder very unpowderlike.

I've never used a liquid foundation, but I do sometimes use non-talc, mineral-based powders and blushes on my face to take away shine and cover some broken capillaries, and also for color. How do you feel about these types of powders? Are they just as pore-clogging as liquid foundation (especially since I seem to have a blackhead problem)?

Recently a new kind of powder has surfaced, called *mineral makeup,* and I believe this is what you are asking about. This type of makeup usually will give you good coverage without causing skin problems, and it doesn't have oil in it. Since you are prone to blackheads, I would monitor your skin closely if you choose to wear this or any type of makeup. And no matter what, doing at-home facials (exfoliating and clay masking) is essential to keep your pores cleaned out. See **Mineral Makeup** for more information.

Proactiv® Solution

I have a mixed report on this infomercial product-by-mail. I have had several clients come into my clinic telling me how Proactiv "tore up" their skin. And I have also had experience with a few people who have had success with it. I am including some stories of how Proactiv helped or hindered the clearing of their problem skin.

What's in Proactiv Solution? This is a benzoyl peroxide-based skin care product line. The most basic Proactiv Solution program consists of four products: Cleanser, toner, moisturizer, and mask. The pH values of all but the mask are acidic, which is good. The mask tested to be alkaline, so if you decide to use this product line, I would be careful about using the mask. As you know, alkalinity can dry out the skin's surface. Proactiv also contains fragrance; something that cannot be ignored once you smell the different products. This should raise a red flag if you have known reactions to fragrance in products, so be aware and be careful.

The Renewing Cleanser has 2.5% benzoyl peroxide (BP). The Revitalizing Toner has glycolic acid as its second ingredient, along with aloe, chamomile, and witch hazel as some of the top ingredients. The Repairing Lotion Acne Treatment (moisturizer) also has 2.5% BP. The Refining Mask Acne Treatment has kaolin (clay) as its second ingredient, which is actually a good thing. Too bad it's an alkaline mask. The ingredients in this system are predominately synthetic, with a few organic ingredients thrown in, mostly in the toner.

Proactiv has definitely worked for many people—although some for just a short period of time. If you are at the end of your rope, you might want to give these products a try. By this I mean you have really looked into your diet and lifestyle habits and cannot determine a source for your breakouts. Or at least no source that you are willing to give up, perhaps. Ingredient for ingredient, I am not impressed with Proactiv, but if it works for you then that is what really matters.

Merry's story. Merry was pregnant with her second baby. (Yes, this is the same Merry from *Timeless Skin*!) Her skin, like with the first pregnancy, had gone completely haywire. No matter how good she was about doing all the right things, her skin was still at the mercy of the baby growing inside her. Hormones are funny things, and when a woman is pregnant, they control just about everything, including her skin.

Merry came in for a facial with what looked like chapped skin all over her face. She was so dried out and dehydrated I couldn't believe it. I asked her what she had been doing, and she reluctantly admitted the truth. She had gone to the store and purchased products that promised to clear up acne. What they had done instead was dry out the entire surface of her face, which did relatively nothing for the infections and cysts coming up from below the skin.

I got her to stop using the harsh, drying products, and considered the options with her. She shyly asked me what I thought of Proactiv. I said I honestly didn't have any personal experience with it, but that several clients in recent years had said it was one of the worst things they had used on their skin.

A month later I saw Merry for another facial and noticed an improvement in her skin. It was perhaps 25% better than the previous month. She went on to tell me she had purchased the Proactiv products and decided to use them and see how it went. She, too, had noticed a difference in her skin; it seemed to be clearing up a bit. Here is what Merry had to say about her Proactiv experience.

Proactiv worked to dry my skin out pretty well, but nothing really helped to clear it up. It definitely improved the bright red, breakout pus things, but didn't help with the blackheads that were so bad. The cleanser and toner are the best products. The lotion (moisturizer) was okay, but the mask was horrific. Let me put it this way, using Proactiv made me feel like I was doing something to sort of help my skin, but nothing really could make it better. It finally cleared up in my fourth month of pregnancy.

One of the side effects I noticed with Merry's skin was dehydration; in fact it was flaky. This was no doubt from the benzoyl peroxide contained in Proactiv. Benzoyl peroxide, although sometimes effective for blemishes, can really dry out the surface skin. Although Merry had some success with Proactiv, she ended up going back to her regular routine with the products she has used for years. Products that don't dry out her skin.

Donn's story. Donn is a beautiful young black man. He is fit, happy, and healthy. He eats a good diet and yet was still experiencing skin troubles—mostly located in his beard area.

Men—especially African-American men—have a propensity to develop a condition called *pseudofolliculitis barbae*. This is where the hair coming up to form the beard cannot find its way straight to the surface. For black men, this is primarily because of the curly nature of their hair. But men of all races can face this dilemma. The result is what seems like acne in their beard area. Some men have so many problems with pseudofolliculitis, they may simply let their beards grow and not deal with the daily hassle of these ingrown hairs.

Donn had to take daily medication for an unrelated condition. Although he was only on the medication for a year, it caused a lot of his skin problems. Once he got off the drug therapy, his skin problems persisted, and all he wanted was clear skin. So he turned to the advice of some people who had used Proactiv and decided to give it a try. Why not? He felt he had nothing to lose. After the first month on Proactiv Donn's skin improved dramatically, and he has enjoyed clear skin ever since.

Donn's is a success story. He approached me one day and asked if I could tell he used to have skin problems. His skin looked clear, without scars, and his beard didn't seem to be housing any infected spots—all looked good. That is when he announced he had been using Proactiv for the past eight months—faithfully and successfully. He was so happy he had found something to help his problem skin.

I include Donn's story for several reasons. First, it is not my goal to knock down every skin care regime out in the marketplace although I don't find many products that are very effective. Proactiv has "torn up" many of my clients' faces, but it has also helped some tough cases of problem skin.

A 20-something co-worker of Donn's also used Proactiv. She said it seemed to work at first, but after a month or so her skin looked dull and felt dry. She didn't get the results she was looking for and was asking me for recommendations.

This seems to be a common comment about Proactiv. It helps, or seems to help, at first. Then it seems to either stop working or the skin just can't adjust to all the drying out and starts to look worse. In my opinion, this isn't a good enough reason to use Proactiv. However, there are many people who swear by it. Try it and see. It's pretty inexpensive, but beware if you don't cancel your required membership after the first shipment you receive, the company will automatically send you a new batch of products on a regular basis—and charge you for them too.

When I started on Proactiv, my skin looked great. It dried everything out. Then I guess as my body adjusted to the new program, I was mega-oily all the time and developed little red bumps. It seemed while I was on the Proactiv products, I had many red bumps all the time. I finally went off Proactiv, and it took my skin about three weeks to get back to normal.

My skin is doing better although I have really been working on eating better. When I choose to be bad and have a treat, there are usually consequences, but they are under my control—I choose when.

That email was written by my client, Tori. She started using Proactiv four months ago. Within a few weeks, she said it was like a miracle. Most of the old spots had cleared up, and there weren't many new blemishes coming up; her skin truly had cleared up. After two months on the program she started noticing an overall oiliness to her skin that hadn't been there before. Her forehead was especially oily and in fact little whiteheads were starting to form there. I told her it was probably the benzoyl peroxide—that it both helped to temporarily clear her skin and was also creating an oil slick on her face. She was essentially drying out her skin, and in rebuttal, her oil glands were pumping more oil than necessary to compensate for the dryness on the surface.

I think Tori's story exemplifies the need to monitor your skin when you are using new products. This is especially true if they are products meant to clear problem skin. If your skin is clearing up, great, but is it also showing signs of dryness? Remember, over time the dryness can have detrimental effects negating anything positive you may have achieved.

> *I thought Proactiv was pretty good when I first used it. Thankfully I never had full-blown acne. It did make my skin look very ragged out, not subtle and balanced-looking. It seemed to enlarge my pores as well.*
>
> *Two of my friends use it and seem to like it. Using the abrasive cleanser every day cannot be good for skin. Proactiv did not make my skin dry, just flat and not very good-looking.*

The flat look is probably due to moisture loss in the surface skin cells. They lose their plumpness and aren't able to reflect light, which does make the skin look dull or flat. This client, like so many people trying to clear up their problem skin, has run into the main problem with using benzoyl peroxide. It dries out the skin and creates its own set of problems. It is great that her friends use Proactiv and like it, but for her skin this product just doesn't deliver the results she is looking for. Proactiv does work for some people. But if the cause of the problem skin is dietary and the diet is not altered dramatically to ensure a healthy body and therefore healthy skin, the problems will continue to occur. You may go through an initial period of clear skin. Then three, four, or maybe six months later (even while still using Proactiv), your problems might seem to be returning in full. This is because you did nothing to stop the acne from occurring in the first place. You took the short cut, which usually leads you in a circle back to where you started. It's about causal healing, not quick fixes. Remember, you must fix the system, not just the symptom.

There are so many product lines available to choose from. Not all products will fit the needs of all people. Proactiv may be what you have been looking for, but be careful and watch the hydration level of your skin. Don't trade one problem for another; trading in blemishes for dehydration. I believe that you can have all good results with none of the bad if you follow my recommendations for healthy skin. Mine is not the quick-fix remedy, but perhaps the long-term solution—the real proactive solution.

Problem Skin

In all the clients I've seen with problem skin, I would have to say that less than 10% of them have problem skin due simply to hormone imbalances. Almost all of the problems I see are directly related to diet. What you put into your body is going to be eliminated; it will be processed first, then discarded. The truth is you have the power on a daily basis to see how what you eat affects your body in general and your skin specifically. You can do this by becoming aware of your skin and your breakouts. As always, you have the answers within.

I am 32 years old, and a few years ago blemishes and acne start-ed to bother me, especially during my monthly cycle. The blemishes I have are mostly red and swollen spots that do not have a white head or open pore. I have tried many acne treatments, but the results have not been good. The red and swollen spots just stay there and do not go away—even with days of treatment. If I leave them untreated, these red spots will shrink a bit and turn dark red but remain there. Then dead skin starts to build up and cover the spots like a scar. The blemishes are bothering me a lot and new ones are popping up before the old ones go away. It's like a non-stop cycle. I am interested in knowing what would help me.

Skin care isn't just topical (product driven), it is initially and primari-ly internal—reflecting how your body is handling food, hormones, stress, and environment. Do you eat sugar, and if so, how much? Do you have a balanced diet filled with healthy foods? Do you drink much water? Sodas? All of these will affect the state of your skin. Products can be quite effective on problem skin. But what you must truly understand is unless the root cause is found and fixed, the skin care problems can and probably will continue.

The first thing I want to know about her skin is why did it change a few years ago? Did something change in her world or her body that caused her skin to suddenly become a problem? For example, did she have a baby? Did she move, change her diet, or start taking medica-tion? There are endless possibilities as to what might have changed (been added or taken away) in her life.

It is not unusual for blemishes to present themselves or worsen during a woman's monthly cycle. Taking evening primrose oil would be something to consider to see if it helps keep the symptoms of PMS to a minimum. This supplement will probably not keep all breakout from happening, but hopefully it will help to lessen skin problems as well as ease the other symptoms of PMS at the same time. (See **Evening Primrose Oil**.)

Making the distinction that her blemishes are red and swollen but without a head is important. Without a white or yellow pus-filled head, these types of blemishes are not extractable. If, in an attempt to get rid of them, you try to squeeze or otherwise self-extract, you will pay for your actions. Since there is no opening for the infected debris to exit the pore, when pressure is applied (through picking or squeezing), the infected mass has to go somewhere, so it breaks through surrounding follicle walls underneath the surface, which unfortunately spreads the infection. This means the blemish will look bigger and take longer to go away. In the case of blemishes like this client's, without a clear and defined head, using clay and/or essential oils is the best and only recommended course of treatment.

I will assume she was using the traditional treatments available over the counter, which include benzoyl peroxide products and perhaps products with salicylic acid and possibly even alcohol (the bad kind). If so, this is probably why she has found little or no relief. Drying the cysts just isn't going to get rid of them. Drying out this already irritated, infected skin can cause the blemishes to become even more red and sensitive than if you didn't treat them at all. When it comes to clearing up breakout, benzoyl peroxide products usually come up short.

That the spots just stay there and do not go away may be helped by increasing your water intake. Water flushes toxins out of the body, and since blemishes are a sign of toxic overload, drinking more water is always a good course of action. In terms of the spots taking so long to go away, the depth of the cysts will be exemplified by the length of time it takes for them to clear. Simply put, the deeper the damage, the longer the healing time. This is not unusual, it is just the frustrating part of having problem skin.

The mention of a nonstop cycle of blemishes is the second clue that something is amiss. The first clue is the actual breakout. Something inside your body is out of balance, and your skin's reaction is the proof. This says to me that something is constantly or consistently being introduced into her daily life that is affecting her skin; it might be through food, drink, stress, or perhaps even products.

Knowing the details of her diet including water intake and of course how much sugar she has in her diet will help me know how to guide her into better lifestyle habits. Then, after finding out what products she uses and making any adjustments there, I would explain how to treat the blemishes themselves—topically. These suggestions include geranium oil for the spots, regularly exfoliating dead cells, and using a clay mask several times a week. I would suggest also using a regular daily program with pH balanced products meant for problem skin.

I usually break out one week before and one week after my period, mostly on my chin along with some blackheads there and on my nose. I use a topical acne medication (Benzamycin®*), which I would love to eliminate completely. I cannot use products designed specifically for acne. They are too drying and irritating and actually cause major breakouts. I tried Proactiv—what a horror show my face was!

*Benzamycin is a gel that combines benzoyl peroxide with erythromycin, an antibiotic.

I think these comments represent a lot of people's experiences. She gets some breakout and has a slight blackhead problem, but her skin is not in a constant problem state. She's used prescription and over the counter products and has even tried products seen on TV infomercials. From what she said, she hasn't found anything that is really helping.

Taking evening primrose oil may help to even out her pre- and post-menstrual breakouts. If the medication is doing more harm than good, or if it is simply ineffective, using other spot treatments might be the answer. For the blemishes themselves, I recommend geranium oil with or without dotting with clay mask. I would also caution her to be very conscious of her sugar consumption leading up to and following her period. Sugar is just going to create more problems with her skin. Generally, sugar cravings increase near a woman's period. It's a cruel joke of nature, really. We reach for the very thing that will cause problems with our skin.

> *My skin has been a daily task to keep clear for the last ten years. I have a very mild acne problem, and it bothers me. I have tried everything in creation to keep my skin clear, but there always seems to be a spot or two at any given time. I have very sensitive skin that does not respond well to AHAs or other acid products, and most oils found in many products bother my skin. I use Cetaphil to cleanse with and it works wonders. I love that product. I need an exfoliator to use before I wash with my cleanser. I have also used your gommage and was happy with the results and how it didn't bother my skin. I appreciate any advice or comments you may have for me.*

Since her breakouts are ongoing, she is definitely doing something on an ongoing basis to encourage her problem skin. Her use of the term *acne* may be an overstatement, but that is my own opinion. The acne I call acne is the full-blown cystic type.

AHAs and other strong acid products don't work for many people. And if you have any sensitivities and especially if you have redness in your skin, I don't recommend them.

Cetaphil works as a good cleanser for many people. It is inexpensive and easy to find. *I need an exfoliator to use before I wash with my cleanser.* You actually want to cleanse before you exfoliate. Cleansing first gets the debris off the surface of the skin, giving your exfoliator a better chance to do its job. The gommage is a great way to get rid of a lot of dead skin while not irritating or otherwise causing problems for sensitive skin. She could use this product several times per week.

I would advise her to really take a long, hard look at her diet and see if she has hidden or even obvious sugar that she may not be counting as contributing to her ongoing problem skin. Many people just haven't yet come to this realization about diet (especially sugar) and how it affects skin, which is why I talk so much about it.

> *I have used Clinique but am not very happy with it. I am a new mom, and I think it's time for a new me and a new skin care regimen. I am 39 years old. My skin is oily in the t-zone but dry everywhere else. Thirty minutes after I wash, it still looks like an oil slick, yet my skin feels taut and dehydrated. I have lines around my eyes from previous sun damage. My skin breaks out a lot, which I think is unusual for my age.*

These comments are very common, so I will breakdown this email and explain what she could do.

I have used Clinique but am not very happy with it. My intent is not to tear down other product lines, but in this case I can't help myself! Clinique is thought to be a great product for problem (especially teenage) skin, but in my professional experience, I have found it usually causes problems.

Many of the Clinique products have turned out to be alkaline on the pH scale. As you know, you want to use pH balanced products (acidic) on your skin and avoid products that are alkaline. As a teenager I remember using Clinique as my first formal skin care product line. And I also remember having to apply the yellow moisturizer twice before my skin felt moisturized. At this young age, I didn't know the reason for this was because everything I had used up to that point (the soap cleanser and the Clarifying Lotion toner) was alkaline, basically drying the surface of my skin out and encouraging more oil to be produced to compensate. So beware if you are a Clinique user.

My skin is oily in the t-zone but dry everywhere else. Technically, you are probably oilier in the facial axis or t-zone and normal everywhere else. You feel dry because alkaline products (like Clinique) remove too much from the surface of the skin. *Thirty minutes after I wash, it still looks like an oil slick.* This is because your oil glands are compensating for the loss of oil that was stripped from your skin by these alkaline products. *Yet my skin feels taut and dehydrated.* Exactly. This is the normal response to using alkaline products. Your skin feels dry but is truly just dehydrated—it has lost all the surface water and oil that normally holds moisture in making your skin feel soft and supple. Instead your skin feels tight and dry (dehydrated).

I am 39 years old, and I have lines around my eyes from previous sun damage. At 39 you will definitely start seeing the effects of the natural aging process. That you have had a lot of sun exposure will only increase the lines for sure. But 39 is normal to start seeing lines.

My skin breaks out a lot, which I think is unusual for my age. The reasons for your breakouts need to be found before passing judgment. Until you are no longer alive and as long as you have started puberty, you are going to be subject to full-functioning oil glands. So at 39, it is not unusual for you to be breaking out. Why you are having skin problems is the more important part of your question.

I recommend getting pH test papers (see **pH**) so you can test all of the products you are using on your skin. Without this data, it is hard to determine if a product is pH balanced. Then, armed with this knowledge, you can be sure to use products that won't strip the oil and water from your skin or otherwise cause many of the problems you are concerned about.

If you are not already, you must start using eye cream—sparingly but frequently. Only through the use of eye creams will you be able to moisturize the area where your crow's feet are forming.

By changing your skin care products and looking at your diet and how that may be contributing to your problem skin, hopefully you can start experiencing skin that reflects the proper care you are now giving it.

On my upper chin (below the lip area) I have these little bumps that have been there for as long as I can remember, and they won't go away. I can't see them (unless under a particular light, close up in scrutiny), and the area is smooth when touched. However, when the area is stretched (as when making a face) I can then feel these little bumps. What can I do?

My first recommendations to not focus too much on those little, undetectable bumps. I do know what you are talking about, however. They are probably little pockets of oil sitting just under the surface of your skin. And sometimes even the clay mask cannot get rid of them—they have too much dead skin grown over them.

One thing you can do, but you have to be gentle, is to use a scrub in that area. I emphasize gentle because in my experience, people who focus on these sort of undetectable places tend to be a bit too gungho about getting rid of them. Also using a clay mask will or should help to minimize the size of these little pockets.

In the past few years, I have had many breakouts. Mostly in weird spots like my neck and behind my ears. I always drink 8-10 glasses of water each day. I also work out on a regular basis. Within the last year I have increased my fruits and vegetables significantly. I am also cutting back on sugar and am trying to eat more organic foods to limit the number of toxins in my body. However the changes haven't seemed to help my blemishes.

This problem could simply be a matter of not getting the sweat off your face after working out. The location of the problems is the first clue. The neck isn't a very likely place for breakout to occur. Maybe occasionally, but not on an ongoing basis. Then behind the ears is equally unusual. Sweat, however, is commonly found in both of these places.

If sweat from exercise is the culprit, you want to always be sure to splash-rinse your face and neck with water after you stop exercising. If you aren't near water, be sure to splash or wash your face as soon as possible. Don't let sweat dry on your skin. It is irritating and can cause problems, especially in these odd areas.

Sweat may not be the problem, and your blemishes could be due to hormones. There are many factors to consider when it comes to skin breaking out.

Keep analyzing your life, in general, and specifically on a daily basis to become aware of what you may be eating, doing, or engaging in that might be making your blemishes worse. I will say time and again, problem skin is caused by something. It is up to you to decipher all the elements and components that make up your life and be the sleuth, helping to figure out why the problems are occurring.

Product Recommendations

I found your book to be very helpful, and my skin has improved a great deal using your suggestions. However, unless I missed it, you didn't provide recommendations for what specific product brands to use.

I realize you are turning to this section in hopes of finding specific product recommendations with the brand names listed. But you won't find that list here. As much as I understand why you want specific product names, my gift to you is to help you understand your skin and about products in general, so you can be armed with knowledge when you go to purchase your products. Sure, it would be great if I would name specific brands, especially inexpensive products, but even then, those products wouldn't be right for everybody. In *Timeless Skin* I mention a few cleansers by name, then I received emails from many readers who couldn't use one or both for various reasons.

Although many people have contacted me to purchase the products I sell, some of my favorite emails have been from those of you who took the information you learned in *Timeless Skin* and went out and purchased products (wherever) that ended up helping your skin. Not because of the product line per se, but because you knew what type of products to look for, when to use what, and what ingredients to seek out or avoid. I want to educate you, the consumer, on the finer things to look for and to know about your skin. Then, armed with this information, you can choose what to use. Yes, this can be a daunting task, but I have empirical data (from you!) that proves it can be done.

I am looking for a hydrating night cream that will also provide some exfoliation or cell renewal. My skin is reasonably sensitive, so I can't use retinol products. What would you recommend for face and body?

The conventional approach for this person would be to put her on an alpha hydroxy acid (AHA) cream that would both moisturize and have some exfoliating abilities. But conventionally is not the way I would help her. She has already told me her skin is sensitive, so any of the acid products (including AHAs, vitamin C products, and products with retinol in them) would not be wise for her to use. These types of ingredients will simply further her sensitivities.

I am not a fan of a product having several jobs. I think a moisturizer should moisturize and, in this case, a separate exfoliator would be in order to give this woman the exfoliation and cell renewal she is looking for. Why is it that we want all-in-one products? Because exfoliation is so important to all skin and ages, it is imperative to do this step separately, rather than use a moisturizer with exfoliation capabilities. Those abilities are limited, I assure you.

My recommendation for this person would be to get a good night cream that is appropriate for her particular skin type, and also purchase a good exfoliator that she can use on her sensitive skin. This is where a gel-type peel or gommage comes in handy. It will do an excellent job of getting rid of the dead cells, which also helps to step up cell renewal, while at the same time not irritating her sensitive skin.

My skin seems to be a little red lately on the cheeks. I am 55 years old, so my skin needs some firming abilities and a good moisturizer. Can you give me some ideas?

Do you use AHAs or Retin-A on your skin? The cheek area usually seems to show the signs of capillary damage more so than other parts of our faces. I think this is primarily because when we get flushed, it usually shows up in the cheeks. So be sure not to use AHAs or any other irritating ingredients, including retinols and topical vitamin C products. Also if you get your face in the hot shower water, over time this will definitely cause redness in the cheek area, among other places.

As far as firming, there is nothing short of surgery that will truly lift the skin or firm it up. At 55 you are probably showing the signs of what 55-year-old skin looks like. This may not be consistent with how you want it to look, however.

There really is no cream that will tend to all of the needs of this client. She wants something to help with redness, sagging skin, and hydration. As an aesthetician, I would try to tackle the most prominent problem first. If, for instance, this person really did have a lot of redness, that is what I would concentrate my efforts on. Any cream she uses will have moisturizing abilities, but no cream will really have firming abilities. I would counsel her on the need to keep hot and cold water off her face and to be aware that sun exposure also affects capillaries, along with alcohol, smoking and caffeine. These can all affect the redness on her cheeks.

If her skin was dehydrated and dry and the redness was minimal, I would probably concentrate on having her exfoliate to alleviate any dead cell buildup that may be inhibiting superficial hydration. If her skin was true-dry, I would give her a hydration booster (a glycerin or even oil-based liquid) and an overall good moisturizer for her skin—one that had the capability to help the redness.

Why should I use some expensive cream when I can buy one for a few dollars at the grocery or dime store?

If you can find inexpensive products that work well for your skin, that's great! You don't necessarily have to spend a lot of money. Experience has shown me that most inexpensive products don't work for people with problem skin, whether it be breakout or redness or sensitivities. So if you have no-problem skin and find dime store products that work, use those if you want to.

Ingredients can make a difference, depending on the product they are in. I like essential oils, and usually the products that contain essential oils are more expensive than what you would find in a grocery or dime store. The bottom line is always to find what works best for you. Maybe you can use inexpensive products; maybe you can't. Your skin will always let you know what you need to do.

I find many skin care systems a little pricey. However, I do real-
ize if you want a good product you have to pay for it. But what
do normal, working class women do if they want great skin? I
have tried many products and most seem to do well on my skin. I
just hope I don't have to mortgage my home to continue to use a
good product!

I realize products can get expensive. However, if you find something that really does work and is something that you can continue to use for a long time, I would imagine you will save money. How? Because you won't be wasting your time and money on the myriad products out there—many of which I am sure you have purchased, and perhaps without much effect on your skin. In my opinion, when it comes to your skin you may have to pay a little more to get good products. It can be a hard road finding something that works. Sampling is very important. Then you can try any product in the privacy of your own home and see how it works over several days.

Depending on your skin, you may be able to use an inexpensive product. Just be sure to monitor your skin to be sure whatever you are using is doing a good job, and of course not causing any problems. You don't have to spend a lot of money, but percentage-wise, better products do tend to cost more.

A friend and I just purchased your book and love it! We are won-
dering what you think of Neutrogena® products. I am currently
40 and using the cleanser, pore minimizing toner (alcohol-free),
and also the regular oil-free moisturizer. I have been told that I
look much younger than 40 so I am thinking so far the products
seem to be working. I also have some broken capillaries near my
nose. I use Bobbi Brown® cosmetics and those seem to be able to
cover up the capillaries. I do exercise quite a bit outdoors, but

always use a sunscreen. Any thoughts would be great. My friend wants to purchase the Neutrogena products and also wanted your opinion.

It sounds like you don't have any real problems with your skin other than broken capillaries. And if you are happy with the results from the products you are using, I would tell you to keep using them if you want to. It is when people have problems with their skin, and therefore specific needs, that a product line like Neutrogena probably isn't going to go the trick. But if you like your program and don't see any adverse effects from the products, I say continue on. And if your friend wants to try what you are using—great. Her skin will be different, but these products may work for her too. Then again, they may not. She will just have to experiment and see.

This is not earth-shattering information. Your skin is always going to let you know about what is good for it and what isn't. It's when you don't listen that you can run into problems. But as I said, if you have no-problem skin, you will be able to use products people with problem skin probably cannot. Consider yourself lucky.

Is it true that after using the same products on your face for about 6 months or so, your skin gets used to them, and they tend not to work?

I've been using the same product for several years. I have read it is good to switch products now and then so your skin doesn't get used to them. Is this true?

My response to these kinds of questions is an emphatic no! There is no reason why you can't use a product indefinitely. The idea that you have to change products due to your skin getting used to them, rendering them ineffective, is a myth. Perhaps this way of thinking is used to promote a new product, or it is simply a misnomer that has never been challenged.

Products you use should work *period*, not just for a period of time. Case in point: I have been using one product line for over 20 years. They are the products I sell and use in my practice. I have never had a feeling I needed to switch brands. The products work great, so why change? Through the years I have used many different products within the line, but I see no reason to switch lines altogether when I have absolutely no reason to. I have many clients who have used this product for years and years, and because their skin continues to do well and look great, they continue on with the same product line.

So the answer to "Can I use the same product for a long time?" is yes, if you are doing well with that product or that line of products. There is no good reason to switch if you don't need to. You may want to, but that is a different story altogether.

I am interested in a night cream. I am 27 and very age conscious, so the product needs to be anti-aging. I have combination skin— dry cheeks and a slightly congested t-zone area with some broken capillaries throughout my skin.

The first thing I would say in response to this email is this person needs to give up the anti-aging concerns, at least at first. Let me reiterate: you need to prioritize how to treat your skin. The first and foremost concern is the amount of oil in your skin. This emailer has combination skin, which means that she has a little too much oil production in the common areas of her nose, forehead and chin. Her cheeks probably aren't truly dry; they may feel that way, but I imagine the skin on her cheeks is normal. She may, however, be even slightly dehydrated, making her skin feel dry where she isn't as oily.

Starting with combination skin is really where she needs to focus. The concern she has about aging is justified, of course. She is 27 years old and is just at the beginning of seeing the aging process start. What I want to tell her is: just wait! The lines and wrinkles that you may just have inklings of now will deepen with time, no matter what you do (short of cosmetic procedures).

If she was to go to the department store looking for anti-aging products, she would probably leave with things that would cause problems and not help her skin. No doubt "anti-aging" products would contain ingredients for true-dry skin; ingredients that would work for that type of skin, but on her skin they could cause congestion at best, and at the worst, breakout.

Can you see how you can't get caught up in the marketing words used in skin care products? You must stick to your guns and buy products based on the number one priority: oil or lack of oil produced by your oil glands. If you veer off course, you will be emailing me with a concern about your problem skin, when it could be something as simple as using products that aren't appropriate for your skin type. Even if this person was 57, she still might not need a product that has a lot of oils and emollients. It all would depend on the amount of oil in her pores.

Her second concern would be the broken capillaries. This probably causes her skin to be a bit sensitive. But again, she doesn't necessarily want to buy products specifically for sensitive skin. It all depends on if those same products will work for her combination skin. Even in the line I sell, many of the products for sensitive skin are better utilized by those who have normal to dry skin. If a client has oily or combination skin and is also sensitive, I will always treat the oil first. Products—any products—shouldn't cause irritation or aggravate sensitive skin. So using products for combination skin shouldn't cause her skin to react. If she can find sensitive skin products that don't also create more congestion in her pores, great. As always, it will be a trial and error process, no matter whose products you are using.

Based on this emailer's comments, this is how I would prioritize what she needs to look for in skin care products. First, treat the combination skin. Second, know what to do and what not to do for the broken capillaries. There is a lot of information in both of my books regarding this condition. Lastly, if aging—or aging well—is a concern, be armed with knowledge about the truth and the myths of products and procedures in regard to aging. She would do well to watch the amount of sun exposure she is accumulating as well as look at her diet to see where she may need some adjustments that could help her body in the short and long run.

Miracle cures can be found in someone else's books or products. With me you will get the truth, and the truth is we are all aging every *second* of every day. How are you going to use your time?

This next email is from my step-niece, Nicole. I wanted to include it because Nicole was 14 when she wrote this, and I think she exemplifies a lot of teenage girls. She is using a skin care routine, but doesn't have a lot of guidance as to what to use other than from magazine ads and TV commercials. Here is her email, with her teenage humor intact.

So about my skin, it is pretty good. It's normal and "well." The only places that I have problems and have to watch are around the creases of my nose and the "middle line" on my chin. My forehead isn't really a problem, and my skin is all around okay.

I wash both morning and night with Oxy Balance® Deep Penetrating Facial Cleansing Wash that contains 2% salicylic acid. It is a gel cleanser and it works pretty well. I also use a Clearasil Stay Clear Zone Control Clear Stick. It also has 2% salicylic acid. Now that I am thinking, the rest of the ingredients (which aren't on the package) are probably just alcohol, which is really cute.*

So if anything I am doing is like horrible, or if you have any suggestions I would love it, because my system is of my own making, and I know that a little advice could probably go a long way.

Oh yeah, I do use a fruit scrub from Origins®, and I really like it. I also use a charcoal and white China clay mask, which I like also. If you have any ideas I would welcome them with open pores. (Ha ha.)

*These exact products are no longer available. They have morphed into new and slightly different salicylic acid and benzoyl peroxide products.

Nicole's program is pretty typical for a teenager. She is probably getting most, if not all of her skin care information from TV and magazines. Neither one will give her much more than product marketing with a lot of advertising dollars behind them.

She seems to have a really good routine. She washes morning and night and uses exfoliators and clay masks. Overall she seems to have done a really good job of divining her own system, and as long as her skin stays clear, she can continue using what she's using.

Although she is using products that might be drying out her skin, it doesn't seem to be bothering her at the moment. My advice would be to monitor the situation, and if she starts to develop problems with her skin, I would get her on some better products that don't contain drying ingredients.

Of course diet is also going to play a key role in Nicole's skin. Maybe not now, but at some point. As a teenager I had a horrible diet filled with sugar galore, and I had great skin until I turned 21. Then everything caught up with me, and I developed acne. To tell a teenager not to eat sugar and other junk food is sort of ludicrous, but do watch the intake of certain foods if problems start occurring with your skin. Otherwise, enjoy your teen years!

I am writing from Florida. I have received many facials over the years, but I don't really know my skin well enough to choose products myself. I have sun-damaged skin with large pores and premature aging. I am 32 years old and look much older. I want to start getting facials again but don't know how to go about finding one locally. Also, how do I start using products when I don't know what my skin needs?

One thing I want to say is next time you get a facial, and every time you get one from a different aesthetician, ask them about your skin. If you are getting or have had a lot of facials, you really should know a little bit about your skin. Perhaps at the time you were in treatment, you didn't really care—but now you do. Asking the professional working on your skin, especially if the same person is giving you facials over time, will give you the information you need to choose products. Every aesthetician may say something a little different from the next, but overall you should get the same general analysis.

I wrote an entire chapter on finding out where to get a professional facial in *Timeless Skin*. Here I will just list a few of the questions you can ask to get a general feel for the salon you are thinking about going to. Without asking questions, you are taking a risk going in somewhere cold. For more details, refer to *Timeless Skin*, but for now here are some questions to ask:

What type of business is it? Mostly hair, a large spa, or skin care only? Which products does the salon use? Are samples available? (This is very important!) How long has the aesthetician worked there? How long has she been an aesthetician? Does she use the product herself? How long is the facial? Does the salon use machines? Which ones? What about extractions? How much does the facial cost? Is the price all inclusive or can extras be added? What will my skin look like afterwards? Will makeup be applied after the facial?

This emailer mentioned sun damage and enlarged pores, but said nothing about oiliness or even dryness. Knowing the oil content will help determine which products she should use. She first needs to determine her skin type, which she can successfully do on her own or with the help of an aesthetician. She needs to assess the oil or lack of oil in her skin by checking in the mirror to see if there is any congestion like blackheads or whiteheads in her pores, along with flakiness on the surface of her skin. All of these are factors in choosing the right products. Coming from Florida, she no doubt has, does, and will continue to get a lot of sun and therefore sun damage. Premature aging is a common occurrence in year-round sunny climates like Florida. Getting regular facials and consistently using products for her skin type will be the best ways to keep her skin in good shape. If she truly is aging prematurely, topical products aren't going to give her the youth she has lost through overexposure to the sun. However, I'll bet she enjoyed all the activities and time spent in the sun, and that has to mean something.

I have spent a small fortune on skin care products over the past 20 years, most of which didn't work or agree with my skin. I have tried every major department store line along with many "natural" lines via mail order. I am about ready to give up! I am 44 years old and have oily skin that is easily irritated. I have large pores, blackheads, and am now getting slightly dry on the surface. My skin never feels comfortable. I have to wear foundation, which I hate. Otherwise as soon as the oil builds up on the surface, my skin becomes reddened and irritated. I have never felt pretty and have always been very self-conscious about my skin. Although I do experience an occasional pimple, I refuse to use those harsh acne product lines. Can you recommend products that will help to balance and clear my skin? I would love to find a line that I could stick with that I was certain would be beneficial and not harmful to my skin. I really don't know what to do with my skin.

Unfortunately, these comments are true for many people. If you have problem skin, it may be very difficult for you to find relief in the land of department store products. These types of products are for the masses and don't necessarily have the capability to deal with real skin problems. Additionally, the people selling the products aren't necessarily the most knowledgeable when it comes to skin and how to treat it.

I am 44 years old and have oily skin that is easily irritated. I have large pores, blackheads, and am now getting slightly dry on the surface. My skin never feels comfortable. The oiliness and irritation are the most important things to treat with her skin. To reiterate, department store products probably aren't geared to help this skin type. The dryness she is experiencing may be due to ingredients in her products meant to help with the oil by drying the surface skin out. Again, something I talk about as being a poor way to treat a problem, and consequently, causing her more angst.

I have to wear foundation, which I hate. Otherwise as soon as the oil builds up on the surface, my skin becomes reddened and irritated. I have never felt pretty and have always been very self-conscious about my skin. I'm not sure how foundation is helping her problem. To me, using a powder would be more appropriate. Powders contain talc and talc helps to absorb oil. Regardless of the past, I truly believe she can get to a place where she feels good about her skin.

Although I do experience an occasional pimple, I refuse to use those harsh acne product lines. This is a smart, intuitive response that I'm glad she is listening to!

Can you recommend products that will help to balance and clear my skin? I would love to find a line that I could stick with that I was certain would be beneficial and not harmful to my skin. I really don't know what to do with my skin. I would like to know the nature of the irritation. Is it always there or do products incite the irritation to appear? If the irritation is being caused by products, try to figure out a common denominator and look for products that don't have the known irritants in the ingredient list. As far as the blackhead problem, doing The Extras (exfoliating along with using a clay mask) at least once per week (two or even three times may be necessary) will go a long way to help your skin stay less congested, which is important to help eliminate blackheads. Foundation, depending on its ingredients, may be furthering your blackhead problem. Since it is sitting on your skin all day, foundation can create not only blackheads but enlargement of the pores too. Using geranium essential oil on the spots (infected blemishes only) will help them to go away faster.

In short, use products for oily skin that don't have drying ingredients in them. Try using powder instead of foundation. Along with The Basics for your skin type, do The Extras. This program isn't complicated, it just gets complicated by the enormity of product choices available on the market. Narrow down your choices (using products for your skin type only) to simplify your program.

> *I am using a moisturizing lotion for all skin types. It says that it is "a light, non-greasy, easily absorbed lotion for daily use," "pH balanced," "fragrance free," "dermatologist tested," etc. I always thought a lotion was very light, but after I put it on, my face becomes so shiny. Why is that, and should I use oil-free products and non-shiny?*

My first instinct is that this lotion has mineral oil or some type of petroleum as a top ingredient. These types of products don't penetrate well because mineral oil tends to sit on the surface of your skin without being absorbed.

Technically, I suppose, lotion does connote a lighter texture, whereas a cream has a heavier consistency. This might not always be the case, so be careful when choosing products.

Rather than oil-free products, I would recommend using creams (or lotions) that contain vegetal oils vs. mineral oil or petroleum. You may not find such an animal at the drug store, but most other places (department stores, health food stores, salons) should provide many choices of mineral oil-free moisturizers. (See **Oils in Products.**)

I have found out that if I do too much for my skin it becomes dry, red, and I get more small pimples. If I do nothing then I occasionally get pimples. What do you recommend?

You may be using products that are actually irritating your skin. Normally when you do extra steps to take care of your skin, it will reflect this care and look more radiant and healthy. That you are having the opposite experience may reflect poorly on your products, but then again, it may just be how your skin is. I recommend finding a place to get a facial in your area. Then you can have someone take a good look at your skin and give you advice on how best to take care of it. Be sure to take your products in to show the aesthetician. She may have some insight as to the types of products you are using and why you are having such negative results.

Doing "too much" in almost any area can do more harm than good. Too much exercise (especially done incorrectly) can cause injuries. Eating too much food can overload your digestive system and cause anything from indigestion to constipation, weight gain and more. Too much stress? We all know about that! And when it comes to your skin, doing too much may indeed cause problems. But this is especially true—and inevitable—if the products you are using are inappropriate and/or meant to "dry things out." Quite simply, I recommend **The Basics** and **The Extras** (see sections).

I am 36 years old and have lots of sun damage. I have had several precancerous moles removed from my body, so I know my face has really gotten it too. I am starting to notice deep furrows between my brows (it's hereditary), large pores on my cheeks and forehead, as well as lines on my forehead, sun (or age) spots on my cheekbones and around my eyes, loss of elasticity around my eyes and a thinning of the skin around my eyes, and these horrible cords are starting to develop on my neck!

I am confused about what to do in the morning. I want to wear sunscreen during the day because of all of my sun damage, but I also want to address my age-related concerns. How many of these products can I combine together? Will putting too many layers on my face start to clog my pores? Would AHA products help with my sun damage? See how confused I am?!

Since this person has already had precancerous growths removed, I would absolutely insist she wear sunscreen every day, rain or shine. There is no point in trying to reverse the signs of aging while at the same time throwing caution to the wind and not inhibiting further damage.

The changes in her skin she is noticing are the signs of aging. Lines deepen, pores may tend to enlarge, and the skin can definitely start to thin. Addressing the age-related problems is not so easy. What I would address is her acceptance policy on the inevitable. I realize that is not what she or any of you want to hear, but that is the truth as I see it. You will age and she is starting to really see the changes that are occurring in this natural process. Of course, she may be experiencing some acceleration in the aging of her skin because of past sun exposure.

She's right—if she piles on too many creams to handle all of her concerns, she will probably end up with rebellious skin—breakout. My recommendations would be to wear a good sunscreen daily and absolutely use eye cream if she isn't already. If pore enlargement is a problem, using a clay mask will at least keep the pores cleaned out but won't shrink her pores. The age or sun spots she is complaining about will fade if she keeps direct sunlight off her face, and wearing daily sunscreen will help to a small degree with that.

She could go the route of surgery for her neck concerns. A cosmetic surgeon seeing the actual person will be better able to assess the situation. She could use Botox for her furrowing brow and maybe even a peel or laser for her aging concerns. All of these procedures and more are available to all of us if we want to change our appearance. However, this surgical approach is not my approach.

I've started noticing a couple of (gasp!) wrinkles around my mouth and eyes. Any suggestions? Yes, I am wearing sunscreen and a hat!

Yes, wrinkles will come, and there is only so much you can do. When you have the first inklings of lines appearing, it may be disconcerting. You're going from nothing to something. Hopefully, you'll get used to the lines because they will get deeper with time.

Sun plus time equals aging. This equation is age old and undeniable. Yes, wear sunscreen and sunglasses to prevent excessive squinting; all those things you know to do—do! Eye cream is vital if you aren't already wearing it daily, and hats are absolutely necessary. If you find a good one, let me know—I'm always on the lookout. And exfoliating is crucial to help keep the dead cell buildup off your face, making the lines look less severe.

I'm sorry I don't have a miracle cure for you. But you can always go to the department store—they are full of miracles! It'll cost you, and it's doubtful you'll see any big results, but they *are* selling miracles! Decide what is important: how you look or who you are.

I found a product from Neutrogena that is a spot treatment for blemishes. Do you know this product, and what are your views?

The product is Neutrogena's On-the-Spot Acne Treatment. The package says "maximum strength," and "less irritation, won't dry out skin." It contains 2.5% benzoyl peroxide. This is far from "maximum strength;" however, this lesser percentage of benzoyl peroxide, which is a drying ingredient, is actually preferable to the higher 5% and 10% versions. Looking at the inactive ingredients, bentonite clay is listed second after water. That means this product is primarily clay along with the benzoyl peroxide. I tried it on a few blemishes, and although I find geranium oil and/or clay mask dotted on my skin helps to diminish the spots more effectively, I did find this product to be OK. It was also without the usual drying effects of higher strength benzoyl peroxide spot treatments.

Note: This Neutrogena product will leave a whitish film wherever it is applied; dotting clay will leave a greenish color (or whatever the color of the mask is); and geranium will leave no visual sign you are wearing it, just a strong aromatic.

The following is a book review I am including to help make a point. Excerpts of Customer Reviews © Amazon.com, Inc. All rights reserved. Used with permission.

Reviewer: A reader from Dallas, Texas USA. I was looking for products Ms. Ash recommends and I was disappointed. She gave some ideas on what to look for in products, but it requires me to spend a lot of time looking. She even says it's a difficult process (unless you go to a professional spa). I looked at her website and as I suspected you'll have to spend a lot of money (at least $30 per product). I bought this book to try and find a way to spend less money—but I found out I have to spend at least $120 for *cleanser, toner, moisturizer and a mask—this doesn't include the other stuff she recommends! Ugghh...Please someone recommend another book!*

No one likes a bad review. I remember the day I read this on the Internet. *Timeless Skin* had just come out, and I was getting so much positive feedback, and then boom! This review hit me like a ton of bricks. That it came from someone in the city I was living in at the time (Dallas) was yet another blow to me. If only I could contact this reader and at least extend an invitation for a complimentary consultation so I might help this person better understand his or her skin and any problems that might be occurring, or at least steer him or her in the right direction.

I included this email to reiterate my stand on product recommendations. Of course if you go to my website, I am recommending the products I know in depth and have been using personally and professionally for over 20 years. I purposely do not mention in this book or in *Timeless Skin* the product lines I work with. I want to give you, the consumer, information so that *you* can pick and choose the products you want to use that will benefit your skin. Certainly, it would be impossible for me to try every single product line available and make my recommendations based on hard and fast research. So instead I am attempting to give you pointers as far as what to look for as well as what to avoid when looking for products so you can make educated decisions. Perhaps the writer of the above review would be better off purchasing a book like *Don't Go to the Cosmetic Counter Without Me* (Beginning Press, 2003) in order to get specific product recommendations.

I make no apologies for the way I disseminate information. No book or skin care product is for everyone, and I certainly hope this reader and any others who were looking for name brand recommendations have found what they are looking for. I only recommend products that either I or my clients have experience with. So for me to recommend an entire book filled with brand name products would take the rest of my natural life to research. I truly believe you can find products out in the marketplace that will work for your skin. And judging from the comments I have received from my readers, I know it is possible.

Puffy Eyes

What causes puffy eyes? Basically it is edema (fluid retention) in the fat tissue above the bones encircling your eyes that causes puffy eyes. Those pockets fill up with fluid causing puffiness, probably due to inflammation. Inflammation comes from many different things: food allergies, alcohol consumption, smoking, sugar, among others.

How can I treat my puffy eyes? Prevention or avoiding the causes of puffiness are the first steps to alleviating puffy eyes. But since we live in the real world, I'll give you a few things you can do to treat the puffiness you may be experiencing.

First, if you wake up in the morning with puffy eyes, before jolting out of bed, take it slow. Sit up in bed supported by your pillows with your back straight. Just sit there for a few minutes and give your body a chance to adjust to this more vertical position. If you get up quickly, the fluids that have settled around your eyes don't have a chance to drain from this area, or at least not as efficiently as they would if you sit up and let them drain first.

Using something cool on the eyes will help to reduce some of the puffiness. Do not use ice or anything extremely cold—you can damage the capillaries. But ice with a heavy cloth over it or some of the gel packs available for the eyes would be OK. You just don't want to use anything ice cold directly on your skin; cool is acceptable.

There are eye creams on the market that address puffy eyes. They contain specific ingredients meant to help with the drainage around the eye area. Rosemary, for instance, has a constricting action, which can help to ease puffiness that results from fluid retention. Be aware that no matter what a product claims to do, it's doubtful anything is going to "cure" or totally eliminate the puffiness around your eyes.

Cosmetic surgery is the only way to truly get rid of the fat pockets underneath your eyes. If you are through having to deal with excessive puffy eyes, you may want to consult with a few plastic surgeons and see what your options are. If you contend with puffiness every day and you are eating foods that are inflammation-inducing, I highly recommend starting with your diet before you consider going under the knife. It is the harder road, but truly it is the one that your body will benefit most from in the long run. Keep in mind, foods that are causing puffy eyes are creating an inflammatory response in more than just your eye area. Any book by Nicholas Perricone (a now famous author and public speaker—and dermatologist) will talk in detail about the body's inflammatory response to foods along with dietary recommendations. I think his first book, *The Wrinkle Cure*, is his best and most cogent effort. Also see **Allergies & Skin** and **Dark Circles**.

Preparation H®. I'm sure many of you have heard about a "miracle" treatment for puffiness around the eyes: *Preparation H*, the hemorrhoid cream. I have read about this in a few books and magazine articles, and I'm frequently asked if it works, so I had to find out for myself what the truth is.

I went to the store and looked at all the different ointments and creams meant to shrink the pain and itching of hemorrhoids. There are a few brands available, Preparation H being the most well-known. Like many medications, there are generic brands that have virtually identical ingredients for less money. In order to do a "controlled" study, I purchased the Preparation H brand, but any of them would have worked the same I'm sure.

The ingredients listed in the cream as "active" are glycerin (12%), petrolatum (18%), phenylephrine HCI (0.25%), and shark liver oil (3.0%). Glycerin is one of the main components of most creams due to its water-binding abilities. It is a humectant and therefore attracts moisture (water) to itself. How this is going to help with puffiness I can't imagine. Petrolatum, which is just Vaseline or petroleum jelly, is another ingredient that helps to make the cream smooth and spreadable. How this particular ingredient helps with puffiness is also a mystery to me. If you were to put Vaseline around your eyes, it would probably cause puffiness due to its ability to retain moisture. I also wonder what the active component is in this very inert (inactive) substance. Petrolatum is also going to clog your pores. I could not find phenylephrine HCI, but found phenylephrine HCL in my ingredient book lists. Also known as hydrochloride, it is used in some nasal decongestants to contract blood vessels or in medications to take the red out of the eyes. This would be consistent with a cream meant to shrink tissue, in this case, hemorrhoids. Shark liver oil is loaded with vitamin A and is used to lubricate many creams and lotions. Out of all these "active" ingredients, the only one that seems to be acting on reducing inflammation is phenylephrine HCI. The inactive ingredients listed on the package are mostly fillers, lanolins, and preservatives; they are nothing special, and certainly nothing harmful.

Like many of you, I wake up in the morning with moderate puffiness under my eyes. Throughout the day, the puffiness naturally diminishes, if only due to gravity and the fluids draining from the eye area. I used the preparation under only one eye so I could see if there was a difference between my two undereyes. After using Preparation H (under one eye) for two full weeks, I can honestly and unequivocally say that this product didn't do a thing for my undereye puffiness. I just didn't see any appreciable difference. I would even ask those people I saw in that time frame, and they couldn't see a measurable difference between my two eyes.

I went back to the store and purchased the ointment and the gel, thinking maybe I had used the wrong form of Preparation H. Neither of these made any difference either, further cementing my belief that Preparation H should be used as it was originally intended and not for puffy eyes.

Perhaps in a situation like a makeup artist working on a talk show guest or a model in a runway show, the Preparation H does work wonders. But my experience using it didn't prove to be as beneficial. Try it for yourself. See if using this hemorrhoid cream around your eye area helps to reduce puffiness you may experience. I'd love to hear your own results.

R

Relaxation

Life is a balancing act. If you continue to lead a stress-filled life without incorporating stress-reducing activities, your body will eventually falter. Sometimes getting sick is your body telling you it's time to slow down. That is why balancing the stress in your life with relaxation is so important. Without the two in balance, it's doubtful you can remain healthy for the long haul.

Relaxing—every day—is the stuff health is made of. Relaxation can come in many forms. It could simply be becoming aware of your breathing by taking a few deep breaths, which immediately helps to calm your nerves. Relaxation could be getting a massage or a facial. It could be drawing a nice hot bubble bath, climbing in the tub and shutting the door to the world for a few minutes. Reading is relaxing for many people.

There are hundreds of books on the subject of relaxation. Audio cassettes and CDs are available that have either meditation exercises or simply quiet, peaceful music that can be helpful tools for relaxation. Exercising is widely known to help many people relax. For me, exercise definitely helps to release stress and get my circulation going, but I don't really find it relaxing. I am more of a massage or facial person. Give me a day at a spa, and I am a happy camper. Most of the time, though, I create my own relaxing spa-type experience in the comfort, convenience, and free environment of my home.

Some nights if I am in need of balancing, I will make some tea or perhaps pour a nice glass of wine. I have a lot of candles throughout my home that I like to light. Candles not only give off wonderful relaxing aromatics, but I think the kind of light they put out is relaxing on its own. I like to relax in the bathtub—especially if it's full of bubbles. Having soft music on in the background lays the groundwork for my body to fully let go and relax into the hot, bubbly water.

If I'm being extra good, I will exfoliate before the bath then put on a clay mask to wear while in the tub. This way I am not only creating a relaxing environment for my body, but I'm treating my skin to a facial as well.

When I'm in the bath, I will do some deep breathing to ensure my body gets a good supply of oxygen while letting all my muscles release at the same time. I don't have children, but if you do and you want to relax in the bath (or wherever), arrange to have your husband (or wife) or a friend take care of them—even for just 30 minutes once in a while so you can take care of yourself.

Without relaxation in our lives, we could not exist—not for long, anyway. There has to be a balance in order for the body to keep going. Whatever it is that is relaxing to you, work on incorporating one, two, or more of these activities into your life to create the balance your body deserves. Relaxation is not just a frivolous waste of time; it is a necessary component of a healthy life and a healthy body—and therefore, healthy skin.

Restylane®

Restylane is basically used as a wrinkle filler and is made from hyaluronic acid. Hyaluronic acid is an amino acid (a protein) found naturally in our own skin. It is suggested that Restylane is going to take over for collagen as the number one choice for plumping up depressions in the skin, aka wrinkles. Unlike collagen, which has an animal origin, hyaluronic acid is made in the chemistry lab, alleviating the possibility of allergic reaction like with animal-derived collagen.

Restylane received FDA approval at the end of 2003. This product is used in many countries in the world and has been for some time. The FDA was no doubt feeling pressure to approve this latest "miracle cure" for wrinkles, since everyone (almost everyone) was champing at the bit to start using it.

The results of a single injection can last anywhere from six months to even an entire year. Prices will vary according to whom you go to and what they are charging, but the basic cost per syringe is around $500. Collagen, on the other hand, costs about the same but only lasts half as long.

As far as I am concerned, the jury is still out on this latest and greatest "miracle" to remove the life and lines that are on your face. I'm in my 40s and am resistant to changing what is now the beginning of my own aging process. I suppose it is the scientist in me that is looking forward to seeing exactly how I will age; I want to see what lines will show up, how gray my hair will get, and what I will look like—untouched—at 50 years of age. Perhaps once I have arrived at 50, I will partake in all the things that now I am rebelling against. I give myself the leeway to change my mind, knowing that I might just keep traveling on the very same path I am on now. Time will tell.

Rosacea: Mystery Skin Disease

If you have rosacea or think you might, luckily you are living in a time of research and discovery about this mysterious, sometimes debilitating disease. And yes, it is a disease, defined in Merriam-Webster's dictionary as "an abnormal bodily condition that impairs functioning and can usually be recognized by signs and symptoms."

Well over 14 million people in America have rosacea, and probably more are not diagnosed who have it. In contrast, however, I have had numerous clients who either thought they had this skin condition or were diagnosed with having it who, in my opinion, did not have rosacea at all. Perhaps this has happened because up until now there has been limited information about rosacea, so it has been lumped in with other (sometimes overly diagnosed) skin problems. Some feel that because they have certain symptoms, they must truly have rosacea. In my experience this is not always the case.

What is rosacea? The National Rosacea Society defines rosacea, pronounced rose-ay-shah, as "a disease affecting the skin of the face— mostly where people flush. Rosacea usually starts with redness on the cheeks and can slowly worsen to include one or more additional symptoms and parts of the face, including the eyes. Because changes are gradual, it may be hard to recognize rosacea in its early stages. Unfortunately, many people mistake rosacea for a sunburn, a complexion change, or acne and do not see a doctor."

It is considered to be a chronic condition that if left untreated, tends to worsen over time. At the beginning of the disease, rosacea may come and go in cycles with occasional flare-ups and then improvement as though it has gone into remission. Over time, if given a chance (by not avoiding your triggers), the symptoms can worsen, causing possible permanent redness and swelling, namely in the cheek area.

The cause of rosacea is unknown, and there are several reasons floating around as to why it occurs. I believe it is first and foremost a vascular condition. Other opinions are that skin mites cause rosacea. These mites are said to find a home in the capillaries of the face, nest and then proliferate and cause swelling, redness, and the bumpy skin associated with rosacea. That skin mites exist is a fact. That they are found in large numbers in the affected skin of rosacea patients is also true. That these mites are the cause of rosacea is where I disagree. I believe that through vascular changes occurring *first*, the conditions are ripe for these mites to exist and proliferate.

Who gets rosacea? Rosacea can occur in adults as young as 20 years old although it most often occurs in men and women well into their 30s up to their 50s and beyond. Women generally experience rosacea more than men, but this could be due to the fact that men tend not to complain or seek treatment for disorders with the same frequency (and tenacity) that women do.

Rosacea frequently appears in the classic "butterfly" pattern on women, with redness fanning out on the cheeks and the nose; men usually find their noses to be the most affected and red place on their face.

People with lighter complexions (fair skin) are more prone to getting rosacea. Fair skin types are more susceptible to many skin troubles just based on their coloring. UV rays, for instance, can penetrate much more readily into skin that doesn't produce much pigment. Therefore redness and sunburn are more common for those of you with light skin. Your skin tends to be more sensitive than someone with more natural sun protection (melanin). The redness of sunburn, breakout, and other skin maladies are more noticeable on light skin due to the contrast.

Let's find out what some of the common symptoms are. If you have rosacea, you already are all too familiar with some or all of these symptoms.

Symptoms: How do I know if I have rosacea? The symptoms of rosacea vary from person to person just like the triggers* will vary for each individual, but there are certain common symptoms that are characteristic of this disease. Separately the symptoms don't necessarily indicate rosacea, but if you have several together they can add up to rosacea. Not always, but potentially.

*A trigger is something that causes the classic red face or flushing associated with rosacea. For instance, using hot water on your face could trigger deep redness to cover your face—especially the cheeks—if you have rosacea. See **Triggers** later in this section.

The number one symptom is **flushing**. This is where you are blushing, but in the case of rosacea it is not necessarily just when you are embarrassed. Flushing is when a large amount of blood flows through the capillaries very quickly and the vessels expand (dilate) in order to handle the load. This causes a definite redness to come over your entire cheek area, making you look flushed. If flushing occurs a lot over a long period of time, the capillaries become damaged and blood will stagnate within the vessel, giving you a permanent redness in the cheeks.

Flushing in a rosacea candidate can occur at any time and due to any number of reasons, only one of which is embarrassment. You can become flushed when you are hot; especially while exercising, receiving sun exposure, or sitting in a sauna, steamroom, or whirlpool. Driving with the top down or sailing (sun plus wind), cooking in a hot kitchen, or sitting by the fire can also cause you to flush. You can also flush for no apparent reason at all.

Some other common symptoms of rosacea are **telangiectasia** (capillary damage), **swelling or puffiness in the cheek area**, sometimes **blemishes** where the swelling is, and always **sensitivity**. This redness, more than anything, is due to flushing. A swelling of the nose can also appear due to rosacea, more commonly occurring in men, which is a condition called **rhinophyma**. Not only the skin on the face but sometimes the eyes can become affected, causing them to become irritated, red, and bloodshot. This is called **ocular rosacea**.

The most unusual characteristic I have consistently seen with rosacea is the aforementioned swelling—something you really don't find with telangiectasia, simple breakouts, or even acne (other than the swelling at the site of the actual blemish). The type of redness is also distinct: deep red, almost bluish.

Another symptom I have found from working on clients with rosacea is their skin in the affected area (namely the cheeks) is hot, or at least very warm to the touch, and it is different in temperature than the rest of the face. It is like when someone has a fever, but the warmth is only on the cheek area. This is a condition I used to call **hot, red skin.** Now I think what I had been seeing in years past was actually rosacea.

With couperose, you can see the capillaries; they look like spider legs—thin, red, and defined. The redness I see with a rosacea client is more mottled, not defined, and the area around the capillaries is red as well. The redness is widespread and not confined to the capillaries like it is with simple couperose.

Why am I making such a big deal about whether or not you have rosacea? If you think you have rosacea and you don't, you will be mistreating your skin based on an incorrect self-diagnosis. You may be missing out on finding what is causing the problems you are experiencing with your skin. Even if you have incorrectly diagnosed yourself as having rosacea, hopefully you will pay close attention to your daily intake of food along with other factors linked to rosacea. In the long run, this awareness may pave the way for your skin to clear up.

Triggers: What causes rosacea? If you have rosacea, you will want to take stock of several things in your life that may be affecting your condition. And remember, what bothers you may not bother another rosacea sufferer. However, finding out what causes other people to have flare-ups may help give you ideas. Let's go through the triggers.

The most common trigger is **vasodilation.** This means anything causing the capillaries to expand. Known vasodilators include: **alcohol, caffeine, hot water, hot weather, flushing/blushing, spicy foods, sun, tanning beds, steam rooms, whirlpools, hot drinks, anger, exercise, menopause** and the flushing associated with **hot flashes,** some **medications,** especially **stimulants** like **ephedrine** (found in many cold and allergy medications), **herbal energy pills, stress,** and **extreme hot or cold.**

I also think **vasoconstrictors** are potential triggers, here again backing my theory that rosacea is first and foremost a vascular condition. Vasoconstrictors include: **smoking, air pollution, cold weather, cold water**, and **ice (applied to the face)**.

A mistaken link to rosacea is alcoholism or simply drinking alcohol in any amount. This, no doubt, comes from W.C. Fields who had a form of rosacea that affects the nose (it causes severe redness and swelling) called rhinophyma. And although alcohol can cause all kinds of problems including vascular changes, it is certainly not the only cause of this disease. Alcohol is a common trigger, but there are lots of people who suffer from rosacea, even rhinophyma, who have never touched alcohol in their lives.

I have a client who was having her hardwood floors refinished. She has what I consider to be a mild case of rosacea. She came in for a facial during this floor refinishing phase, and I could see a noticeable flare-up of her rosacea. Not only had the redness in her skin increased, but the poor-quality air in her house was causing severe sinus problems as well as a developing cough. I mention this case study to illustrate how things that might not be on the trigger list may still be culprits in causing your rosacea to flare up. Be consciously aware of your environment and what may be affecting your body and therefore your skin.

Treatment: How do I fix/control/treat rosacea? Instead of thinking of eliminating rosacea, start thinking of managing it. Rosacea can't be cured, but it can be controlled. If you are constantly looking for the symptoms of rosacea to completely go away, you may be setting yourself up for disappointment. I am in no way saying that it isn't possible for your rosacea to disappear, but realistically it might be more advantageous for you to see rosacea as being an ally, continually relaying messages to you about the state of your internal health. This of course includes the amount of stress in your life. I am not trying to trivialize something that is serious. I am really trying to guide you to a new way of thinking; I also want you to understand that your body is constantly sending you signals about what it likes, what it doesn't like, and how it is handling everything you are feeding it and asking it to do for you.

This relationship (between you and your body) needs to be a close, committed marriage of awareness, acceptance, and responsibility. Otherwise symptoms will go unnoticed until, perhaps, it is too late. And I'm not just talking about rosacea. I am speaking on a broader platform about every conceivable disorder caused by a body imbalanced. Rosacea may be burdensome to handle on a day-to-day basis, but if you figure out your body's language you can cut down the amount of symptoms and therefore the look of rosacea.

Professional help. The experience many of my clients have had at the dermatologist is not a great one. Commonly, dermatologists do not spend much time delving into your history, and rarely if ever do they ask questions pertaining to your diet, skin care regime, and other factors that may be affecting your skin. In part, I think this is because many dermatologists simply don't believe that you are what you eat. Yet to me, this is one of the fundamental truths about life, and I apply this principle to my work in skin care with all of my clients (and now you). What you eat and drink does affect you, but decide for yourself if you experience this to be true in your own life. I am starting to hear of more dermatologists being alert to the food/body connection, but more often than not it is a quick in-and-out of their offices. You may have to do a lot of the research and investigation yourself.

What I have divined from my clients is summed up with the words "patient, heal thyself." This is not to say that your skin problems should always be self-diagnosed or go undiagnosed. On the contrary, if you think you have rosacea, I highly recommend a check-up with your dermatologist.* But don't expect a very long consultation or a great deal of helpful information. Generally, you will get a prescription for medication, oral and/or topical. Topical medications like MetroGel® or MetroCream® may indeed help to keep the redness down to a minimum. As with so many aspects of rosacea, the efficacy of these medications is individual. Some people have great success with them, while others said these products didn't seem to help. It's worth a try to see if you can keep your rosacea at bay.

You know more than anybody else about how you are affected by food, drink, activity, stress, etc. So truly, I give you the responsibility to get to the root cause of your rosacea more than I expect a dermatologist to do so for you. You know better than anybody what works and what causes reactions. A dermatologist cannot follow you around all day to see what you do, but you are there with yourself and therefore can gather a wealth of information on what creates reactions and what creates a calming of rosacea. "Patient, watch thyself and thy habits, then go forth, and avoid thy triggers!"

*Be sure to get your moles checked while at the dermatologist!

Photoderm is a laser therapy that has been found to be effective for rosacea. Photoderm uses an intense pulsed light source that tunes into the blood vessels and can potentially clear up rosacea—capillarywise. Dr. Geoffrey Nase, author of *Beating Rosacea*, says "Photoderm was the single best treatment for my facial flushing and rosacea symptoms. Six full-faced treatments resulted in dramatic improvement in flushing, skin sensitivity, chronic facial redness, swelling, burning sensations, rhinophyma, and pupils. I cannot recommend this treatment any more highly." See **Intense Pulsed Light (IPL)**.

What is *not* rosacea? Some books note a shiny face as one of the symptoms. People who use Retin-A many times appear to have a shiny quality to their skin. This, coupled with the redness that can accompany the use of Retin-A and the sensitivity that inevitably follows using this acid, means you have already racked up three symptoms of rosacea. But do you have rosacea? You certainly would not be able to use something as irritating as Retin-A if you truly had rosacea.

A common skin problem that is often mistaken for rosacea is couperose. Couperose, as you may know, occurs when the capillaries, which are very weak by nature, are broken or rendered dysfunctional for various reasons. This condition looks similar to rosacea in many ways but capillary damage is only one symptom of rosacea and couperose should not be thought of as full-blown rosacea.

I have seen many clients over the years who have severe couperose but not what I consider to be rosacea. And some people with rosacea don't have noticeable couperose. Rosacea and couperose are, however, linked in a way because both of these skin conditions reflect problems with the capillaries.

Another skin condition that is commonly thought to be rosacea is acne, or even simple breakout. I think the confusion is due to people wanting to label their unknown problem as a known entity. If someone is breaking out and can't figure out why, then labeling it rosacea, adult acne, or a host of other titles may bring about a feeling of control, a concrete resolution. Unfortunately, this labeling process might cause a person to not scrutinize lifestyle habits (in search of probable causes), and say, "Oh, well, it's rosacea, and there isn't anything I can do about it. I'm doomed."

Wrong! Even if you truly do have rosacea, you certainly are not doomed! You are just a person who has to be more diligent than the next guy and consciously aware of what you are eating, drinking, and putting on your skin. And I've got news for you: other people should be as diligent as you have to be. Although they may not be seeing outward signs of internal problems, if they are consistently eating a poor diet and/or under stress almost all the time (even if the skin is not reflecting a state of poor internal health), the body's organs are taxed and someday, somewhere they will have to pay a price. It is just how the game of life is played. And that is why I tell my clients who have problems with their faces that it is actually a blessing in disguise. Their faces are telling them that something is wrong *inside* and that action needs to be taken. Inevitably this means a new view on how and what they are eating.

Products and rosacea: What to use? Your daily routine won't really change; you will still do your cleanse, tone, hydrate (The Basics 1-2-3) program morning and night. *What* you use will be the biggest trial and error experiment you have had to date. Even if I could give specific product recommendations here in this book, they wouldn't work for everyone. I know it is frustrating not knowing what to use, and no doubt you have already gone through a lot of different products—hopefully finding some that work for you and your rosacea.

When it comes to what products to use on your face, **mild** is the one word that comes to mind. You want to find non-irritating, mild products to use on your rosacea. You will want to avoid anything that is going to irritate your skin. This may seem like an obvious recommendation, but I still get people who come into my office who don't heed the most obvious advice. Even if they know they shouldn't do something, many times they do it anyway. Thus the saying, "Throw caution to the wind."

Soap may be an irritant if you have rosacea. I'm not a very big fan of soap—in fact I'm not a fan at all. I recommend using liquid cleansers (milks and gels) over soap any day—every day. The ingredients that make soap soap are too harsh for the skin on the face, especially if you have a condition like rosacea. In other words: Don't use soap!

Although I never recommend anyone use products that contain alcohol (the bad kind: SD and ethyl), rosaceans want to be especially careful to avoid this harsh and reaction-causing ingredient. Your toner should not have alcohol in it. Again, this is true for anybody, but especially for those with rosacea. Look for soothing ingredients like allantoin, camomile, lavender, and stinging nettle as good ingredients to have in a toner. Some natural-type products may say for sensitive skin, which would be the toner you would naturally reach for, right? But still, look at the ingredients. The toner for sensitive skin in the line of products I sell is also for a drier skin type. It contains special ingredients in it to moisturize a true-dry skin, which would be a disaster for an oiler skin type. So if you tend to have an oiler complexion, you will want to use extra caution when choosing a toner for sensitive skin. If you do end up with a toner that is too much for your skin, take it back and try one for a skin type more closely related to your own. Remember: your skin type is first and foremost based on oil content.

Moisturizers will vary, and the trial and error method may be what you have to go through in order to find the perfect moisturizer for you. Know that you will want to avoid AHAs (alpha hydroxy acids). I would also avoid glycolic peels in a facial, retinoic acid products like Retin-A and Renova, and most vitamin C products, which will probably be irritating to your skin.

Basically acid compounds, like AHAs, citric, and retonic, will worsen the symptoms of rosacea. Acids tend to dilate and irritate skin they are used on, so avoid them in the products you use. If you get facials, make sure the aesthetician has an awareness about rosacea and how to treat it in a facial.

In my facial, there are certain products I won't use if I have a client with rosacea. Instead of the citrus gel peel (gommage) I have, I use one with stinging nettle and other ingredients meant to soothe redness. There is a mild liquid peel that I won't put directly on the affected areas where the rosacea is located. I have several clients with rosacea who come in for regular monthly facials without any problems. If you have rosacea, you can carry on a regular skin care treatment schedule;

you just want to take extra care to make sure where you get your facials is helping to calm your skin down rather than causing flare-ups.

Probably by now you have gotten accustomed to what you have to do to keep your flare-ups to a minimum. But in case you don't know this yet, sun exposure is one of the worst offenders and promoters of flushing and flare-ups. So, to the degree that you can, avoid sun exposure—especially direct sunlight, and always have sunscreen on your face. Everybody needs to wear sunscreen, but those of you with rosacea (especially active rosacea) need to wear it always. Any amount of protection from sun exposure will help to some degree. There are several companies who make tinted sunscreens. If you feel the need to hide the redness that comes with rosacea, you might want to try one of the these products so you get some coverage for the redness and sun protection at the same time. And certainly if you are going to be out in the sun for a long period of time, be prepared and have a hat handy. If you don't have a hat, you will be sorry, and the extended sun exposure will probably inflame your rosacea.

What about medications? Topical medications that you may be given a prescription for at the dermatologist include MetroGel, MetroCream, and MetroLotion®. These all contain an antibacterial, antifungal agent called *metronidazole*. There are other companies who make similar products, but these (especially MetroGel) seem to be the most commonly prescribed.

Oral antibiotics are generally given to treat inflammation and possible bacterial infection in the form of pustules and pimples. Tetracycline, a common antibiotic prescribed for acne, is sometimes recommended for rosacea. Personally, I disagree with taking antibiotics in general and specifically in the case of rosacea.

Treating a problem with oral antibiotics does two things that I have a problem with. First, not only are you treating the problem, in this case rosacea on the cheeks of the face, but you are also feeding all the cells in your entire body the same medication. Second, treating with oral drugs does not generally promote self-responsibility in regard to your problem, but rather promotes a quick-fix mentality, not to mention the effects from long-term use of oral antibiotics. (See **Acidophilus/Acidophilus and antibiotics**.)

Rosacea cannot be treated with a quick fix. It requires paying attention—daily—to what you are eating, and drinking, and the environment you are allowing your skin to be exposed to. Taking a pill may give you temporary relief from the problem, but it will do nothing for long-term solutions. Rosacea may go into a remissive state while you're on oral medications, but generally it will return if the triggers are not eliminated from your life.

What *not* to use on rosacea. While reading several books about rosacea, I kept coming across the words "ice," "cold packs," and "cold water" to help control the redness associated with rosacea. I realize how frustrating having rosacea can be, but please heed this warning: Extremes in temperature, whether hot or cold, can and do have a negative effect on rosacea. Why? Because capillaries are immediately and adversely affected by temperature extremes, which can cause breaking or dysfunctioning of the capillaries, in a word—damage.

Because I believe rosacea is a vascular condition, you want to minimize dilation and constriction of the inherently weak capillaries. Therefore, using moderate temperatures on your skin is a must. Use tepid, lukewarm water on your face and use nothing in extreme (hot towels, steam, cold water splashes, and especially ice). If you have rosacea and you need to cool down your flushed face, by all means do what you have found to be effective. But if possible, steer clear of extreme cold and reach instead for something cool. As much as possible, go for moderate rather than extreme.

Case study: Ida

Many years ago my friend Ida came to me with an unusual skin condition. I honestly wasn't sure what was going on with her skin. I guessed it was rosacea, but ten years ago, I don't think I had ever (knowingly) run across this skin condition.

Ida first noticed the redness in her skin after an arduous job she was working on one summer. Ida is in the film industry and was working on a Movie of the Week special being filmed in the Mojave Desert. The Mojave, by the way, is very close to Death Valley—the hottest place in the United States. Needless to say, Ida was in the sun—a lot. She wasn't very careful about keeping her skin protected with either sunscreen or just standing in the shade. To top this off, she was on an espresso rampage, drinking several of these coffee drinks every day. At night, she would have some alcohol—after all, she was working 16- to 18-hour days! Ida, unknowingly, was subjecting her poor capillaries to many of the triggers known to create rosacea: sun, caffeine, and alcohol.

When she returned home from her out of town job, she noticed her red cheeks just didn't go away. In fact, when she drank coffee—especially—her face turned bright red. The same was becoming true when she ate certain things, especially spicy foods, which before the Mohave Desert adventure didn't bother her.

Through trial and error Ida finally figured out what she could and couldn't eat, drink, and use on her skin. And through her research, I learned a lot about this mysterious disease. I owe my initial interest and investigation of rosacea to Ida. She has it under control, now that she understands her triggers, although admittedly it has been a long, hard, and often frustrating road.

I have fairly normal, very fair skin, but at age 38 and with two young children, the skin on my nose, cheeks, and chin gets red and hot. Do you think it is rosacea and if so, do you have any recommendations?

Usually hot and red are indications of a possible rosacea condition. My first recommendation is to read up on the subject and educate yourself. After reading enough material, you may find that you have many of the symptoms of rosacea. If so, you can get diagnosed by a dermatologist—to be sure—and then try the different topical medications that may indeed help your red and hot skin. Some people find the topicals effective, others do not. Reading and understanding more about your triggers and how to manage this disease (if you indeed have it) is the best first step to helping to control the symptoms.

Case study: Suzanne

Suzanne was diagnosed with rosacea over five years ago. Her dermatologist has her on a program of MetroCream, which is a topical medication, and the oral antibiotic tetracycline. She has tried to go off each medication separately, but whenever she does, the rosacea returns in force. She called to ask me where in her skin care program should she apply her MetroCream—before or after her moisturizer?

Whenever you are incorporating topical medications into your regular skin care regime, you want to get the medication on your skin first before you put your moisturizing cream on. If you put the medication over your moisturizer, it will have less contact with your actual skin. So Suzanne would cleanse, put the MetroCream on and let it settle on her skin, then use her spray-on toner, and apply her moisturizer last, which should be a sunscreen during the day.

I wondered why Suzanne had been on an tetracycline for five years. She did question her doctor about the long-term use of this medication, and he told her it was OK to take these low-dose antibiotics even over a long period of time. My question to the doctor is how long can or should she take them? Forever? Was the dermatologist ever going to end Suzanne's use of tetracycline? In the meantime, I highly recommended she start taking acidophilus (see section) to help her colon increase the healthy bacteria that had no doubt been affected from all those years of oral antibiotics.

I asked Suzanne if she knew her triggers (the foods and lifestyle habits) that caused her rosacea to flareup. She said, "Hot and cold, right?" Yes, extremes in temperature definitely exacerbate any redness in the skin and especially rosacea. But there is so much more to know about what causes your own rosacea to pronounce itself. I felt that if she could educate herself a bit more, she might be able to lessen the rosacea and potentially go off the oral antibiotics. I encouraged her to read *Rosacea: Your Self-Help Guide*, the best book currently out on this subject (also listed in the **Resources** section). I asked Suzanne to stay in touch so I could track her progress and find out if she discovered anything new from reading the rosacea book.

My face is not permanently red, but it tends to blush easily when I'm in a hot room. Sometimes when I'm with a lot of people my face goes red, and I find this very embarrassing. Can you suggest a good face cream that can cover this? What about creams with fruit acids?

I wonder if this woman has ever been diagnosed with rosacea. She said the redness was not permanent, but is triggered by circumstances—this could very well be the beginnings of rosacea. I realize she wants a solution. I doubt she can cover up that kind of all-encompassing redness that is probably just a temporary response to heat. Plus, using a covering cream would be treating her skin all the time for a response that only happens occasionally.

I would recommend she stay away from anything with fruit acids (AHAs). These ingredients will only serve to aggravate and possibly incite rosacea to appear. Even it she doesn't have rosacea, she has a propensity for redness. AHAs will only worsen this problem.

Because rosacea can worsen over time, she might go to her dermatologist and, if diagnosed with rosacea, try using the topical medications and see if in the long run it helps her skin. Left untreated, a minor case of rosacea can turn into a chronic and never-ending concern.

Rosacea is a very frustrating skin condition. If you do indeed have it, hopefully you have also discovered what your particular triggers are. They will be individual to you, but it is imperative that you know what causes a flare-up so at least you can be somewhat in control of this skin affliction. You may have to let go of or alter anything that you find aggravates the situation. Read as much as you can on this subject. Remember, knowledge is power.

Running & Skin

If you are a runner, undoubtedly you are usually exercising outside. Your skin, therefore, is going to be exposed to the sun for long periods of time, which is problem number one. Problem number two: so far, there have been no decent solutions to the dilemma of hats to wear while running. Your choices are either a visor or a baseball cap, neither of which offers your face much coverage. If you stand outside wearing a baseball cap or visor and go somewhere where you can see your reflection, you'll see that only your forehead and parts of your upper cheeks and nose are shielded from the sun. The rest of your face, the bottom two thirds, is exposed.

Are you a runner who has discoloration on the lower half of your face? Since you are exposing your face to sun when you run, even if you are wearing a cap, you are going to see the discoloration increase over time. This condition is called hyperpigmentation (see section), and avoiding direct sun exposure is truly the only way to keep the dark color away. There are bleaching creams and products that are meant to help even out the skin tone, but if sun exposure continues, so will the pigmentation irregularities.

Always wear a waterproof sunscreen when you run. It will stay on your skin through all the sweating that occurs as you exercise. You still need to wear a hat that shades as much of your face as possible, and waterproof sunscreen on your exposed body as well.

Anytime you sweat, you want to be sure to get the sweat off your face and neck before it dries on your skin. If it dries, it can cause little irritations on the surface of the skin. If nothing else is available, at least splash rinse at a drinking fountain or carry extra water in your car for this purpose. Don't allow the sweat to dry or you may have to contend with small breakouts as long as you are exercising hard enough to sweat.

Be aware of your skin. Since you are exercising outside and exposed to the sun, know your moles so you can see if any of them change over time. I highly recommend an annual visit to your dermatologist so they can keep tabs on the goings on of your skin as well.

*D*on't just count your years, make your years count.

— Ernest Meyers

S

Seborrheic Keratoses

Seborrheic keratoses, sometimes called seborrheic warts or even *barnacles* (I've heard a few dermatologists use this term) are simply skin growths that show up due to age or sometimes for no reason at all. They come in the form of darkened skin, occasionally flesh-colored or brown or black, that resemble small, raised moles or are flat like a wart. They can also feel scaly, although not always.

I have several of these "barnacles," mostly concentrated around my lower jawline and one above my eyebrow. They all have a scaly texture, and because of this I went to have them checked out by my dermatologist. I just didn't know if they could be trouble (cancerous) in the future, and I wanted to find out for sure. They turned out to be seborrheic keratoses.

Seborrheic keratoses are noncancerous skin growths. In other words, they aren't a problem, they just aren't very attractive. They can be burned off at your dermatologist, or liquid nitrogen might be used. But please know, if you remove one of these spots, you run the risk of having a white, non-pigmented spot where the keratosis was.

I plan to just leave my seborrheic keratoses alone. Sure, once in a while if I pay too much attention to them in the mirror or touch them on my face too much they bother me. But then again, they aren't anything to worry about healthwise and I know if I mess with them (try to have them removed), it will just be trading one thing (keratoses) for another (possibly noticeable white spots or pigmentation spots). They really aren't worth the trouble.

Shelf Life

What is the shelf life of products?

Every product is different, and every shelf life is different, so the answer to this question varies and is based on several factors. First, has the product been opened? Depending on how they are sealed, unopened skin care products have (or should have) a long shelf life. But at the same time, you don't want products that have been on the shelf forever. Opened, it is really anyone's guess how long a product will last without losing its potency. Second, has the product been exposed to heat or sunlight? This can dramatically decrease the life of a product.

Products in tubes tend to have a lower rate of bacterial infestation than products that come in jars. With jars, you are usually putting your bare fingers in each time to get out product, which may allow a lot of bacteria to enter the cream or lotion. Even though many companies provide a spatula or some type of applicator, I don't know if anyone really uses them. In general, your opened skin care products should last at least six months to a year or even more.

Sunscreen is different. I recommend throwing any sun product away after a year. Why? I want the potency of these sun protective products to be at their peak. There is no way for the consumer to test sun products to make sure they are still potent and therefore actively helping with UV radiation. Why take the risk?

Also, if I find a sunscreen in my car and it's not summer, I automatically toss it. Summer is over and who knows how many days this product has spent in a hot car. Buy new sun products at the beginning of spring or summer. This way you will ensure fresher ingredients in these all-important products. If you wear sunscreen on your face on a daily basis, it won't be an issue as to whether the product is potent or not. You will naturally be going through a tube or jar of sunscreen within at least six months time.

Do be sure to keep any and all products away from direct sunlight, which can cause damage to anything if given enough time.

How can I tell if my products have "gone bad?" How long do products last?

Just like food, organic ingredients in skin care products do go bad and will let you know by emitting an unpleasant odor. The more organic and natural the ingredients are in a product, the more likely it will go bad at some point. This also depends on the preservatives used (all products contain preservatives) and if your product has been exposed to heat or direct sunlight over a period of time. So if a product smells funny, rancid, or in any other way "bad," I wouldn't use it anymore.

Ingredients sometimes separate (for instance creating a runny consistency), and this may be a sign that your product has gone bad. If the texture has changed from its original state (if it is now runny when it wasn't before, or if it has hardened when it wasn't before), it is probably time to toss it in the garbage.

The shelf life of products vary, and there is no ironclad answer as to how long a particular product will last before going bad. If products have a seal and this seal hasn't been broken, they could last several years on the shelf without altering the ingredients. This is not always true, but I have had experience with taking products home and forgetting I had them. Then, when I moved to a new home, for instance, I found them again, unopened, and started to use them even though they were a few years old. I had no problems and the products seemed (and smelled) as though they were from a brand new shipment.

Less organic, more synthetic products (inert or inactive) could last indefinitely on the shelf. They don't have many bacteria-forming ingredients that could cause potential damage to the product.

Obviously we all want the freshest, newest batch of products to use on our skin. But the shelf life of most products (unopened) is probably longer than you would imagine. As a general rule of thumb: Let your nose be your guide.

Skin Cancer ABCs

This section should really be *Skin Cancer ABCDs*. I recommend you memorize and use the following information to help determine questionable moles or spots on your skin. Please remember this: **When in doubt, get checked out!**

A stands for **asymmetry**. A circle is symmetrical; it has an evenness to it and is perfect in its round shape. Therefore asymmetry is a circle that isn't fully and completely whole. One half doesn't mirror the other half. It is uneven.

B stands for **border**. The border or outline of the mole has irregularities, either a ragged edge or notched—not smooth.

C stands for **color**. Moles and spots on your skin should have an even color to them. If they are two-toned, for instance, having one shade of brown mixed with a darker shade of brown or even black, that is not a good sign. Along with differing shades, sometimes even patches of red, white, or blue are present. Color differences within one spot means it's time to get your mole checked out by a dermatologist—now.

D stands for **diameter**. In the American Cancer Society's literature they describe the diameter of anything bigger than a pencil eraser (wider than 6 millimeters or about one-fourth inch) is cause for concern. From my own personal experience, I had a precancerous mole removed that was less than a quarter of the size of a pencil's eraser. But this mole also had color variation ("C"), so it was biopsied and removed. Size alone is not necessarily a negative, but if a smaller mole has any of the other ABCDs, don't wait to have it checked out.

Next is a different set of ABCs used by permission from the American Academy of Dermatology. I am including it because it offers just that much more information that can help you remember how important protecting yourself in the sun is.

A*void the sun especially during midday between the hours of 10 a.m. and 4 p.m.*
B*lock the sun by applying sunscreen with Sun Protection Factor 15 on children 6 months or older.*
C*over up with long-sleeved shirt, sunglasses, and wide-brim hat if going outdoors.*
S*hade; keep infants out of direct sunlight. Infants younger than six months need special protection because their skin is so delicate. They should be kept out of direct sunlight as much as possible. Sunscreens that contain para-aminobenzoic acid (often shortened to PABA on labels) or oxybenzone are not recommended for infants. Sunscreens that contain zinc or titanium oxide are a possibility, but check with your baby's doctor before using them.*

The main thing to remember when it comes to sun exposure and your skin is **don't wait until it's too late** to get checked out by your dermatologist. Skin cancer is preventable and curable if caught early enough.

Smoking & Skin

I'm a daily smoker. Honestly, I'm not going to stop smoking, but I am concerned about what it is doing to my skin. Is there anything I can do to get rid of the redness in my skin?

You don't need me to tell you that smoking isn't good for you. There are no two ways around it: smoking cigarettes causes numerous physical problems. I do appreciate this woman's honesty, although I hope she is concerned about what smoking is doing to her entire body—not just her skin.

When it comes to smoking, there are definitely effects to the skin, long- *and* short-term. Smoking causes a constriction or closing of the vascular system, including the already weak capillaries that transport blood to and from your face. What you are doing by smoking is, in essence, suffocating your cells by causing less oxygen and vital nutrients to be transported throughout your body. Less oxygen to the cells means less nourishment and a decreased ability to get rid of toxins. This can show up as gray-looking skin—skin that is lacking oxygen.

Smoking affects collagen, and if you've ever seen a heavy smoker's skin up close, they tend to have a lot of fine lines and wrinkles. Smoking causes a loss of healthy collagen, which creates wrinkles through collagen breakdown. Add to this the constant pursing that occurs around the lips as the mouth hugs the cigarette, and you have a recipe for increased wrinkling; it happens partly from the cigarettes themselves and partly due to the constant motion smoking causes with the facial muscles.

As if this wasn't enough, nicotine is a neurostimulant, which can cause problems with getting sound sleep, yet another potential consequence from smoking. Not getting adequate rest brings with it a whole host of problems, not the least of which is that the body doesn't have enough quality time to recuperate and regenerate. This can age you whether you smoke or not.

The tar that accumulates in your lungs inhibits their natural ability to self-clean. Do you get sick frequently? Perhaps smoking is to blame. Not only does smoking deplete your immune system, inhibiting its ability to fend off foreign invaders, it also causes excess mucus to form, narrowing the air passageway and leaving you susceptible to infections like bronchitis, colds, and the flu.

Smoking is one of the leading causes of coronary artery disease, lung cancer, and emphysema. Even if you don't smoke but you live with a smoker, you are not immune to the effects of his or her cigarette smoke. You are still breathing in the toxic chemicals that are being thrown off by the burning tobacco and paper. Although you are not drawing the same amounts of tar and nicotine into your lungs, make no mistake about it—you are exposing your body to the harmful effects of smoking. This of course is known as secondhand smoke.

As far as the emailer's concern with redness, depending on the severity of her condition and the doctor she goes to (what lasers they have available), getting the broken capillaries lasered may help her skin look less red. Obviously, as long as the cause (smoking) is ongoing, so too will be the aftereffects (redness, among other things).

If you are going to do things that are known to be harmful (or less than healthy) to the body, at least get familiar with the side effects, whether from alcohol, medications (prescribed or not), or cigarettes. No matter your habit, be smart and know how it is affecting your body. Then take measures to try to make up for the imbalance by trying to balance things out nutritionally and supplementally.

Of course, the best course of treatment would be to remove the offending habit, and in this case it is smoking. Luckily, there are many different programs available today to kick the habit and enable you to enjoy better health—and skin.

SPF

If my moisturizer has SPF 8 and I put my foundation on that has SPF 8, does that mean I am protected like an SPF 16 product?

I love this question—and the answer is no! The highest SPF of whatever you are wearing is the sun protection number you are getting. In other words, if your moisturizer has an SPF of 15 and your foundation has an SPF 8, then you are getting SPF 15, not 23.

I read in your book that you don't think it is necessary to wear a sunscreen higher than SPF 15. Are you saying that SPF 30 isn't worth wearing?

No! What I explained in *Timeless Skin* was that many times people feel falsely protected when wearing high SPFs. This is precisely why the regulations for sunscreens may be modified in the future, and SPFs higher than 30 may not be allowed. Absolutely, wear as high an SPF as you want to, but know that with the higher numbers, you also get more sunscreen chemicals, and some skin may be sensitive to these.

I use an SPF 25 sunscreen every day as my moisturizer. Even on a rainy day, or a day I won't be outside very much, I still wear it. I am in no way advocating wearing lower SPF sunscreens, but I am cautioning you to be aware that no sunscreen, no matter its SPF, is capable of protecting you completely for an extended period of time. You must reapply sun protective creams as well as wear covering over your body such as hats and protective clothing. If you have a cream that you like and it is an SPF 30, great! But know that if you will be in the sun for extended periods of time, you must reapply in order to continue the SPF benefits. (See **Ultraviolet Radiation**.)

Adopt the American Cancer Society's slogan, Slip, Slop and Slap. *Slip* on a shirt, *slop* on sunscreen, and *slap* on a hat. Only by wearing sunscreen and covering your skin with clothing and hats are you truly protecting your skin in the sun.

Spirulina

If you are looking for a great all around supplement to take, spirulina would be a good choice. Spirulina is sometimes called "the perfect food." It contains amino acids, vitamins, minerals, and high levels of vitamin A. This vitamin A is in the form of beta carotene from a food source, therefore allowing the high IU content to be safe.

The following is taken from a handout I picked up at a natural foods grocery store many years ago. I could not find a source for this piece and hope that its author will be pleased with its inclusion in this book.

Spirulina: Diet and Energy Aid

Spirulina is considered by many to be an amazing diet and energy aid and is a source of concentrated nutrients that has been used for centuries. The ancient Aztecs thrived on spirulina from Lake Texcoco in Mexico, and for the people who live around the Lake in Chad, Africa, spirulina has been a mainstay in their diet for generations.

Spirulina is a water-grown, 100% vegetable plankton. It is a blue-green algae that grows in fresh water lakes in Africa and Central America. Spirulina has been found safe by the Food and Drug Administration and is now available in health food stores.

Spirulina is an incredible source of concentrated nutrients. It is 65% protein, making it the world's highest known source of protein. Raw meat is only 27% protein, and even soybeans are only 34% protein. The protein in spirulina contains all eight essential amino acids, making it a complete protein. Spirulina is the world's highest known source of B-12, with high concentrations of vitamins A, B-1, B-2, B-6, D, E, H, and K. In addition, spirulina also provides all necessary minerals, trace elements, cell salts, and digestive enzymes. The list does not end here, however, because spirulina also offers an abundance of chlorophyll, ferrodoxins, and other pigments.

One of the most amazing functions of spirulina is its ability to help people lose weight while providing them with nutrition at the same time. Spirulina strikes at the very heart of the problem that plagues all dieters—excessive hunger itself! Usually, as a result of an improper or imbalanced diet, the body is not sufficiently nourished and is constantly giving out signals, which we know as hunger pangs or cravings. This is the point at which spirulina steps in. It can satisfy these hunger pangs by offering the body complete nutrition. The protein in spirulina is much easier to digest than other proteins and as a result, spirulina is absorbed very quickly. This quick absorption in turn signals the body that it has all the nutrients it needs, and thus stops the hunger-pang signals.

Spirulina helps keep blood sugar at normal levels. Since a certain area of the brain will react to low blood sugar levels, setting up hunger pangs, a normal blood sugar level is important for losing weight as well as for general health. Spirulina contains phenylalanine, an amino acid, which some researchers believe acts directly on the appetite center of the brain.

Another advantage of spirulina is that you can adjust dosage to suit your body's individual needs. One program initially sug-

gests the dosage of three 500mg tablets, ¹/₂ hour before meals. If this dosage succeeds in keeping hunger away, you can try reducing the dosage to two tablets or even one tablet. If hunger persists, however, the dosage can be increased. You can take as many as six to eight tablets before each meal. Naturally the use of spirulina is invaluable in modified fasting, but before engaging in any type of fasting, consult your physician.

Along with spirulina's fantastic weight loss effects, it is also able to provide quick and long-lasting bursts of energy. The source of this energy is a starch found in spirulina that is identical to the glycogen used as a carbohydrate storage product in the human liver and muscle cells. As soon as spirulina is consumed, its glycogen content becomes almost immediately available to human metabolism and provides a fast energy boost that lasts.

This fast energy burst is very advantageous to physically active people. If you are involved in an energetic pursuit such as marathon running or swimming, spirulina can give you the extra energy needed to complete the activity without relying on sugar or other products normally used to achieve this result. Spirulina also helps the athlete avoid the use of bulk foods or juice that would slow down the system instead of moving it more efficiently. The dosage suggested for energy bursts is from 3 to 6 tablets of spirulina.

As you have read, you can't go wrong with spirulina. When I first started taking this supplement, one of my regular facial clients started complaining about feeling lethargic and never having enough energy to get through the day. She didn't need to lose weight, but did need an energy boost, so I recommended she experiment with spirulina. She started with 2-3 500mg tablets, 2-3 times per day. The next time I saw her, only one month later, she was amazed at how much energy these little tablets had given her. She didn't go through her normal roller coaster of energy during the day; the spirulina had stabilized her blood sugar and increased her energy level significantly.

I definitely feel an increase in energy throughout the day from this supplement. But it's not a rush or a buzz like some herbal supplements or ephedrine products tend to produce. The energy that I feel is steady and strong and doesn't make me feel nervous or jittery at all. That is because when taking spirulina, I am supplying my body with complete nutrition; it gets all of the essential amino acids that make up a complete protein. I tend toward hypoglycemia and found spirulina helps to keep my blood sugar levels at an even keel.

I like to take spirulina with me whenever I travel. Whether in a car, plane, or boat, spirulina gives me access to actual food; something that may not be readily available during certain stages of a trip. It's an asset on a camping trip, which is somewhere you usually need as much energy as you can find.

Spirulina is a perfect supplement for vegetarians. For obvious reasons, vegetarians are challenged to get enough protein in their diet every day. What could be better than this complete vegetable product that is also a complete protein? I highly recommend any vegetarians consider taking spirulina on a daily basis. Protein is essential to balanced health as well as providing the body with energy and the capacity to heal itself.

Steaming & Skin

At-home facial steamers. These machines may seem like a great item to have around the house, but my recommendations are this: If you have to use it, put a clay mask on your face, and then steam (never steam a bare face) or sell it in your next garage sale.

My main problem with these at-home steamers is they require your face to be fairly close to the machine, similar to steaming over a hot pot of water. Because of this close proximity mixed with the heat of the steam, you can cause capillary damage very easily.

Salon steaming. Many, if not most facial treatments in a professional salon include facial steaming. I am probably in the one percentile of aestheticians who don't use steam. If you find yourself in a treatment and steam is being used, be sure that you can't feel real heat on your face from the steam. If you do, that means the machine is too close to your face. Don't be afraid to ask your aesthetician to either move the steamer farther away from your face, or just do away with this step altogether.

Steaming constitutes heat. And heat dilates capillaries—the delicate and susceptible blood network of your face. Throughout our lives, due to weather, lifestyle habits like drinking alcohol and smoking cigarettes, pollution, and even certain foods, our capillaries are challenged to stay strong. Subjecting them to heat that is unnecessary is not such a great idea. (See **Capillaries**.)

Sugar & Skin

Perhaps you've seen the evidence: when you eat sugary foods, your skin breaks out; when you eat less sugar, your skin clears up. When you know *consciously* that sugar is affecting your skin, you will undoubtedly curb your sugar intake. You will understand the consequences of your actions, and you will take pause before your hand goes to your mouth with that sweet delight. Now you choose and decide whether you want to take the chance and eat the sugar. There's a saying that if you want to keep on getting what you're getting, keep on doing what you're doing. That just about says it all.

For any of you reading this who know me or have come to me for facials, you also know that sugar as it relates to skin care is one of my favorite, if not my biggest, soapboxes to stand on. The reason sprang from my own experiences with sugar and skin problems in my 20s, coming to conclusions, then passing on the information I discovered through trial and error with my own sugar addiction.

I believe beyond a shadow of a doubt that sugar causes skin problems (among other things). Its damage to our bodies is huge, and it continues to amaze me how few people are talking about it. Yet sugar is all-pervasive. It is in *everything!* It's in obvious places as well as places you would never expect. I believe if you get rid of or at least reduce the amount of sugar in your diet, whether you can see, feel, or otherwise know it, your body will be better off.

Sugar by any other name. The following is a list of known and not-so-known sugars. This list is used by permission from an excellent book on sugar and how to get it out of your diet, *The Sugar Addict's Total Recovery Program* by Kathleen DesMaisons. She has also written another great book, *Potatoes Not Prozac*, which I also recommend. And now, the different names for the same thing—sugar:

amasake
apple sugar
barbados sugar
bark sugar (zylose)
barley malt
barley malt syrup
beet sugar
brown rice syrup
cane juice
cane sugar
cane syrup

carbitol
caramel coloring
caramel sugars
caramelized foods
concentrated fruit juice
corn sweetener
d-tagalose
date sugar
dextrin
dextrose
diglycerides

disaccharides
evaporated cane juice
Florida crystals
fructooligosaccharides (FOS)
fructose
fruit juice concentrate
galactose
glucitol
glucoamine
gluconolactone
    (may be found in tofu)
glucose
glucose polymers
glucose syrup
glycerides
glycerine
glycerol
glycol
high-fructose corn syrup
inversol
invert sugar
isomalt
karo syrups
lactose
levulose
"lite" sugar
"light" sugar
malt dextrin
malted barley
maltose
maltodextrins

maltodextrose
malts (any)
mannitol, xylitol, maltitol
mannose
microcrystalline cellulose
molasses
monoglycerides
monosaccharides
nectars
neotame
pentose
polydextrose
polyglycerides
raisin juice
raisin syrup
ribose rice syrup
rice malt
rice sugar
rice sweeteners
rice syrup solids
saccharides (any)
sorbitol (aka hexitol)
sorghum
sucanat
    (evaporated cane juice)
sucanet
sucrose
sugar cane
trisaccharides
unrefined sugar
zylos

Malts, syrups, and most things ending is "ose" are going to be sugar—of some kind. And as you can see by the size of this list, there are numerous variations of what we think of as sugar. No matter what name it goes by, sugar causes skin problems in many people.

Did you know that when you drink a soda, you may be getting as many as 12 teaspoons of sugar? Let me repeat that: *twelve* teaspoons! Why not just take 12 teaspoons of sugar and add them to a glass of water? Of course you would never drink a glass of water with that much added sugar, yet that is exactly what you are doing when you drink sodas. Plus you get the added "benefit" of a bunch of chemicals that may or may not be carcinogenic (cancer causing).

If I drank just one soda per day, by the end of only one week I would have numerous little blemishes on my face. If I continued for one more week, those spots would become larger and more widespread. Finally, after just a few weeks of consuming only one soda per day, I would have a big skin problem on my hands. That's because I am sensitive to sugar. Are you?

Some people are less sensitive to sugar. Men seem less sensitive than women; some women are more sensitive than others. But if you are one of the sensitive ones, watch out! If you continue to consume even small amounts of sugar on a regular basis you will no doubt have the telltale signs written all over your face. Does it matter that many dermatologists say sugar, chocolate, or junk food doesn't cause acne or problem skin? It doesn't matter to me. And it doesn't stop me from trudging ahead with what I believe to be true and with what I see in my clients' and my own skin. Some of you may be getting away with eating sugar and having virtually no problems with your skin. But no doubt you are having unseen or unfelt problems due to this tasty toxin; you just haven't been made aware of it—yet. There is nothing inherently good about eating sugar and sugary foods, symptoms or not.

I'm no angel. I have my moments and can be seen going down the grocery store frozen food isle with a pint of Häagen-Dazs™ ice cream in my cart. (Yes, I eat ice cream!) But that is an exception, not the rule for me. And through years of experiencing how sugar affects my body, I know what will most likely happen when I eat that glorious ice cream. For me, eating sweets is a decision based on awareness. And that awareness has come through trial and error and eventually solid data accumulated through my own life experiences.

By the way, immediately after eating a sugary food, I march into my bathroom and brush my teeth. I'm sure my dentist would be proud of me! We all know from being kids that sugar causes tooth decay, which is a fact that doesn't change when you are an adult. Once I have thoroughly brushed my teeth, I proceed to drink water. Water will help dilute the concentrated sugars, hopefully helping my body to process these toxins more easily. Even though I may have a little break-out from eating the ice cream or other sweet, I want to live a well-rounded life and abstaining from everything all of the time is definitely not how I want to live. I don't eat sugar very often, but when I do, I try to do healthy things to offset the negative effects of my activities.

The following are a few case studies straight from my skin care salons that might shed some light if you suffer with problem skin. I hope these stories will bring more awareness about the detrimental effects of sugar. Although sugar intake causes many ill-effects in different areas of the body, here I am going to explore the problem that I deal with in my profession, which is sugar's effect on skin. Sugar takes an enormous toll on many people. And it is here in these case studies that I hope to open your eyes and help guide you through the maze of sugar addiction, and then to the freedom of clear and healthy skin.

Case study: Sam

I came into the facial room to meet a new client, Sam. I went over her current skin care routine, and any medications she might be on, especially the birth control pill. I asked if she took vitamins or herbs, did she exercise, drink water, and wear sunscreen? As soon as all the questions were answered, I began the facial.

After cleansing her skin, I brought my magnifying lamp over and peered through it at her face. The lamp magnifies about seven times, but in Sam's case I really didn't need the lamp. I could see from pretty far away that her skin was very broken out. She didn't have pustules; her breakout consisted of those hard, red, deep-under-the-skin places. I could also see she was causing some damage from picking at her skin.

Instantly I knew she was ingesting way too much sugar, but I held myself back and proceeded to ask about her eating habits. I told her not to tell me what was good in her diet, but that I was interested in what she was eating regularly that wasn't so good. The good, clean, healthy foods aren't the troublemakers. And someone can tell me till they're blue in the face how much grilled chicken and vegetables they eat. *That* isn't causing their skin to break out, but something is.

I asked if she had much sugar in her diet. She responded the way most people do, "No, not really. Sure, I'll have the occasional bite or two of a dessert I'm sharing with someone, but generally the only sugar I get is from fruit, like apples and oranges." I asked about her menstrual cycles. Perhaps Sam's skin problems were indicative of a hormone imbalance. "No, everything is normal," she said in regard to her periods. So I was back on the sugar hunt.

It looked to me to be so simple: sugar was the culprit, yet she insisted she had very little in her diet, and in fact she ate very similarly to me—simple, clean foods. I explained to Sam that something was causing her breakout. It isn't just happening for no reason or explanation. And it is my job (and Sam's) to decipher her lifestyle habits and figure out what was the offending edible substance.

All breakouts are hormonal. Hormones are little chemical messengers that tell your glands what to do. And in this case, it is the oil or sebaceous glands that are overproducing and causing problems. So to say that her breakouts were hormonal was true, but I wanted to find out *why* the hormones felt the need to exceed their normal and balanced dosage within her body.

Years ago a biochemist friend of mine told me that sugar can sometimes be a precursor to certain hormones in the body. I have absolutely no substantiated studies or clinical trials to back me up on this; I only have hundreds of clients who have been in my care for years who have stopped eating sugar and cleared up their skin. If the precursor theory is true, I would imagine it would be the androgens or male hormones that are being activated by eating sugar.

Since her periods were fine, I didn't think it was a hormone imbalance causing her breakouts, so I went into my sugar speech. I started telling Sam about my own sugar addiction. I told her that I am so sensitive to sugar that if I ate just a small amount of sugar, but ate it *every day*, I would have a lot of breakouts consistently. Bingo. When I said the words "every day" it hit her. Every morning (or almost every day) Sam gets a coffee drink with a shot of vanilla in it. There it is. That vanilla syrup is essentially highly refined sugar—with vanilla flavoring. I told Sam that if I had one of those coffees with just one shot of vanilla every day for just one week, my skin, even in that short amount of time, would be a disaster.

We'd finally hit gold! We had something to work with, and now Sam could start taking control of her problem skin. I recommended she cut the vanilla shot out completely for at least one month to see if her skin did a turnaround. And it did. Admittedly, she also went on the products I recommended for her. But I know it was the sugar that in the end was causing her problems and that it was the avoidance of sugar that ultimately cleared up her skin.

Case study: Gretchen

Gretchen came in for her first facial. She had widespread breakout over her whole face; small red infected places that were persistent. As I examined her skin I figured it was sugar consumption but kept from saying anything until I had more information.

She had recently gone through a round of antibiotics from her dermatologist, which brought her little relief from the breakouts. I explained that she was probably contributing unknowingly to her condition and until we discovered how, antibiotics or any other therapy was only going to be a temporary solution. As long as she was feeding her problem, the problem would continue to grow.

Finally I asked about her diet. I asked her to tell me the bad stuff she ate. She said she didn't really eat bad things, but she probably drank too much coffee. How much coffee? "About 2-4 cups a day— at least." Do you put anything in it, I asked. "Yes, I put sugar, one packet per cup of coffee." Once again we hit the jackpot. Gretchen was ingesting 2-4 teaspoons of sugar (that we know about) every day.

She couldn't believe sugar was causing the problem. She had never heard that sugar was bad for skin and certainly didn't realize it was creating the breakouts she had been experiencing. I hear this from most people I break the news to. They just don't have a conscious awareness of this very simple compound that is creating problems with their skin. Obviously, this is one of the main things I am trying to change. Sugar causes breakouts.

Although she had a tough time reducing her sugar intake, Gretchen did see a change for the better in her skin. At least now she is holding the reins and is at the controls of her breakouts.

Case study: Anne

Anne called me concerned with scarring on her face. She was also concerned about a hormone imbalance she was experiencing. She had deep cysts on her face that itched and hurt and stayed red for a long time. Rather than addressing the breakout as I normally would, asking about a possible link to sugar, I chose to focus on the hormone imbalance.

Another concern for Anne was severe and painful menstrual cramping, and I recommended evening primrose oil to help. She was very well-versed in homeopathy and other natural studies. She had worked with a kinesiologist and believed in muscle testing. Anne had been muscle tested for evening primrose in the past, and her doctor's test results always came up with a "no" for using it. I asked her if she was willing to bypass the muscle testing and just try evening primrose oil for a course of treatment for at least one month, although three months would be better. This way her body would have time to show some results. The primrose might help with the painful menstruation as well as her skin problems.

I finally asked Anne about sugar, and she said some amazing things. She intentionally did not read the chapter in *Timeless Skin* on sugar (Chapter 13). She skipped it on purpose because she figured it would have things to say about sugar she didn't want to hear. She proceeded to tell me her sugar intake was immense and intense. I told Anne I would be happy to help her with her sugar addiction, but first she should read that chapter. I also recommended reading *Sugar Blues* by William Dufty, an excellent book about sugar addiction. After that, I thought she would have some background and that she also might be ready to make the necessary changes.

Christiane Northrup, in her brilliant and essential book, *The Wisdom of Menopause*, talks about how sugar can cause cramping. Sugar was no doubt the key to unlocking Anne's problem skin and possibly her problems with severe cramping during menstruation. With all the knowledge she had about how to take care of her body and what to do and what not to do, Anne still chose to ignore the most obvious culprit contributing to her problems: the Evil Sugar! Are you avoiding the obvious? Take a look and see.

Case study: Sue

Sue came in complaining of new breakout (new within the last six weeks), concentrated mostly on her chin and around her nose. She couldn't think of anything new she had been doing; she had no real changes in her hormones or menstrual cycle, and no unusual stress.

After I got her in the facial chair and looked at the problem at hand, I asked if she had been eating any sugar or more sugary foods than normal. "No. I don't think so," she insisted, "except for a new protein shake I've been making each morning." She was putting soy milk, a soy protein powder called Soy-lycious®, and a banana in her drink. This sounds pretty harmless, doesn't it? *Wrong!* Soy milk, some more than others, contains quite a bit of sugar. Plus, anything that tastes *'licious* is always suspect to me.

In order for the manufacturers of these protein powders to make their product palatable, they tend to add quite a bit of sugar. And so was the case with Soy-lycious. In researching this product I found that one serving has 15 grams of sugars. That is a lot of sugar and too much for a protein drink that you're drinking once a day. Occasionally you could get away with it, but not every day—if you are sugar-sensitive. If you check the labels, you can find a low- to no-sugar protein powder. In my kitchen I currently have a powder that has 8 grams of sugar, which is still high, but just over half the amount of Sue's protein product. I also have a protein powder that has a sugar content of zero. These lower versions do exist; you just have to read the labels.

I believe the biggest contributing factor to Sue's skin problems was sugar. Later that day Sue called me after speaking to her gynecologist. Her confirmation was complete: even the doctor, after finding out Sue was drinking soy milk, agreed it contains too much sugar.

Case study: Kim

After spending about 15 minutes on the phone with Kim, who was complaining about having breakout that wouldn't go away, she finally told me about her huge sugar intake. Every morning she has the equivalent of two cups of coffee with two tablespoons of sugar—not teaspoons (which is bad enough), but *tablespoons*. That is a lot of sugar! Day in day out, it is bound to eventually cause problems. Do you put sugar in your morning coffee? Do you experience frequent breakouts? Maybe there is a connection here for you too.

Kim said the breakout started about six months ago, yet she had been drinking sugar in her coffee for longer than that—for years. My theory is that about six months ago she crossed the threshold of her body being able to tolerate excess refined sugar. This may not be the sole cause of Kim's skin problems, but her coffee drink is probably not the sole source of her sugar intake.

This is what I instructed Kim to do—if she was willing. First she needed to understand there is a psychological (as well as physical) addiction to sugar. Kim's coffee probably won't taste very good if she goes cold turkey and stops adding sugar to it. So I recommended she be patient with her breakout and to slowly taper off the sugar. I told her that tomorrow she should start to put $1^1/_2$ tablespoons of sugar into her morning coffee. It would only be a 25% reduction and probably wouldn't affect the taste of the coffee too much. Once she was used to that less-sweet taste, then she should go to one tablespoon. Once she was used to that, cut the amount in half, and then half again. Finally, Kim could try to totally eliminate it from her coffee. In this trial period of sugar reduction, she would probably see a difference in her skin and the breakouts.

What I have found in the past is clients will speed up this elimination process because they see a positive difference in their skin. Knowledge is power, and once you know that sugar is contributing to your problem skin, you can decide to stop eating sugar, or at least you will know why you have breakout.

Note: Kim has read my book and has heard me, through several consultations over the phone, talking about sugar and skin problems *for years*. She just didn't make the connection. My guess is she just didn't want to, so the sugar snuck by her consciousness. That, by the way, is a common occurrence. You love your sugar, and you certainly don't want me trying to take it away from you! I tell you this so you will look a little deeper at your sugar intake and maybe come up with sugar you were ignoring that is a mainstay in your diet. So be honest. You don't have to stop eating sugar completely; I just want you to take ultimate responsibility for your clear (or problem) skin!

A sugar alternative for Kim or any of you trying to reduce sugar in your diet (coffee, tea, baking, etc.) is to use **stevia**, an herbal substitute for sugar. Although you probably won't find it readily available in grocery stores, coffee houses, or restaurants (yet), you can purchase stevia at health food stores in either a powder or liquid form. If you have to have sweet in your coffee (or wherever), give stevia a try.

Case study: Jody

Jody came in to see me after reading my book and realizing we lived in the same city. She is a 23-year-old with problem/acne skin. When she first walked in, it was obvious she had skin troubles; the whole bottom half of her face was red from blemishes and sensitive, irritated, skin.

As I always do, I asked her a series of questions ranging from what her skin care routine consisted of to how much water she drank, what if any vitamins and herbs she might take, and what type of exercise she was committed to. She was aware of sugar in her diet, and in fact Jody said she had just given up putting two teaspoons of sugar in each of the 2-3 cups of coffee she drank daily. That she stopped this daily sugar habit is something to be congratulated. And because is was a recent change, her skin hadn't had enough time to clear up significantly.

What Jody hadn't given up (yet) was a sugary cereal she was eating every morning for breakfast. At this point, she wasn't able to make the switch to more non-sugary breakfast foods. She felt she would have to get up earlier in order to have time to make a good breakfast, and she didn't want to be late for work. This is understandable, but I also believe eating a healthy breakfast can be accomplished without taking too much time. I encouraged Jody to consider changing and to incorporate making a healthy breakfast just one day per week to start, and see how that went. I think taking small, baby steps leads to permanent changes.

Jody left my office with some challenges in terms of changing her dietary habits—even more than she already had. Without getting more sugar contributors out of her diet, her skin problems would persist. I encouraged Jody to realize that when she was ready to commit to a more complete dietary change, bigger improvements would happen. I told her to remember every time she ate sugar, she increased her chances of breaking out.

Taking a more subtle approach rather than something more drastic may work better for you in terms of eliminating sugar from your diet. Even small steps, over time, can produce big changes. First, set your sights on where you want to be, and then take small steps, focus, and attain your goal. You absolutely can reduce or eliminate sugar from your diet; you just need to make a plan. Once your skin starts clearing up, you will have the impetus you need to complete your goal.

The following is just one example of how sensitive I am to sugar. One holiday season I was given some delectable chocolate-covered almonds. Dark chocolate, to boot—my favorite. I didn't want to throw the gift away, so I put them in the freezer, hoping I would forget about them. Of course, in a pinch, there they were—just waiting for me to come eat them whenever I chose to. And I did. If you have read some of my previous writings, you know I have said, to the best of my ability, I don't eat sugary foods two days in a row. But I had a deadline and was working long hours at home, and by the end of the day I just wanted a little taste of sweet—so I reached for these freezer goodies. I ate only three candied almonds each night, for three nights. By the third night I had breakout that was obvious and also a few places inside my mouth that were sensitive—just waiting to become canker sores.

I'm telling you about this in the hope of illustrating how sensitive to sugar some people can be. And if you are one of those people and you eat the equivalent of what I ate or more, then the skin problems that you are currently experiencing are very likely the product of your sugar addiction. I make no bones about it—sugar can wreak havoc with your skin.

What about wine and its sugar content? Can drinking it cause breakout?

I have rarely had skin problems due to drinking wine. And I am one of the most sugar-sensitive people I know. When grapes are picked, they contain about 24% sugar by weight. That is a lot of sugar! During the fermentation of wine, yeast eats up this sugar and expels alcohol. So the process of making wine does reduce the amount of sugar in this alcoholic beverage. Sweeter wines will have a higher sugar content, drier varieties will have less sugar. Dessert wines, of course, will have the highest sugar content of all. Because grapes are some of the sweetest, most sugar-concentrated fruits, and wine is made from grapes, you will find a higher sugar content in wine than other alcoholic beverages. If you are sensitive to sugar, you may break out from drinking wine—it's not out of the question. If you do notice a breakout after drinking a particular wine, it may have too high of a sugar content—so avoid that one.

> *I try to be aware of what I put into my body. I drink a lot of water, take vitamins, and I really watch my sugar intake. I am 24 years old and am struggling with acne along my jawline and chin. I definitely see an increase in the breakout around my period, so I think it is mostly hormone- and stress-induced.*
>
> *Since reading your book, I am extra aware of sugar in my diet. But I will be honest—I do give in to the occasional chocolate fix (and those Girl Scouts are around again). I also know there is a lot of hidden sugar in my diet. My daily intake consists of two teaspoons of sugar in my coffee in the morning, a mid-afternoon yogurt (which I know is high in sugar), a peanut butter and jelly sandwich, sometimes a cookie or small piece of chocolate, and then wherever sugar is less obvious in other things in my diet.*

If this is an example of watching sugar intake, it is about watching a lot of sugar going into her mouth. No wonder she is having skin problems! Usually when people come to me for advice, they don't have so much obvious sugar in their diet. But here, with this example, I hope you can see how much sugar this client is eating—every day. If she would simply and totally rid all of the above mentioned sugary foods from her diet, I would be very surprised if her skin didn't clear right up.

The sugar in the coffee *alone* is too much sugar—especially on a daily basis. That this client is experiencing any problems with her skin, severe or not, is absolutely no surprise. Yogurt, plain with nothing added, is the only yogurt I recommend eating. You can always add fresh fruit, like bananas, apples, etc. But if you eat yogurt with fruit added during manufacturing, just look at the label—you are getting a lot of "hidden" sugar. A peanut butter and jelly sandwich may be a great meal on the run, but it is loaded with sugar. The jelly is obvious, but I'll bet the peanut butter has sugar in the ingredient list too. If it is from a health food store, perhaps not. It may just be peanuts and oil. But a grocery store product will contain sugar. Cookies and the "occasional chocolate fix" are only going to compound this young lady's problems.

Her program is simple: eliminate at least all of the above-mentioned items from her diet. In *Timeless Skin*, I recommend going on a three- to ten-day sugar fast. Sometimes limiting the amount of time you will abstain from something makes the process a little easier to get through. I don't advocate reintroducing the same amount of sugar into your diet that you were eating before the fast. But sometimes just taking a break from sugar completely will give you the extra willpower you need to begin to reduce the amount of sugar you are getting on a daily basis. Once you stop feeding the problem, your blemishes will (hopefully) be a thing of the past.

Chapter thirteen [in Timeless Skin] was helpful as were the articles I read on your website. While I don't eat a lot of refined sugar, I do frequently eat a salad that, among other things, has carrots and raisins. I have come to see that raisins have a ton of sugar. Also, I get a Frappucino® three of four times a week.

It's not the raisins that are the biggest problem, it's the *coffee drinks!* If this reader is able to just give up the Frappucinos—completely—she will see a huge difference in her skin.

I don't eat a lot of refined sugar. This illustrates once again that many times we neglect to see the obvious, blatant sugar in our diets. (Is it denial?) Of course it is the high-sugar content coffee drink that is the most egregious offender in this client's problem skin. Caffeine is addictive, so is sugar. So removing this three to four times a week habit will not be easy, but if clear and healthy skin is her main goal, it *is* possible!

Raisins (and carrots, too) *are* high in sugar. If you are eating a lot of raisins and have problem skin, try reducing or eliminating the raisins from your diet for a week or two, and see if your skin clears a little—or a lot. This client recently gave me some feedback:

> *Since the last email, I have been monitoring my sugar intake. I have eliminated the Frappucinos, much to my chagrin, and I am definitely seeing some positive changes. I also eliminated the raisins. Not only is my skin prettier, but my mood seems to fluctuate less.*

Sugar in Unsuspected Places. The following examples are of less obvious or even hidden sugars that you may be consuming on a frequent or even daily basis. Hopefully this information will help you determine sugar in your diet. When a client tells me they "don't eat sugar" yet they have (what looks like) sugar breakouts, I start down a list of possible problem foods that perhaps they have overlooked as being "bad."

Be honest. I find that after asking lots of questions, a client will eventually tell me about some sugary food they are eating—knowing that it is probably a bad thing. Don't waste this time, just cut to the chase and be up front about how much sugar you are eating. If you have a breakout that seems "unexplainable," go back in time and see if you can discover how you might have eaten something incidentally that could have caused your skin to erupt, even if it is just a slight breakout.

Do you **add anything** to your coffee or tea? Some sugar substitutes can have the same effect on your skin as table sugar.

Do you use **non-dairy creamer**? The first ingredient is corn syrup solids (sugar) and the second ingredient is hydrogenated soybean and/or canola oil (both of these are the bad kind of omega-6 fatty acids). If you are using a non-dairy creamer to avoid the fat of regular half and half cream, or maybe you can't have dairy products, just know you are consuming "hidden" sugar, among other things.

Do you eat **yogurt**? Yogurt with fruit already added contains a lot of sugar. Yogurt in and of itself has natural sugars in it, but if you want something added to plain yogurt, add your own fruit like bananas or apples. This way you won't get all the added sugar except the most natural kind: fructose from fresh fruit.

What about **muffins**? Every time I walk into a coffee shop, I am amazed at all the "cake" they are selling. All of those muffins and croissants are loaded with sugar—hidden and obvious. If you partake in these types of breakfast foods, you are essentially having a piece of cake with your coffee. Non-fat? Usually non-fat foods are extremely high in sugar.

Japanese rice cracker snacks are salty-tasting snack crackers that are loaded with sugar, even though it doesn't seem like they would be (and they don't taste very sweet). The first part of the ingredient list goes like this: sweet rice, sugar, soy and tamari sauce, salt, sweet rice wine, corn syrup, natural wasabi snack seasoning [that has sugar and dextrose in its makeup]. Further down the list, sugar and corn starch are mentioned again. As you can see, this is a very high-sugar snack. In fact for a $1/2$ cup serving it contains 8 grams of sugar, which is a lot.

Ketchup contains tomato concentrate, high fructose corn syrup, corn syrup, distilled vinegar, salt, natural flavors. In other words: tomato, sugar, sugar, vinegar, salt, and possible sugar. This seemingly harmless condiment can add lots of extra sugar grams to your daily diet—if you eat ketchup with any frequency.

Propel® Fitness Water is, to me, an example of sugar water. The first three ingredients are water, sucrose syrup, and natural lemon flavor with other natural flavors. ("Natural flavors." What's *in* that?) The amount of sugar—by grams—looks incidental; this 8 ounce drink has only 4 grams of sugar. But considering you are drinking "water," this seems like an easy (and unnecessary) way to get a lot of ancillary sugar in your daily diet.

Protein bars are very close to regular candy bars in terms of their sugar content. Even though you are getting better ingredients overall, you still need to look at the sugar grams on the package. Protein bars may make a good meal replacement once in a while, but if you are having problems with your skin and you eat these bars regularly, perhaps you need to rethink their health value for you.

If you are taking **Tums®** to supplement your diet with calcium, or for whatever reason, have you ever looked at the ingredients? Sucrose [sugar], calcium carbonate, corn starch [sugar], talc, mineral oil, natural and artificial flavors [no doubt containing sugar], adipic acid, sodium polyphosphate, plus various color additives. As you can see, when you eat Tums, you are essentially eating candy, and is Tums really a good calcium supplement substitute? I include it here because one of my clients who was having problems with small, but continual breakouts, was an avid Tums taker. It took a long time to figure out she was getting sugar from this source. I recommended finding alternative ways to get more calcium in her diet.

I don't eat a lot of junk food, but I like to have crunchy munchies every now and then. One day I chose to get some **baked potato chips** because they are healthier than fried chips, they contain less fat, and they are crunchy. At the grocery store, I neglected to check to see if there was sugar in the ingredient list. Believe it or not, just a few short hours after I ate those chips, my skin broke out a little! I was disappointed to find that these chips are yet another product I wouldn't be able to eat due to their sugar content. The possibility of breaking out by eating them offsets the pleasure in crunching down on these chips. The ingredients include dehydrated potatoes, modified food starch, sugar, corn oil, partially hydrogenated soybean oil, salt, soy lecithin, leavening (monocalcium phosphate and sodium bicarbonate), and dextrose.

Soy milk is my favorite example of a product that you don't think of as being sugar-laddened. Soybeans, soaked, ground fine and strained, produce a fluid called soybean milk, which many people consider a good, healthy substitute for cow's milk. Plain, unfortified soymilk is an excellent source of high quality protein and B-vitamins. Soymilk is most commonly found in aseptic containers (nonrefrigerated, shelf stable), but also can be found in quart and half gallon containers in the dairy case at the supermarket. Soymilk is also sold as a powder, which must be mixed with water.

I looked at all the soy milk I could find on the market and morphed their basic ingredient lists (they all have very similar ingredients) to prove to you nonbelievers that soy milk is loaded with sugar. Please note all of the following are ingredients for plain or original soy milks, not the kind containing added flavors. Purified water, organic soybeans, naturally malted corn and barley extract, Job's tears, organic barley, Kombu seaweed, sea salt. If you look at the earlier section, **Sugar by any other name**, you will find malted barley and, short of finding malted corn, it lists "malts (any)" as being another form of sugar.

Recently, at a specialty store, I did find unsweetened soy milk. Its only ingredients are filtered water and whole organic soybeans. If you drink soy milk, I highly recommend switching to the unsweetened variety.

Rice milk doesn't seem to have added sugar, but on the nutritional facts label it lists the sugar content as 15 grams per serving; four servings per one liter container. Rice milk also has virtually no protein, where soymilk does have a good protein to carbohydrate ratio. Rice milk is almost all carbohydrates. The rice milk I found had these ingredients: purified water, brown rice, sunflower oil, tricalcium phosphate, lecithin, sea salt, vitamins A and D2.

Here's another personal story to further illustrate my own sugar sensitivities, and perhaps yours. I ordered out from a new Thai restaurant. I usually order chicken and broccoli. The food looked and smelled good, but after the very first bite I could tell there was sugar somewhere in the mix. The broccoli could have been soaked in sugar water (it tasted sweeter than broccoli normally does) or sugar could have been (and probably was) added to the sauce. What a shame. This dish was so sweet that I didn't want to eat it. I added some tamari sauce to get a saltier taste, but I was still eating a lot of sugar with that meal—a meal that was not dessert.

I remember years ago when I was eating at a popular pizza restaurant, I took one bite of the pizza and couldn't believe how sweet the dough tasted. I knew I couldn't eat it. I asked the waitress if they used sugar in the recipe. She checked with the chef and was told they use honey, not sugar. Well, even if that is true, honey is basically the same thing to your skin: sugar.

So if you are eating something that really shouldn't taste sweet but does, more than likely it has some form of sugar in it. And if you are sensitive to sugar, your skin may react. It may be a small, hardly noticeable reaction, but take note so you can avoid this food in the future or at least know why your skin is broken out. The more aware you become of sugar in your diet, the more aware your taste buds will become.

Don't discount the fact you may be eating a food that "shouldn't" be sugar-laddened, but is. This is especially important if and when you are trying to figure out why your skin is breaking out. Perhaps you don't eat a lot (or any) obvious sugar, but that doesn't mean sugar isn't creeping into your life. Start reading labels of the foods you have at home, and don't be afraid to ask questions when you are eating out. Find out if there is sugar in your prepared foods and ask for them to omit this problem-causing ingredient—at least in your "regular," non-dessert foods.

HOT TIP: Do you have kids? Is there candy laying around, like M&Ms® or another kind of bite-sized candy? Try putting out baby carrots or cherry tomatoes or the soy product, edamame. They are healthy snack foods that don't contain artificial sugars.

> *You're right on about sugar. I'm not much of a sweet eater, but if I do indulge in something sugary, I notice the pimples in a day or two. Thank you for your help!*

Not everyone will have sensitivity to sugar that causes breakouts, but my experience with my own skin and hundreds of clients I have shared this information with is that cutting out sugar reduces or eliminates breakouts altogether. Experiment and see for yourself. Then you will know, and you can take responsibility for the state of your health. Then you won't be puzzled by frequent breakouts that seem unexplainable. All breakout has a reason for coming about. It is up to you to determine what you are doing consistently that may be contributing to your skin problems.

HOT TIP: You don't need sugar—you are sweet enough!

Sun

I was standing at the counter of my dermatologist's office, paying the bill for a mole check. Next to me was an older gentleman, probably around 65 years old. I assumed he had skin cancer because he was having Mohs' Surgery, which removes malignant (cancerous) growths. After a few minutes, another gentleman walked through the door who I guessed had skin cancer too because half of his face was covered with a bandage, and he didn't have an appropriate bulge for a nose.

These two gentlemen apparently knew each other, as they said, "Hey, Charlie," and "Hi, Jack." The image I got was of two golfing buddies who had spent their youth throughout adulthood out in the sun, unconscious of the disastrous effects of all that (probably unprotected) sun exposure. And now, years later, here they are as older men, both at the dermatologist's office, and both having cancers removed from their faces. This is a sad story, but more disheartening because it is a common one.

"I never get in the sun." Usually I hear this in my treatment room when I'm asking a client about sun exposure. Many times I'm asking because I see the signs of overexposure. True, I may see sun damage on a client's skin long after he or she has stopped baking in the sun. But to say you never get in the sun is untrue. Each and every time you walk outside you are getting sun. Sun exposure is accumulated from birth, so every hour, every minute, every second is adding up on your sun exposure report card. Why am I being so adamant about this seemingly picky detail? Because if you are not aware of how much sun you are getting, you are not going to be as careful as you need to be.

Hyperpigmentation (see section) is a big reason for being truthful about the incidental sun you're getting, but may not be acknowledging. Hyperpigmentation comes in the form of dark spots on your face (or anywhere) that some people describe as blotchiness or uneven coloring. As harmless as it may seem, even small amounts of sun exposure do add up. And that is why when a client is bewildered because dark spots have appeared on her face while she claims to "not have been in the sun," I go into my speech saying the only place you are not getting sun is inside (four walls and a ceiling), away from a window.

Obviously hyperpigmentation is not the only problem sun exposure produces. The most obvious and sometimes fatal condition is, of course, skin cancer. You (we) must start now or continue to aggressively protect your face and body from sun exposure. Even sunscreens are no match for the powerful rays of the sun. They are helpful but not foolproof, and are truly only meant to keep your skin from burning in the sun. Wear hats whenever possible, sunscreen always, and enjoy being out in the sun—*protected*. Don't become one of these gentlemen at the being of this section. Protect your skin now and always!

Sunscreen

When I say *sunscreen*, I am referring to either a sunscreen or sunblock. I don't differentiate between the two because neither a sunscreen nor a sunblock is keeping all the damaging rays off your face. So for simplification, I lump all sun protection products under the heading of sunscreen.

How long should I wait to go outside before my sunscreen is effective?

Generally, dermatologists recommend applying sun products to the skin at least 20 minutes before going outside. Without giving the cream or lotion enough time to soak in and penetrate the skin, the effects of the actual sun protection may not be as good. If you have forgotten to apply sunscreen once you are outside, go ahead and apply it—better to have it on than not. For optimum benefits, try to remember to apply it before you go outside.

My day cream doesn't have a lot of SPF. Is it OK to use sunscreen on top?

I'm not a fan of layering your creams. If you have true-dry skin, it may be OK because your skin is lacking in natural oils and may need the extra layer. But if your skin is oily, problem, or even combination, putting two layers of cream on may be excessive and cause further problems (primarily blackheads and a shiny look to your skin).

Since sunscreens are creams or lotions and have emollient ingredients that help them spread over your skin, I would recommend simply using your sunscreen *as* your day moisturizer. This way you will get the full benefits of the sunscreen (SPF), and it should be moisturizing enough—especially if you have an oilier skin type.

I've started doing some work with a dermatologist at a VA Clinic and in just the short time I've been there, I've seen so many pre-cancerous and cancerous lesions. The doctor I work for tells his patients to put sunscreen on twice a day, every day, even for just walking to and from the car because damaging sun rays penetrate the car windows. I never wear any kind of sunscreen during the week (since I'm at work all day), and I would like to start. After seeing all the skin cancer, I realize putting a sunscreen on every day is worth lessening my chances of getting skin cancer.

Here is more confirmation that you need to wear sunscreen—every day—no matter what activities you are engaged in. If you work inside an office and truly don't leave the building except to get there in the morning and leave after the work day is finished, a light-textured SPF 15 is probably all that you need. For outside activities, you want to wear something that is applicable for that kind of exposure. A waterproof or water-resistant sunscreen would be most appropriate.

Even though you're wearing a waterproof or water-resistant sun product, you still need to reapply after you have been in the sun for over an hour. When you initially apply the cream, don't forget to put some on your ears, behind your ears, and in that ridge between your earlobe and cheek. If you have short hair or are wearing it up under your hat, don't forget the back of your neck, which is a common place to get sun exposure and sunburn.

I want to emphasize this point: whether you are wearing a sunscreen or a sunblock, whether they block UVA, UVB, or both, and even when you reapply frequently, you are still receiving sun exposure. There is no way to block out all of the sun's damaging rays unless you are inside a building, away from a window. Wear sunscreen and get your moles checked at the dermatologist. Take care of your skin—and your future.

Supplements

What vitamins are good for skin?

Many people ask me about vitamins and other supplements. What should they take and which ones are good for skin? Although there may be certain vitamins and minerals that are specifically good for the skin, eating a well-balanced diet is the best way to get them. With that said, in our world today getting everything from the foods we're eating may just be a fantasy. First, because we don't eat as balanced a diet as we should, and second, because the good foods we do eat may not be as vitamin-rich as they once were. This is partly because of the harvesting techniques, and the soil used isn't as nutrient-dense as it once was.

Originally, I was going to include an expanded section describing most of the vitamins, minerals, and other supplements that can be taken to support health. Because there is so much information out in the world about every supplement known to man and therefore I would essentially be reinventing the wheel, I have decided to forgo writing an entire passage on vitamins and minerals. Check the **Resources** section for some of my favorite book recommendations about nutritional supplements. Also see **Antioxidants** for additional supplement recommendations.

My feeling is that all vitamins and minerals are important and that no one or two should be taken in lieu of the others. The best way to get your vitamins is through the food you eat. Barring being able to do this, taking a wide range of supplements is probably a wiser idea than just focusing on one or two. You can really throw off the balance of nutrients in your body by taking large amounts of one vitamin or mineral. It is a very complicated process how everything is digested and assimilated in your body, so use caution when seeking out vitamins to help your skin specifically. Research supplements that will build a strong and healthy body; unquestionably this will also help your skin.

I have had several clients, myself included, who found that taking certain supplements including herbs, actually caused problem with their skin. Monitor what supplements you are taking and any changes, for better or worse, that are occurring in your body in general, your skin specifically, or even your energy level. Before deciding to take any supplements listed here or wherever you may find them, check with your health care provider to see if there are any contraindications that you may not be aware of.

Doing all the right things all of the time. I don't want to portray myself as a yoga-practicing, acupuncture-receiving, perfect-diet-eating, do-everything-right-all-the-time person. I am far from that! All of those things and more are the things I aspire to do. Life, as we all know, has other plans for us from time to time.

Take my diet as an example. I know a lot about nutrition and what to eat and what to avoid. There are times, however, that I let go of that knowing and literally let myself go. It may be a shock for some of you who have decided that I am a certain kind of person, but I do eat sugar and "bad" foods on occasion. And sometimes I do so in excess, especially when I am under stress or have a large project that takes a lot of my time to complete.

I am sharing this with you so you will afford yourself the same leniency of being human as you no doubt extend to others. I think we are hardest on ourselves and give a lot more leeway to our fellow humans when they falter. Be kind to yourself and do try to do the right things most of the time. When life takes over and you can't do it all, be sure to have supplements that will give you the vitamins and minerals that your body needs even though you may not be able to eat your way to this level of nutrition.

Drink your salad. Because eating all the right foods and getting all the vitamins in the course of a day can be (or at least can seem) impossible, I do rely on several things that give my body the nutrients I should be getting from my food. I consider these supplements to my diet "foods."

Something I started to take once my deadline was drawing near for this book is *Green Foods' Veggie Magma*. They call it, "Your salad in a glass." It contains broccoli sprout powder and 16 other vegetables and herbs that make an excellent addition to my daily intake of food—especially if that intake isn't so nutritious. Basically it provides a wealth of vitamins and minerals in a powder. I take the recommended dosage, two teaspoons dissolved in a glass of clean, unfiltered water. I fill the glass halfway, stir in the powder, then try to get all the lumps out. Next I add the rest of the water, and drink it down. It tastes really good, and I know it is good for me. Yes, it would be preferable to be getting all that nutrition from eating vegetables, but sometimes I just don't have time.

Another way to drink your salad is to juice. I am an avid proponent of juicing as a way to ensure I am getting a good supply of fruits and vegetables, thus their nutrients, into my body on a daily basis. See **Juicing**.

Spirulina (see section) is a great energy booster for me. So much so that I won't take it after 5 o'clock in the evening. Otherwise (I found this out accidentally) it tends to keep me up at night. If you know you're not getting enough protein and other vitamins in your diet, I highly recommend spirulina. And if you're looking for something to give you extra energy without the side effects of caffeinated drinks or supplements containing stimulants, try spirulina.

A calcium story. Robyn, like many women, is prone to the blues from time to time. She read a magazine article that said high doses of calcium could help curb depression. She was also concerned about calcium loss and osteoporosis. Robyn already drank a normal amount of milk (not excessive), but thought taking calcium supplements might help her on several levels (bone loss as well as occasional depression). So she purchased Caltrate®, an over the counter calcium supplement, and started taking about 4-5 tablets per day. Unbeknownst to Robyn, she couldn't process this synthetic calcium quickly enough and it was beginning to collect in her kidneys, eventually (and painfully) creating kidney stones less than a year after starting to take the calcium supplements. Unfortunately this condition would prove to be hard to diagnosis at first.

Robyn had to go through the painful process of having the stones removed surgically. To add insult to injury, literally, the surgeon found one of the stones had such a sharp edge to it, it had gotten stuck in the lining of her ureter. The surgery was successful, and after a lengthy recuperation, Robyn had a full recovery. She doesn't, however, take calcium supplements anymore. She now relies on calcium-rich foods to supply her body with adequate natural calcium. As a side note, Robyn recently moved to a new city and says she no longer experiences even occasional depression. Environment really can adversely affect our lives—or enhance it.

I wanted to tell you this story just in case you are taking a lot of calcium supplements. Although calcium is important to support healthy bones and shouldn't be ignored as an important part of your nutritional supplementation, be aware of any changes in your body and keep your physician apprised of any supplements you are taking or choosing to not take.

Many vitamins, minerals, and other supplements get their turn at having notoriety and public acclaim. I would read up on any and all supplements you decide to take. Also remember that the body is a machine and works in a particular balance with everything it is given to work with, whether that be food or supplements or both.

Swimming & Skin

I swim a lot. Is there something special I should do for my skin? Is there anything I can put on my face before I swim to protect it? What about after I swim?

If you are a swimmer, you don't need me to tell you how hard the chlorinated water in a pool is on your skin. I have lots of clients who are avid swimmers (several are on Masters swim teams), and I sometimes swim several times a week myself. So I know firsthand about how hard chlorine is on skin.

Chlorine, as defined in Merriam-Webster's dictionary, is "a nonmetallic chemical element that is found alone as a strong-smelling greenish yellow irritating gas and is used as a bleach, oxidizing agent, and disinfectant." It renders anything it is added to free from any type of antibodies and/or germs.

Someone once asked me if she should put Vaseline on her face before swimming in order to keep the chlorine off her skin. Well, that is an interesting idea, but unfortunately I think it will do more harm than good. Yes, the occlusiveness of pure petroleum jelly will keep just about everything off your skin. Whether or not it will keep the chlorine from going right past the petroleum and into your skin is hard to say; maybe the Vaseline is not a complete barrier. One thing it *will* do is clog your pores and cause the potential for congestion. While you are swimming you may keep the chlorine out, but how would you get all that jelly off your face afterwards? The only option that has the potential to do the job is using a scrub. This might be OK for some people but not for everyone. And you would certainly want to get all of the petroleum off your face immediately after your swim. I suppose those of you who are adamant about keeping chlorine off your face could take this extra step, but even for skin-conscious people like me, it's too much trouble. Therefore, in conclusion, I do not recommend putting Vaseline or any other thick, petroleum product on your face for swimming.

But I am going to give you some suggestions on how to take care of your skin *after* you swim. Some of these things can be done at the gym, or you can wait until you're home. But whatever you choose to do, make sure to tend to your skin as soon as possible. It has just been immersed in a harsh chemical for however long you've been swimming. Give your skin a break and take care of it ASAP.

Your number one concern is to replenish the moisture that has just been stripped from your skin. But first, you want to **thoroughly cleanse your face**. Do not use soap at the gym! If you forgot your cleanser, just rinse in the shower and remember to go through The Basics 1-2-3 as soon as you get home.

After cleansing and if you have the time, **exfoliating** would be beneficial. I would choose a light-textured scrub in a moisturizing base as opposed to a scrub that is thick and doesn't have a lot of filler cream in it. Using a gommage would be great because it is gentle, with no abrasive particles, while at the same time it is hydrating. Either one of these exfoliators will help get rid of some of the dried out surface cells. If you swim every day, you may not want to scrub this often. If a scrub is all you have to use, use it as often as you can without causing irritation to your face.

Next, use your **spray toner**. Even if you are just getting dressed and planning on doing your skin routine at home, spray the toner on your face before leaving the gym. The moisture from this product will superficially hydrate your outer skin and help to replace the proper pH after being in the pool.

Try applying a **hydrating booster** underneath your moisturizer. A hydration booster can include a hydrating gel mask, glycerin, or even an oil mixture that you have either made or purchased. For those of you with normal to oily skin, I recommend using a gel-type hydrating mask or glycerin instead of an oil. True oils are tricky to use because you don't want them to cause breakouts or clog your pores. For true-dry skin, using light-textured oils under your moisturizer after swimming can go a long way to rehydrating your skin. If you have one of these booster products to use, simply apply it to your face and neck, taking a few extra seconds to massage it in really well, and let your chlorine-drenched skin soak it up.

Last but not at all least, use your **moisturizer**. Finally your skin will get the needed hydration it has been looking for ever since you set foot in the swimming pool! Don't forget to use eye cream as well. After applying both of these moisturizers, you are ready to go.

If you are swimming at a health club and plan on taking a whirlpool or steam bath after your swim, there are a few extras you may want to do in order to save your skin.

In previous writings I have talked about how you don't ever want to go into a steam room with a bare face. It is damaging to the delicate capillaries, potentially causing couperose (broken capillaries). My solution is to put on a cleansing clay mask. This will keep your capillaries protected from the hot steam, and the steam will keep the clay moist, which is better than letting it dry on your face. If not clay, use a hydrating mask instead. You will be helping to get the moisture back into your skin and at the same time keeping your capillaries protected with the mask on your face.

When I do a whirlpool, I don't always have a mask on my face. The heat is not as intense as in the steam room, but if you do a whirlpool more than occasionally, I would recommend protecting your face. Use either a clay or moisture mask, hop in the whirlpool and relax after a hard workout in the swimming pool.

Swimming in a chlorinated pool can be hard on the skin, but if you take care of your skin afterwards, you should be OK.

T

Tanning Beds

Telling you that tanning beds are harmful is like saying that smoking is not good for you. Aren't the health risks obvious? If you still think lying in a tanning bed really isn't all that bad, please hear this: Going to the tanning salon can increase your risk of melanoma (the deadliest form of skin cancer). But, like smoking, I'm sure hearing that isn't enough to keep you from these cancer beds.

Your argument may be that the owner or employees at your tanning salon say that no matter what you may hear, tanning is actually a safe thing to do. What a surprise that someone selling you a service is going to do what they can to promote that service. It is doubtful, because you want to believe tanning is safe, that you will do any more investigating than that. And that is where you are making a big mistake. All you have to do is ask a doctor—a dermatologist—to hear how dangerous these tanning salons really are. Make no mistake about it: *Tanning beds are hazardous to your health*.

Here is another point to stress: **There is no safe tan**. If you are getting UV exposure, no matter how you are receiving it, it is causing the potential for skin cancer. The American Cancer Society's "Fry now, pay later" dictum says it all. And although you aren't literally getting a sunburn when you go to a tanning salon, you are causing damage from the inside out. That is the inherent danger of these beds. You receive a lot of damage that you don't immediately see.

The primary reason you don't see the damage is these beds use mostly UVA radiation. UVA is the longest ultraviolet ray and goes deep beneath the skin's surface. UVB radiation is the shorter ray and is the one that gives you a tan or even a sunburn. You may not think of a tan equating to damage, but that is exactly what it is. The color changes you see in your skin after using a tanning bed or just regular sun exposure are your skin's response to danger. The color of a tan is a sign the skin has been damaged. Of course, getting that tan color is the whole point of getting sun, because we intellectually equate a tan with healthy-looking skin. If you changed your paradigm about what a tan means from something sought after to a possible health risk, maybe this would keep you out of the tanning salon.

Which is worse, lying out in the sun without sunscreen or using a full spectrum (UVA/UVB) sunscreen in a tanning salon?

One of the benefits of sun exposure vs. tanning bed exposure is you will get a sunburn if you stay in the sun too long. Sun rays emit a lot more UVB (the rays that tan and burn the skin) than a tanning bed does. In fact, this is one of the selling points at a tanning salon—there is less of the UVB radiation, so your skin won't burn. But burning is your body's natural warning mechanism, telling you to get out of the sun! Whenever you've gotten sunburned, it is doubtful you went out for more sun immediately afterwards. More than likely, you protected your sunburned skin and avoided further exposure until the burn went away. With tanning beds you don't burn, so you could conceivably stay in them much longer and create much more damage than if you were in the sun.

The answer to this question, although I wouldn't recommend either scenario, is to stay out of the tanning beds under any circumstance. Why? Tanning beds are worse than sun exposure. You get accelerated UV damage, and no matter how you slice it, tanning beds should be avoided at all costs.

You may be going to a tanning salon to get a "base tan" before a vacation, or to get some color in the winter when you feel like you look too "white." You may be trying to avoid getting a sunburn while on vacation, but if you get color from the beds, in theory protecting your skin, doesn't that mean you'll be prone to spending more time outside in the sun—perhaps even unprotected? In theory, this preparation mentality is understandable; in practice, it just means more sun damage—first from the tanning bed, and then from more exposure than you would normally be able to tolerate from the sun.

Obviously, I am not trying to sugarcoat the truth of going to a tanning bed. It is dangerous and will have long-term and long-lasting effects. Any pleasure you get from the change in your skin's color is far outweighed by the fact you are damaging otherwise healthy cells. If you want to age faster and create an environment for cancer in your skin, go to a tanning bed as often as you can. Why wait? You could cause all kinds of damage sooner rather than later.

TendSkin® Lotion

This product is made to help reduce the pain and inflammation of razor bumps, ingrown hair, and razor burn. The main active ingredient in TendSkin is aspirin (acetylsalicylic acid). Aspirin, of course, is an analgesic (pain reliever) as well as an antiinflammatory agent. Next on the ingredient list is isopropyl alcohol. This, as you hopefully know, is the "bad" kind of alcohol. Isopropyl alcohol is very drying to the skin. Water is the next ingredient, so the fact that alcohol comes before water means this product is almost entirely made of alcohol.

However, many people have seen results with their ingrown hair by using TendSkin. Sometimes even I have to bypass the information I know to be true in lieu of getting results, as long as there are no adverse effects to the skin when using this product. In other words, if you can use TendSkin successfully without experiencing any problems as a result of using it, you may be able to help your ingrown hair problems. But if you use TendSkin and it causes reactions or just doesn't help your problems, I don't recommend using it. This is a specialized product and because of the alcohol content, it won't be for everybody.

Titanium Dioxide

Does titanium dioxide clog pores?

Titanium dioxide is a common ingredient used in sunscreens. It is opaque (vs. see-through) and acts as a physical block against UV rays. Because of its inability to penetrate the skin, it does sit on the surface and therefore can have the potential for clogging the pores. Not all products with titanium dioxide will clog your pores; it really depends on the surrounding ingredients. It might be yet another trial and error test to see what works for your skin.

One of the benefits of titanium dioxide is it helps to reduce the amount of UVA radiation reaching down to the lower parts of your skin. It is by no means a complete deterrent, but it does have some blocking abilities. Why is this important? Because it is the UVA rays that are the aging rays (UVAging) and also the type of sun damage that causes cancer. By wearing a full spectrum sunscreen (one that protects against UVA and UVB), you are better equipped to fight off the harmful effects of the sun. No sunscreen is total protection, but look for titanium dioxide as a beneficial ingredient in your sun products.

Triphala

You may not have heard of triphala until now. I hadn't either until a few years ago. I was having some trouble with my colon (chronic constipation with on again off again pain) and my acupuncturist recommended triphala. It is a digestive tonic, helping to tone and strengthen the lining of the colon. It is also a digestive aid, helping to gently purge waste and debris stagnated (stuck) within the large intestine. It is nontoxic and non-habit forming, making it an ideal supplement for anyone having digestive problems, most notably constipation.

Triphala is an Ayurvedic formula from India. Ayurvedic medicine is the most ancient form of medicine documented. It revolves around three different constitutions of the human body: pitta, vata, and kapha. Ayurvedic medicine has become more popular in recent years here in the West, and for good reason, but rather than go into a lengthy explanation of Ayurveda, I will simply tell you this approach offers a fascinating view of the body. If you are interested in finding out about yourself through the eyes of this ancient medical way, there are many books on the subject.

You may be wondering what triphala has to do with your skin. The reason I have included it in this book is due to the constipation connection. If you have chronic or even occasional constipation, you are not eliminating toxins efficiently. If your body's toxins are not being released on a daily basis, most notably from the large intestine, this can and will affect the health of your skin. If you suffer from problem skin and you also experience constipation, triphala may be able to help.

What is triphala? Triphala, which means three trees or fruits, is a preparation that combines three of India's premium herbs into a traditional Ayurvedic formula; amalaki (*emblica officinalis*); haritaki (*chedulic myrobalan*); and bhibitaki (*beleric myrobalan*). It is so popular in India that doctors recommend it for many other maladies other than constipation. Although triphala is sold over the counter, it won't be found in the grocery or drug store. I have only seen it in health food stores.

What results will I achieve? Triphala is traditionally used to treat constipation. Not only does it offer a laxative effect, but triphala also supports and actually strengthens the digestive tract, especially the lining of the colon walls. It has tremendous detoxifying qualities yet does not deplete the body of essential nutrients. In fact, triphala offers a wide range of beneficial vitamins and nutrients that add to the health of your entire system.

Purgative laxatives (such as Ex-Lax®, for instance) speed up the elimination of debris by irritating the lining of the intestines. Over the counter laxatives like these are not recommended to be used on a regular basis. Herbal laxatives like psyllium husks and flax seeds work by swelling and absorbing the fluids in the intestines and moving stuck mass along in the large intestine and are generally called bulking agents. Triphala works by toning and strengthening the entire large intestine and helping to deep clean the G.I. tract. This helps to alleviate all kinds of built-up toxic residue. This cleansing will give you more energy and help with the overall health of your entire intestinal system.

Triphala is known to improve digestion, has been found to reduce serum cholesterol, and can improve liver function. It has proven anti-inflammatory and antiviral properties, contains linoleic acid (a component in essential fatty acids (EFAs) important to cell integrity and overall health), and may help lower high blood pressure.

Why wouldn't I take triphala? The only contraindications I could find for this supplement are pregnancy and diarrhea. Otherwise, at least in India, triphala is taken by most people since it is so good on so many levels for supporting health. Check with your healthcare practitioner to be sure triphala is right for you.

Do I need to take triphala? If you suffer from chronic (or even occasional) constipation, you might want to at least try triphala for a period of time to see if it does indeed help you eliminate more efficiently. If you are not getting the garbage out of your body, you are inviting trouble. Toxic waste that is reabsorbed into the bloodstream can bring about a whole host of problems, short- and long-term.

If you don't suffer with digestive trouble, you could still try triphala simply because it benefits the system on so many levels. Based on my own experience with taking this supplement, triphala will certainly help support and promote your health.

What is the dosage? You will want to experiment with dosage when using triphala. When I first started using it years ago, I had chronic constipation. I started with a low dose (1-2 capsules 2x daily) to get it into my system and let my body get used to its tonic effect. After a week, I upped my dosage since I wasn't getting any appreciable effects from taking the lower dose. I went up to 2-3 capsules morning and evening. Three seemed to make my bowels too loose, so I went down to 2 capsules twice a day. This seemed to be my personal best dosage.

Experiment for yourself and find the dosage that works for you. The recommendations I have found range from taking 4-6 capsules daily (2-3 each with morning and evening meals) to taking large doses at night (3-4 capsules) to help cleanse and detoxify and then 1-2 capsules with meals for the health building and rejuvenating effects.

How long should I take triphala? You can take it for a course of treatment to help the constipation you may be experiencing once in a while. But if you have chronic constipation, I would consider taking triphala as a daily supplement to help tone and condition your colon as well as keep your bowels moving. Triphala is actually intended to be used as a regular supplement to your diet, rather than just when symptoms of constipation are present. And the longer you use this tonic preparation, the greater the benefit you will receive.

Ultraviolet Radiation

428

Ultraviolet Radiation

People are always asking me what they can do to keep their skin from aging. The simplest answer to that question is to avoid overexposing your skin (your face, in particular) to ultraviolet radiation (sun). I know this is not an easy task, especially when so many activities are enjoyed outdoors in the sun, but if your goal is "anti-aging" you will have to adopt behaviors which support that goal.

When some clients hear me talk about sun exposure and how to protect their skin, I think they hear me saying, "Never go out in the sun." And that, obviously, is simply not possible—or desirable. It is not about avoiding all exposure, it is about understanding the short- and long-term effects of exposure and how to avoid damaging your skin while enjoying a life spend out of doors. As we all know, too much of a good thing can turn bad. And so is true with sun exposure. Anytime you receive ultraviolet radiation (UVR), you are exposed to the negative effects of the sun: waves of radiation coming down from millions of miles away, adversely affecting your skin.

Protection, reapplication, and wisdom are at least three of the components to keeping your skin from getting too much sun. Protection comes through the use of sunscreen, staying in shaded areas when possible, and keeping a hat on and/or protective clothing— especially when you know you'll be exposed over a long period of time.

Reapplication of sunscreen is so important, but I believe this step is usually avoided or ignored. If you are going to have extended time in the sun, taking along your sunscreen is a must. This way you can reapply frequently (and liberally).

Wisdom comes into play because without it, UVR will get the best of you. How many summers have you seen people who either fell asleep in the sun or otherwise ignored the fact they were getting overexposed? Now they are walking around in pain and hosting a deep red sunburn. (Aloe vera would really save their skin!) Be smart. Don't get overexposed. Don't get caught without protection (whether clothing or products) and keep your UVR exposure to a minimum. Remember: Sun damage is cumulative. Each year (each day) you rack up more sun damage points, which down the road could equal skin cancer.

The following was adapted and used with permission from the American Academy of Dermatology. This information is important to keep in mind in your day to day life, even if you aren't "sun bathing."

- Shade only *lessens* UVR exposure. Sunburn from scattered or reflected UVR can still occur in shaded areas.
- Certain surfaces reflect UVR. Water reflects up to 30% of UVR; dry sand up to 18%; concrete 12%; and grass 5%.
- UVR increases with altitude.
- 70-80% of the total UVR from the sun on a midsummer day is received between 10am and 4pm.
- UVR damages the eyes. A wide brim hat reduces the amount of UVR reaching the cornea of the eye by 50%. Sunglasses, if UV protective, can filter out as much as 95% of UV rays.
- SPF 15 sunscreen protects against 93% of UVR. SPF 30 protects against 98%. As you can see, the difference between the two are not great. Therefore don't be *as* concerned about the SPF number on your bottle of sunscreen; *do* concentrate on applying enough sunscreen and, if exposure is prolonged, you must reapply *frequently*.
- Medication can make your skin more sensitive to UVR.

You can prevent (or at least curtail) UVR exposure. Please take this information to heart, and always wear sunscreen!

*P*erhaps one has to be very old before one learns
to be amused rather than shocked.

– Pearl S. Buck

Whiteheads

What is a whitehead? *Milia* is the technical term for whiteheads. Some people think the term is pronounced *Amelia*, but it is not. Milia are found when dead skin has grown over a pore that has become congested (filled with oil and debris). Whiteheads need to be professionally extracted—even more so than pustules. Why? Because even though you can see the whitehead on the surface of your skin, it takes someone who really knows whether or not it can be extracted. Just because you can see the milia doesn't necessarily mean it is ready to come out.

> *I am 50 years old and have pretty good skin. It is best described as combination skin—a little drier along the cheeks and under the eyes but a little oiler around the forehead and nose. I do not have breakouts to speak of. I do have a few spots that might be whiteheads, but I'm not sure. They are relatively hard to see (unless you are really looking for them), but they are almost like tiny cysts under the skin. They are white, but the clog itself is like a little hard bead, not a fluid. I do not typically try to extract these myself. Over time some go away. I do not know if they can be extracted during a facial or if a dermatologist would be required. Like I said, though, they are few and small so it's not a big problem.*

The way she described her little white bumps is a good description of a whitehead. This, in a nutshell, is a whitehead. It is like a seed or bead nestled inside a closed pore. Some are easier to see than others, but sometimes they really can't be detected.

Because there is skin grown over the opening of the pore, the debris (oil) can't just come out if you squeeze like a blackhead will. An opening has to be made (in the salon, a lancet is used) in order for the actual extraction to take place. Then if you don't have knowledge about what is extractable and what isn't, you may go after a whitehead that won't come out no matter how hard you try. What comes next is possible capillary damage (couperose) and almost definitely a small infection.

Since the whiteheads are few, small, and hard to see, I would leave well-enough alone. If you go in for a facial, see what the aesthetician thinks, and if possible have them extracted. Know that if you are prone to whiteheads, they will more than likely return.

Wholistic*

*I chose to spell this word wholistic verses holistic. It immediately connotes whole, as in the whole body.

This word has gotten a bad rap. I think for certain people it connotes some sort of airy-fairy, nonsensical, even religious meaning that has nothing to do with its actual definition. The base word is whole. This, as anyone knows, means entire, all, or everything. So *wholistic*, in relation to the human body means taking into account the body in its entirety.

A wholistic approach to medicine or a medical condition simply means looking at the body as a whole instead of just focusing on the affected area. I use this wholistic approach as a rule whenever I am treating someone with problem skin. It's never just about the breakout and how to make the blemishes go away. For me, and thus my clients, it is about looking at the individual as a whole person, breaking down their diets, their exercise programs (or lack of one), and looking at how much stress is in their lives. I also look for other factors such as things that are new. New laundry detergent, a new living situation (new house, new apartment, new housemate), new foods, (eating unusual food while on vacation, for instance), a new workout routine—new anything that might be contributing to their skin problems.

If you are only treating the symptom, or just one part of the body (in this example, the skin), I believe you are missing out on the total and long-term solution. Try this word on for size next time you are faced with a skin condition or other problem with your body. Don't just focus your attention on the symptoms; truly look at all aspects of your life as holding answers to the potential cause or causes of your health concerns. Take a wholistic approach.

Witch Hazel

A client asked me if witch hazel was OK to use as her toner. I asked what her experience was when she used it, and she said it really dried her skin out. She would have to quickly put her moisturizer on afterwards because her skin felt so dried out. Her experience is also her answer. Drying out the surface skin is not an ideal outcome, so I wouldn't recommend using witch hazel. As you know, drying the skin out is counterproductive and not conducive to healthy skin.

The type of witch hazel you find (very inexpensively) at any grocery or drug store is actually witch hazel *water*. It has been distilled and stripped of all the benefits of the natural herb. I do not recommend using witch hazel water on your skin as a toner. Although it is primarily water, it contains as much as 15% ethanol alcohol, which is the bad type of alcohol.

The herb witch hazel can be very beneficial. The extracts from the leaves and bark of the *hamamelis virginiana* plant have anti-inflammatory and wound healing properties. So, as an ingredient in a skin care product, witch hazel is probably going to be OK, but I don't recommend using it straight on your face as a toner.

434

Y

Yoga for Health

David Sunshine, my friend and owner of the Dallas Yoga Center (www.dallasyogacenter.com), wrote the following about the importance of yoga. I highly recommend finding a class in your area (see **Resources**) and giving this type of exercise a try. Yoga is wonderful for young and old alike.

The classroom is packed with people of all shapes and sizes. A teacher walks through the rows of brightly colored sticky mats as students move through a variety of yoga postures. The teacher calls out the next pose, "downward facing dog," and suddenly from all fours, hips lift into the air and bodies shift into the position that is similar to the way that dogs stretch into after waking from a long nap. Forearms quiver as the instruction is given to extend their hands into the floor and ground their heels, and skin glistens with sweat.

Until recently, the term yoga *brought to mind images of a bearded man sitting on a mountaintop in a posture resembling the shape of a pretzel. However, over the past five years the popularity of yoga has grown so much that presently more than eighteen million Americans consider themselves yogis. People of all ages, backgrounds and body types are singing praise for what has now become a common household activity.*

Yoga originated in India over 4,000 years ago. The term yoga *means "union." The essence of yoga is the unification of mind, body and spirit. Our modern day lives are fast paced and filled with often overwhelming stress. We are overtaxed mentally and physically as we try to make it through our endless lists of things to do. Though its roots are ancient, yoga brings harmony even to* our modern fragmented turbo drive inner state of being. And yet, yoga is not just a path to inner health, but glowing healthy skin as well.

The yoga sage, Patanjali, wrote that each person has a light within and yoga brightens that inner lamp. However he also noted that some people, like some lamps, have dustier covers than others. Patanjali explains that yoga is a life long journey that removes the dust enabling the lamp to shine brighter. Through the practice of breathing techniques, physical postures, positive thought and behavior, and proper diet, yoga reduces stress, detoxes and strengthens the physical body, calms and clears the mind as well as uplifts the spirit. Even after a single yoga class one will notice a deep sense of wholeness, harmony and well-being. Eventually with continued practice, a soft innocence returns to the face and the inner light grows bright emanating outward in a sweet warm glow and youthful appearance.

In addition to inner radiance, yoga promotes an intimate mind/body connection. Yoga expands our consciousness with an acute awareness of each inhalation, exhalation, movement and stretch. As tension in the mind and body disappear, a deeper inner awareness arises, and we begin to appreciate life anew for the marvelous interconnections that make it up. Cultivating our inner awareness creates a feeling of balance, freedom and joy bringing a special sweetness to life known as "rasa."

Within yoga, "rasa" refers to our "inner juice," which is associated with health, joy and flexibility. We are born from a place of water, and youth is characterized by both fluidity and resilience. As we age, we often loose that quality of rasa, and life becomes dry, rigid and routine. The different phases of our lives are reflected in changes to our skin. As we grow old, wrinkles appear, and the skin thins and becomes less elastic. Yoga is designed to reverse the aging process and replenish our rasa.

Specific yoga postures bring fresh blood and oxygen to the skin, remove toxins and restore elasticity. Yoga provides the tools necessary to diminish the effects of aging so that a healthy inner and outer complexion is achieved naturally.

In the past 10 years, yoga has grown in the United States with ever-increasing numbers of students and studios. There is every type of yoga class imaginable; from strenuous exercises done in a heated room to restorative yoga classes, which are relaxing and healing to the soul. You can work up a sweat or relax your body into different yoga positions, depending on the class you take. Personally, I like the more traditional yoga classes vs. high energy types. I find the more traditional type classes help me make the body, mind, spirit connection easier than classes where I am sweating my sox off. The bottom line is do what works for you and your body, but do try yoga—for your health! I know you will benefit from this most ancient form of exercise.

Z

Zinc

Zinc, the mineral, is widely known for its healing abilities. Zinc is linked to improvement with acne and other skin maladies. However, as is true with many vitamins and minerals, if you supplement only zinc or take it in high doses you run the risk of causing major deficiencies in other vitamins and minerals, resulting in problematic imbalances in your body. Therefore, taking zinc alone is not recommended, but there are a few food sources for this vital mineral.

Spirulina (see section) is an excellent source of zinc, plus you get the benefit of many other nutrients contained in this sea algae. **Brewer's yeast** is another good source of zinc, as well as almost all B vitamins and an appreciable amount of protein.

Zinc Oxide

Zinc oxide is used in sunscreens as a reflective or physical block against UV rays. You probably remember as a kid seeing (or even wearing) zinc oxide on the nose—it was pure white and very noticeable. Nowadays it is used as a key ingredient in sunscreens.

Zinc oxide is one of only three ingredients that are currently used to block the damaging UVA rays. Parsol 1789 (avobenzone) and titanium dioxide are the others. Please don't misunderstand: in a sunscreen, zinc oxide is not a complete block—nothing short of being inside will keep all the sun's radiation off your skin. But zinc oxide, along with avobenzone and titanium dioxide, are ingredients to look for in your sun products.

If you are a skier (or a sailer) there are zinc products made in wild and fun colors. So you can protect your skin and make a fashion statement too!

Books

A Consumer's Dictionary of Cosmetic Ingredients by Ruth Winter, M.S. (Three Rivers Press, 2005) This is the ingredient book I turn to more than any other.

Beating Rosacea: A Must-Have Guide to Understanding & Treating Rosacea by Geoffrey Nase, Ph.D. (Nase Publications, 2001)

Beauty and the Beam: Your Complete Guide to Cosmetic Laser Surgery by Deborah S. Sarnoff, M.D., F.A.A.D., F.A.C.P., and Joan Swirsky, R.N., M.S. (St. Martin's Press, 1998)

Body for Life: 12 Weeks to Mental and Physical Strength by Bill Phillips. (HarperCollins Publishers, Inc., 1999) This book has great information about diet and exercise. The before and after pictures are truly amazing! His workout program *works*.

Dr. Jensen's Juicing Therapy: Nature's Way to Better Health and A Longer Life by Bernard Jensen, D.C., Ph.D. (Keats Publishing, 2000) A great reference guide to health and healing through juicing.

Evening Primrose Oil by Judy Graham. (Healing Arts Press, 1990) There are several books on primrose oil, but this one was my first and continues to be my favorite.

Fast Food Nation: The Dark Side of the All-American Meal by Eric Schlosser. (Perennial/HarperCollins Publishers, Inc., 2002) This is an interesting book about fast food and how it has infiltrated our American diets.

The Friendly Bacteria: How Lactobacilli and Bifidobacteria Can Transform Your Health by William H. Lee, R.Ph., Ph. D. (The McGraw-Hill Companies, 1999) See **Acidophilus** for an excerpt.

Get the Sugar Out: 501 Simple Ways to Cut the Sugar Out of Any Diet by Ann Louise Gittleman, M.S., C.N.S. (Three Rivers Press, 1996) In your quest to get sugar out of your life, this book can help.

The How To Herb Book: Let's Remedy the Situation by Velma J. Keith and Monteen Gordon. (Mayfield Publications, 1994) This is my all-time favorite book on vitamins and herbs. I highly recommend this excellent reference guide for anyone truly interested in herbs, vitamins, and minerals. If you can't find it, write to the publishers: Mayfield Publications, P.O. Box 157, Pleasant Grove UT 84062.

The Juiceman®'s Power of Juicing: Delicious Juice Recipes for Energy, Health, Weight Loss, and Relief from Scores of Common Ailments by Jay Kordich. (William Morrow & Company, Inc., 1992) As I wrote in the **Juicing** section, this is my favorite book on the subject.

Lick The Sugar Habit Sugar Counter: Discover the Hidden Sugar in Your Food by Nancy Appleton, Ph.D. (Penguin Putnam, 2001) Be sure to check out "110 Reasons Why Sugar Is Ruining Your Health" (page 5).

Milady's Skin Care and Cosmetic Ingredients Dictionary by Natalia Michalum. (Milady Publishing Company, 2000)

The OmegaRx Zone: The Miracle of the New High-Dose Fish Oil by Barry Sears, Ph.D. (ReganBooks, 2002) A good book about essential fatty acids (EFAs) and how important they are for health. I recommend reading any of Dr. Sears' books, including *The Zone, Mastering the Zone,* and *The Soy Zone.*

Physiology of the Skin II: An Expanded Scientific Guide for the Skin Care Professional by Peter T. Pugliese, MD. (Allured Publishing Corporation, 2001) Written for the skin care professional, this book has lots of information about skin and how it functions.

The Pill Book: The Illustrated Guide to the Most-Prescribed Drugs in the United States. (Bantam Books, 11th Edition, 2004) A great little pocketbook chockfull of most known prescription medications, dosages, actions in the body, precautions, and more.

Potatoes Not Prozac: A Natural Seven-Step Dietary Plan to Control Your Cravings and Lose Weight, Recognize How Foods Affect the Way You Feel, and Stabilize the Level of Sugar in Your Blood by Kathleen DesMaisons, Ph.D. (Simon & Schuster, Inc., 1999) If you have problems with sugar and sugar addiction, this is a great book.

Rosacea: Your Self-Help Guide by Arlen Brownstein, M.S., N.D. and Donna Shoemaker, C.N. (Harbinger Publications, Inc., 2001) Even if you don't have rosacea, this book is filled with helpful information about acidity and alkalinity in foods as well as information about supplements and more. And if you do have rosacea, this book is a must-have.

Stevia Rebaudiana: Natures Sweet Secret by David Richard. (Vital Health Publishing, 1999) Stevia makes a great sugar substitute. This book includes sections on the plant's history, botany, pharmacology, usage and safety, with nearly two dozen stevia recipes.

The Sugar Addict's Total Recovery Program by Kathleen DesMaisons, Ph.D. (Ballantine Publishing Group, 2002) Listed in the **Sugar** section, this is another book by Dr. DesMaisons that I highly recommend. The more you know, the more you know how to help yourself. (Also see *Your Last Diet!*)

Sugar Blues by William Dufty. (Warner Books, 1975) This is the quintessential book on the power of sugar addiction and one man's powerful recovery.

Sun Protection for Life: Your Guide to a Lifetime of Healthy & Beautiful Skin by Mary Mills Barrow and John F. Barrow. (New Harbinger Publications, Inc., 2005) This is a great guide to understanding the effects of the sun. It has a large section on sun protective clothing.

Timeless Skin: Healthy Skin for a Lifetime by Carolyn Ash. (Splash Publishing, 2000) If you can't find my book, contact me through my website: www.carolynashskincare.com.

Vitamin C and the Common Cold by Linus Pauling. (W. H. Freeman and Company, 1970)

What's In Your Cosmetics? A Complete Consumer's Guide to Natural and Synthetic Ingredients by Aubrey Hampton. (Organica Press, 2003)

The Wisdom of Menopause: Creating Physical and Emotional Health and Healing During the Change by Christiane Northrup, M.D. (Bantam Books, 2003) If you don't have this book, get it!

The Wrinkle Cure: Unlock the Power of Cosmeceuticals for Supple, Youthful Skin by Nicholas Perricone, M.D. (Warner Books, 2001) This first book from Dr. Perricone has lots of information on inflammation and other interesting matters that affect our skin—and bodies. Dr. Perricone now has many books available, but I think this one is his best.

Your Last Diet!: The Sugar Addict's Weight-Loss Plan by Kathleen DesMaisons, Ph.D. (Ballantine Books, 2001) Dr. DesMaisons has several books, all of which I highly recommend. Here she shares a lot of information pertaining to sugar and addiction, information you need if sugar is a part of your daily life. I recommend this book even if you are not looking to lose weight.

Websites

How to find an acupuncturist. (www.acupuncture.com) Although I really think that getting a referral for a practitioner is your best bet, in case you don't know anyone currently receiving acupuncture treatments, try this website. They have tips for finding a therapist along with general information about acupuncture. You can search the web to find more sites, but at least this is a start.

How to find a dermatologist. (www.aad.org) This is the website for the American Academy of Dermatology. Here you can do a search for a dermatologist in your area.

How to find gommage. (www.carolynashskincare.com) Since so many readers have had trouble finding a gommage product, I am listing my skin care website as a source for the gommage that I use. There may be other gel exfoliators on the market, but if you can't find one—or one you like—you will have this resource.

Information on rosacea. (www.rosacea.org) This is the website for the National Rosacea Society (NRS). If you have (or think you have) rosacea, I highly recommend going on the Internet and reading what the NRS has to say. As with anything, not all the information is going to be pertinent to you specifically, but they do a great job of disseminating important information for rosacea sufferers.

Information on skin cancer. The American Cancer Society (www.cancer.org). This website offers a wealth of information about all types of cancer, including skin cancer. The Skin Cancer Foundation's website (www.skincancer.org) is another good resource for information on skin and all types of skin cancer.

How to find a yoga class. (www.yogafinder.com) No matter where you live in the United States—or the world—this is a great resource.

*Y*ou're not as young as you once were,
but you're not as old as you will be.

– Irish Proverb

The day I heard Mel Ann had passed away, I was flooded with memories of our working together. She had been the primary editor for my first two books, and she'd spent perilous hours working with me to get my writing up to both of our high standards. Her excellence, advice, and technical support proved invaluable, and I believe Mel Ann made me a better writer for having worked with her.

When I approached her to edit this book, she was unable to accept the job. She had so many projects on her plate as her own career as a writer was starting to take off. My disappointment was no doubt audible as we spoke on the phone, but I hung up thinking I would somehow get through without her. I didn't put much effort into finding another editor—I really wanted Mel Ann and was in complete denial about her turning down this job.

A few months later I got the call: Mel Ann would be able to edit for me during a break she had coming up in her schedule. I was thrilled and excited, to say the least! Her tireless efforts and attention to detail are once again reflected in the quality of this work.

I am forever indebted to Mel Ann Coley for giving me so much of herself during the editing of *Timeless Skin* and *Skin Care A to Z.* To her husband Bryan and her children Rachel and David: God Bless you and all of your family. I know this loss was devastating.